WHERE THERE IS NO MIDWIFE

Fertility, Reproduction and Sexuality

GENERAL EDITORS:

David Parkin, Director of the Institute of Social and Cultural Anthropology, University of Oxford

Soraya Tremayne, Co-ordinating Director of the Fertility and Reproduction Studies Group and Research Associate at the Institute of Social and Cultural Anthropology, University of Oxford, and a Vice-President of the Royal Anthropological Institute

WHERE THERE IS
NO MIDWIFE
BIRTH AND LOSS IN RURAL INDIA

Sarah Pinto

Berghahn Books
New York • Oxford

Published in 2008 by

Berghahn Books

www.berghahnbooks.com

©2008, 2012 Sarah Pinto
First paperback edition published in 2012

Library of Congress Cataloging-in-Publication Data

Pinto, Sarah.
    Where there is no midwife : birth and loss in rural india / by
Sarah Pinto.
        p. cm. — (Fertility, reproduction, and sexuality ; v. 10)
    Includes bibliographical references and index.
    ISBN 978-1-84545-310-7 (hbk) -- ISBN 978-0-85745-153-8 (pbk)
    1. Childbirth—India. 2. Rural health—India. I. Title.
RG965.I4P56 2007
618.40954—dc22

                                                            2006100545

British Library Cataloguing in Publication Data

A catalogue record for this book is available from the British Library

Printed in the United States on acid-free paper

ISBN 978-0-85745-153-8 (paperback)
ISBN 978-0-85745-448-5 (ebook)

For Eve

CONTENTS

NOTE ON TRANSLITERATIONS

Transliterating Hindi and Awadhi is a complicated prospect, demanding that one question etymologies, colonial histories, the politics of ethnographic conventions, the way "anglicized" words get "distorted" or remade, regional and "modern standard" pronunciations and spellings, and at times one's own ear. Consistency, even in the most rigorous and thorough of forms, is confounded by the lovely variabilities of human speech—to be truly consistent at least half of the words used here would require a footnote listing possible pronunciations, Awadhi and Hindi variants, and modern standard spellings. Therefore, my approach to transliteration is minimalist. I use no diacritical marks and few elaborations of sounds not distinguished in English. My sense is that for those who recognize terms the presence or absence of diacritics won't matter and context will make certain differences clear enough, while for those who do not recognize terms, diacriticals don't offer much anyway. However, where context alone may not give enough for Hindi speakers to go on in understanding terms and where distinguishing between phonemes is necessary for comprehension, I spell out pronunciation rather than using diacritical marks. Likewise, many Hindi words have entered English usage; terms like "dai" and *purdah* are spelled here in a way that most closely combines their correct transliteration and conventional Latinate spellings—in India as well as in "the West." Where Hindi and Awadhi terms need to be pluralized, I do so in "English," with an added *s* which, while not grammatically correct, makes for more comprehensible and fluid reading in English.

Acknowledgments

It is difficult to pinpoint a beginning to this story, and thus difficult to know where to draw the lines around my scope of gratitude. I suspect that subsequent projects may not have the expansive social lives of the books that begin as dissertations and the dissertations that begin, as mine did, as captivation with a particular category I happened upon long ago—"the dai." I am grateful to have this opportunity to thank the many people who helped me along the long way— opening doors; making introductions; sharing homes; taking care of me when I was sick; helping me learn to speak and to listen; reading the same words over and over and offering new insight. And to say that any mistakes or errors in judgment here are entirely, completely my own.

The research for this project was funded by a generous International Dissertation Research Fellowship from the Social Science Research Council, and preliminary data collection in Bihar by the Princeton University Council on Regional Studies. My final year of dissertation "writing-up" was supported by the Woodrow Wilson Scholars Program at Princeton University. The Sardar Patel Association's generous award in 2004 gave me encouragement in turning the dissertation into a manuscript. While redrafting this manuscript I had the great fortune to hold an NIMH postdoctoral fellowship in Culture and Mental Health Services at Harvard University in the Department of Social Medicine. Many people at Princeton University, teachers and fellow graduate students, were involved in this project at various stages: Carol Zanca, Gananath Obeyesekere, Rena Lederman, James Boon, Carol Greenhouse, Gyan Prakash, Heiko Henkel, Rachel Newcomb, Susanna Trnka, Thomas Strong, Sylvie Bertrand, Kavita Misra, Alison Lake, Lisa Wynn, Elizabeth Hough, Kenneth Croes, Chris Garces, and Alex Edmonds. Emily Martin was a teacher in the best sense of the word, and offered incisive critiques that made me think about the bigger point of things. João Biehl devoted an extraordinary amount of time to reading and engaging with this text, always pushing my analyses to a new level. Isabelle Clark-Decès' confidence in this project and its perspective often felt tireless, and her thoughts on identity, caste, and ritual continue to inspire me.

In India, where research and friendship were intertwined, many people provided insight, conversation, homes, meals, and companionship. In Delhi, Janet Chawla has been an intellectual touchstone, and I have learned a great deal from her important work with dais. She and Kanwarjit Chawla have been generous friends. In Lucknow, I could have accomplished very little without the kind assistance of Tony Castleman, Rajni Castleman, Leah Pareil, Suniti Neogy, KC Tripathi, Sister Brigeeta, Aradhana Johri, and the friendly staff of the Uttar Pradesh State Assembly Library. I am also indebted to Anindita Baidya and Naval Pant for research assistance. Deepak Singh was especially helpful, in research as well as in walking me through various bureaucratic jungles and in the many, day-to-day ways I called out for help. Continuing gratitude is due to Ram Advani, for friendship and concern, first and foremost, but also for making introductions, offering advice, supplying books and many cups of tea, and telling wonderful stories. Nirmala Sharma was a kind and knowledgeable friend, and I enjoyed her company and appreciated her understanding. Other scholars working in Lucknow were important as well—offering advice, helping me figure out archives, and generally sharing the journey: David Campion, Magdalena Inkinen, Anita Anantharam, and Travis Smith. I owe a special gratitude to Ramnarayan Rawat, who has read and commented on large portions of this text, educated me and supported my efforts to think and talk about caste, and who, with remarkable generosity, shared his painstakingly acquired archival material.

In Cambridge, many people read and commented on large and small portions of this text and its various offshoots: Byron Good, Mary-Jo Delvecchio Good, Arthur Kleinman, Chris Dole, Sarah Horton, Everett Zhang, Cesar Abadio, Theresa O'Nell, and Sara Bergstresser. I have also been fortunate to be part of the Friday Morning Seminar and the wellspring of conversation and critique it offers those who gather at its long table under the reserved and watchful gaze of William James. Maya Unnithan-Kumar provided insightful comments and readings, as did, with portions of this text, Josie Saldana and Anne Anagnost. Neil Aggarwal, Audra Ladd, and Bobbie Peyton helped in important ways in the technical work of pulling all of this together at the very end. Gillian Goslinga and Diya Mehra provided important intellectual challenges and insights, and I have, for nearly a lifetime, benefited from the brilliance of Kristina Pinto, the only person who can not only finish my sentences, but also start them.

Ideas and arguments and phrasings are best produced in conversation, and are seldom the work of one. For a few choice moments that enabled me to move further, I owe gratitude to Ram Rawat for his ability to restate my arguments as observations of "remarkable fit" and thereby bring to mind earlier colonial processes, Kavita Misra for the notion that "the outsider" is thematic, Neil Aggarwal for reminding me about *lila* and its potential for anthropological grapplings, James Boon for suggesting that "placentas are good to think with," and Rosalind Shaw for questioning my translation of "him" as "it" in a story of infant death. Likewise, this project is also indebted to several teachers, though their influence on my thinking and questioning predates it: Jack Betterly, Thomas Jackson, and Steve Ferzacca. Mary Pinto and Bruce Pinto, have been encouraging and supportive, sharing their gifts of wonder and outrage (and childcare). I thank them for their many forms of assistance. Clifford Meyer, with his superhuman equanimity, has continued to inspire, provoke, and support me. For putting up with everything, thank you is hardly enough.

Deepest gratitude goes to those who, due to anthropological convention, an urge to protect, and IRB rules cannot be named here, but who showed phenomenal willingness to put up with me and give me a home and all of the warmths that go along with it. This is true of just about everyone in "Lalpur" and "Devia," but especially so of the women I call "Bari Bhabhi," "Choti Bhabhi," and "Pushpadevi." Throughout the drafting of this text, their reheard voices have reminded me in palpable and visceral ways of this web of complicity and chance that makes for the "ephemeral excess of survival," as de Certeau puts it. The other person who continues to remind me of the fragility and beauty of this *lila* is Eve. In so many ways, without her none of this would have been possible. This book is for her.

INTRODUCTION

The issues that emerge from childbearing in India are multiple, and so it has not been easy, at any point, to say succinctly what this project has been about. This is a book about birth in rural India, about women as "midwives" and women as childbearers, about infant death and public health, emotion and citizenship. More broadly, it is a story about the vulnerabilities of new life.

It is also about interventions, broadly imagined—the things people do to make life better for themselves and for others, to protect what is good and hold at bay what is not. It is about the way childbearing becomes a focal point of interventions, and maybe of life; the way it can say so much about one's position in the world; the way birth can mean loss as much as its newness brings something hopeful and auspicious into the world.

Location is also important: this is a story about a rural part of the north Indian state of Uttar Pradesh, a district called Sitapur. This is a place in which a history of intervention has made the female and fertile bodies sites upon which national and transnational interests have been lodged. A longstanding zone of what we now call "globalization," the rural is an overdetermined object of longing and imagination for urbanites, nationalists, colonials, anthropologists, interveners. The "interior"; the "field"; the "target area"; a place one goes "out to," "in to," and "back to"; place of "the backward," "the blind," "the traditional," "the future of public health," and the "remembered"—these are only some of the ways that a sense of "the rural" maps out movements and moral imaginaries of contemporary Indian life. But comings and goings there shake up the core-periphery metaphors that guide so many ways of talking about space and time and the teleologies of sought-for change. In "villages" (as iconic as "the rural" yet bounded rather than expansive) women live at once under the scrutiny of state and transnational forces of intervention and at a remove from the certainties of life captured in the term "infrastructure" or the fantasy of "health care." Social life in such a heavily mythologized locale requires we consider the ways the heres and theres, nows and thens, "uses" and thems that dichotomize life in the name of progress attach themselves to women's bodies and lives and to the diacritics that are part of their own daily imaginings.

The basic argument of this book is that childbirth and infant death provide source material for political subjectivity in places that become loci of change, the arenas of "development" and "uplift." It begins with the long-held feminist position that childbearing is political, and asks how this is so in those contexts too often considered at a remove from political consciousness: in households and homebirths; among noninstitutional and spurious practitioners; through ideas emergent in domestic, familial, and neighborly relations; amid circulations of something like "modernity" that are neither consolidated under the term "modern" nor aimed westward (or even always city-ward); in the nuances of affect that inflect gossip and the rituals of daily life and healing; and, most importantly, in the way losses happen not so much at a remove from institutions as in the skirting back and forth across their unstable boundaries. Births and deaths that take place in zones demarcated as "marginal"—especially the fringes of institutions, health and otherwise—rather than being yet-to-be-reached or beyond the extent of the political are part of experiences of belonging and outsiderness central to citizenship. They shape and are shaped by affects that link people to various forms of power and authority, ways of identifying and distancing oneself from a range of ideas and identities. In these intimate realms, intervention is a broad category of action and interaction, applying to nearly everyone. In such an approach, I hope, we move outside the formalities of policies and programmatics and into the courtyard, the kitchen, the veranda, the street corner, the spaces of the everyday in which and through which people both struggle and survive.

Certain theoretical tensions drive this account: As anthropologists of reproduction in other locales have asked, does reproduction contain the force of the new or reiteration of the old? Is it a time to bolster up what we already know or to reinvent the world and re-world the self? Even as birth provides another way by which "newness enters the world" (Bhabha 1994: 212), by which natality speaks to the core of action that is the essence of political thought (Arendt 1998), the prefixing of "re" onto "production" reminds us that, not only in a Hindu world of karmic cycles, it might also involve reiteration of what has come before. And there are tensions in the way death is related to power: is dying that which unfolds from very specific yet near-universal (at least universalizing) modes of contemporary power (as scholars working from Michel Foucault's concept of biopower suggest—cf. Biehl 2005; Das 2001, 2005; Mbembe 1999). Or is death the final affront to the certainties of the regulation of life, that which contemporary assurances about healing, life, science, and medicine cannot speak (as Michel de Certeau suggests [1994])?

In Sitapur, where infant mortality rates are staggering and health care is dominated by its own temporality and unstable availability in a system underfunded, privatized, commoditized, and outsourced (or in-sourced—that is, shifted to private organizations and transnational projects), engaging with institutions and their imaginaries—hospitals, doctors, pills, needles, operations—on the basis of childbearing entails certain kinds of citizenship. It can consist of deals made, often on a one-off basis, with all that authority and power may mean. In rural areas, often outmoded-sounding (at least to academics interested in the technological insidiousness of modern forms of power) grand visions of progress consolidate in "dai trainings," "family planning schemes," and "health camps" and a range of pedagogical messages themselves involve a sense that progress is interpellated on the body, even as they are also situated amid state failings and lack of basic care. "Access" here is complex, involving unavailability as well as affects associated with hegemonic surveillance and moral subjectivities associated with privatization, commodification, and the flows of late capitalism. Yet the fantasies of outside power on which many interventions rely for their authority demonstrate a deeply rooted locality.

It is for these qualities that childbearing and child death in the postcolonial space of "intervention" tell us something about how marginalized women and rural subjects fit into broader pictures of citizenship, social change, and power. To me, the story that most asks to be told is about how notions of improvement, equality, and "care" come together less for institutions, states, or policies than for people themselves—recipients, as it were, of a range of efforts. In rural north India, multiple crosscutting diacritics (often glossed as "hierarchies") and inequalities emergent within longstanding health intervention expand this key question outward: how are rural women embedded in and *constitutive of* global flows, and how does their place within them shape the unfolding of new life, loss, and critique in their own lives?

Rural women have complex stakes in the promises of intervention, in the ideas and languages that package health intervention.

They are themselves overdetermined by the discourses—in which they participate—which health-care often brings. Efforts to account for their experiences must, if not always intentionally, write within, alongside, and often against the current of clichés and tropes, many of which bear a sneaky inevitability in the way they reemerge. This is true of condensed moments of representation that circulate in India, as much as it is true of the clutter of categories in public health, anthropological scholarship, and accounts of the world speaking of the time-space crunch of "modernity."

This brings us back around to what "the country," the rural, or *dehat* (for some "the countryside," for others something like "the sticks") comes to mean, the way that as a concept the rural collapses complexities into a single geographical-moral entity. R. K. Narayan (1976) wrote, in his novel *The Painter of Signs*, about people—instantly recognizable figures—who move through towns and villages, and from town to village, to carry messages of progress and uplift (especially about "family planning"). His eponymous phrase is both apt and evocative; it captures something about figments of progress in "the rural"—about language as technique, endlessly replicable modes of improvement, and the moral high ground that becomes an entity in its own right/write. "Painters of signs" are part of movements through space that at once constitute and constrain "the rural" within imaginaries of progress. Not exactly "marginal" spaces, as the rural of West Virginia is so beautifully described by Kathleen Stewart, the "remembered villages" (one of the few ethnographies I had with me "in the field") of north India are at once heartlands that live deep inside an imaginary of the modern self and outlying spaces where there is work to be done. To Nandy's "ambiguous journey to the city," there are the countermoves toward *dehat* that are part of mobilities of both intervention and everyday life for "rural people" and "city people" alike. In spite of such fluidity, clichéd difference reappears, re-erupts, remains something always to be accounted for in the ways that births come to stand for something and tell us something. At least, this was the way people spoke to me.

In a recent interview, Gayatri Spivak described rural India as a "new" site of globalization because of technologies of genetic modification (and their potentials for new kinds of ownership) (Sharpe and Spivak 2002). But evocations of newness repeatedly imposed upon the rural reiterate a sense of where *dehat* stands in relation to history, where the bodies of "rural people" are located in relation to the stuff of modernity. As family planning efforts, "dai trainings," and various efforts to engage rural women on the ground of childbearing and the reproductive body suggest in their sheer longevity (over a hundred years and counting), transnational and universalizing flows of commodities, goods, ideas, moralities, and funds have long moved through these locales. The Indian postcolony, especially in the agrarian north and in the "problem states" against which the successes of the south are so often posed (Uttar Pradesh, Bihar), remains dominated by concepts of onward marches, of "development." Even the glance back is part of the way postcolonial identities can be said to carry the tinge of the "not quite" (Bhabha 1994) and postcolonial politics and life a sense of the "just a bit off" (Aretxaga 2000). In such spaces—long globalized—in which meanings circulate, but, more importantly, people and programs and efforts and actions move, what does one of the few intimate things that might (arguably) be thought of as "new"—new life—mean? How are its vulnerabilities and losses managed? What kinds of powers come into the foreground in its flows and forces? More to the point, what does birth tell us about what life is like for rural, poor women? What kinds of power, and accountability, and consciousness, and care, and making-right coalesce in birth and death?

The scene

This project began as a study of dais and dai trainings, but, as I explain in Chapter 1, it became something quite different when I put down roots in Lucknow. It might, then, be prudent to mark the point of "beginning" not so much in my interests and efforts in other parts of India but in my "arrival" in January 2000, on the anticlimactic side of the millennium, in the capital of the state of Uttar Pradesh, a location I selected in part because I was told it was "unthinkable" for me to continue such a project in Bihar (the area I initially studied) and in part because it is a central space from which numerous state and private health schemes extend into rural areas. In Lucknow, rurality as much as intervention is shaped through the nascence of plans and projects and the ways organizations reaching into "the villages" link up with larger, overarching, and fund-channeling organizations in Delhi and beyond. It was in Lucknow that my plan to "study dais" fell through; I now shudder to recall that my initial plan was to "apprentice" with a dai, to record her "knowledge," and along the way learn something about the contestations of "modernity." But I soon learned that local birth procedures in households made "the dai" very much a figment of crosscutting imaginaries. Indeed, "modernity" was not something the people I ended up spending time with cared much about. But the entanglements of "imaginaries" and "reals," entanglements people have with the reifications of their own lives, stayed with me throughout my efforts. From Lucknow, through connections with intervention programs, I moved to a village (which I call Lalpur) in the district of Sitapur, about 80 kilometers north of Lucknow, and spent much of the remaining time (until May 2001) coming and going between Lucknow and Lalpur, with a few trips to Delhi.

Anthropology is overburdened with arrivals, as are my own narratives; I add one more, but leave it to a minimum: I moved to Lalpur, a village of about eleven hundred people, at the end of the monsoon, during the last downpour of the year, with a field assistant who left after ten days. I brought a relatively small cache of stuff, some of which would take on fetish-like qualities in my life and relationships—gas cylinder, borrowed stove, camera, tape recorder, typewriter. I also brought a motorcycle, by which I thought I might supersede the old-fashioned but tenacious tendency to treat a village as *the village*, microcosm of "Indian life." To get to Lalpur (when rain doesn't make the road impassable) from Lucknow, you take a northerly route that passes through a town I call "Munniabad," in which there is a government health clinic, private hospital, several schools, a few large temples, a collapsing palace of a raja who now lives in England, and several bazaars. From Munniabad you take a turn at the *cauraha* (crossroad) on the edge of town, and follow increasingly minor turnoffs, past more bazaars, over a canal, through a small town where the road forks, and beyond it until the track to Lalpur appears on the right.

As a village of mixed caste and religion, Lalpur has twelve *jatis* which, by ethnographic convention, I list here: Brahmin/Pandit, Srivastav, Varma, Gupta, Julaha, Naai, Yadav, Kurmi, Lodh, Teli, Pasi, and Chamar. The Muslim population is about 15 percent, (and overlaps with the Julaha and Naai castes); the rest are Hindus, and the Dalit (or Scheduled Caste, or formerly "untouchable") population is about 17 percent. Land ownership in Lalpur is dominated by Kayasth Hindus who remain the best educated, best housed, and most well-off financially. A government school not far down the road serves children up to class six, though children were often on impromptu *chutti* (vacation), self-taken or "given" when the teacher did not show up. For grades beyond six, there are state schools a bit further away and several private ones on the road to Munniabad. Lalpur has a post office, a central Hindu temple, and a shop that stocks basic items. Most men and women work as agricultural laborers, on their own or on others' land. Some, especially Kayasths, work as teachers in nearby schools, hiring laborers to work in their fields. A few men work in shops in Munniabad or nearby *qasbahs*, in the brick factory down the road, or in a sugar mill. A few live and work in Lucknow as heavy laborers and rickshaw-pullers, sending money home to family.

The colonial and postcolonial history of Sitapur is informed by shifts and persistences in land-ownership patterns and labor relations. From the mid nineteenth century until Independence, the region of Awadh, in which Sitapur District falls, was characterized by a system of *taluqdari* rule, in which tax revenues were collected by the British from landlords with vast holdings, who themselves collected rents from cultivators and held much of the population in relations of tenancy. Within this structure, rigidified by the British through legislative acts meant to stave off rebellion, was a system of bonded labor, in which members of low castes such as Chamar, Kori, Kurmi, and Lodh were kept indebted to cultivators, landlords, or moneylenders (Kumar 1984). In the 1950s the newly independent government of India instituted caps on landholdings and attempted to force landholders to sell their above-limit land to the government at fixed rates. However, these laws went relatively unimplemented, and the slow pace of legislation allowed many landowners to circumvent rulings until 1974, when much lower land-ceilings were put in place centrally and land ownership laws were written into the constitution. Even now many evade land restructuring laws and preserve a status quo of landlessness among the most marginalized. At the same time, inheritance practices have meant increasing subdivision of land, such that by the late twentieth century, many landholdings were too small to support a family, a practice which made borrowing money against land, or from local moneylenders at enormous rates, commonplace. Debt is a pervasive, pernicious burden here.

Some transformation in land ownership has taken place in Sitapur, as land has changed hands to some extent in recent decades. Relationships between landowners and laborers have also changed with the increased education, economic power, and political mobilization of members of lower castes and classes. At the same time, in much of rural India there has been a large-scale relocation of local authority from landlords to the state (Wadley 1994: 165). For the lowest castes and classes the political climate has undergone significant change over the last decade; in the 1990s Uttar Pradesh witnessed the rise of Dalit politics and powerful Dalit political leaders. In spite of these changes, "caste," defined in ways that much of the following chapters aim to parse, remains—and has, perhaps, *become* in new ways—an important symbolic structure in everyday life in Sitapur, even as it comes under scrutiny in political formations. Likewise, while the shape of land ownership has changed, control over agriculture remains largely in the hands of historically land-owning and upper-caste families.

While the shift from landlord to state authority exists in terms of the ideals of government planning, in everyday ways, dominant castes and descendents of landowners have not so much been replaced by state institutions as they have become mediators, pathways *to* institutions. When it comes to health care and adjudication of disputes, many remain sites of authority, either standing in for state institutions themselves, or never having been supplanted in the first place. Men from prominent families settle arguments and suggest when to take matters to court. They advise whether to take family members to hospitals or act as doctors themselves. They help transport people to hospitals in dire cases, and explain how state institutions are best approached. When it comes to reproduction, women and men from powerful families become health authorities, occupying a place the state imagines itself to hold.

In the decades since Independence, agricultural development in India has also transformed social relationships and has made development a common idiom in rural areas, just as it has, arguably, entrenched a certain picture of poverty. Development has become, according to Akhil Gupta (1998), the defining characteristic of postcolonial rural Indian identity. Rural development programs have been implemented by both central and state governments, and the picture of rural development is becoming increasingly disparate as local and global non-governmental organizations (NGOs) implement a range of agricultural, banking, income generating, and educational programs. Where agricultural policies are concerned, growth-oriented programs have dominated development, with a "green revolution" beginning in the 1960s oriented toward technological change, often to the detriment of long-term sustainability and preservation of natural resources (Agarwal 1988). The effects of these programs, where women are concerned, have often been to reinforce gender and class inequalities, especially in situations already characterized by dramatic inequalities in land ownership and work relations, as is the case in central Uttar Pradesh (Agarwal 1988: 96). As Susan Wadley notes of post-1971 politics, "There is a paradox here ... for while the state is now ostensibly supporting the laborer *jatis*, with programs designed to aid the poor, for example, or to ensure the appointment of untouchables to office, its green revolution policies have in fact encouraged the development of a new capitalist landlord" (1994: 164). Thus, while political parties continue to send out populist appeals to working classes and lower castes, benefits of state programs continue to accrue to those in the position of landlords or former landlords (Gupta 1998; Wadley 1994: 164).

In Lalpur I lived, against my initial interests, with one such family, Kayasth Hindus. I spent mornings in the household, in fields, and around the village, my afternoons on trips to other towns and villages, to NGO and state "programs." Or I hung out in Lalpur with the women in my house or with neighbors, walking with children in the fields, entertaining and being interviewed by curious "outsiders" who had come to "see" me. In evenings I was always torn between typing notes and the more attractive option of sitting in the courtyard with other women. In the early mornings I sipped my instant coffee, sat on a stool in the outer yard, and wrote, watching and hearing and smelling the day begin around me—sounds of coughing and hacking, babies crying and children yelling, smells of onion frying, haze and mist slowly evaporating and the day coming into sharper focus as the sunlight eventually pushed me into the shade and "to work."

My analyses, my ways of writing and describing, and indeed my sense of the scope of "reproduction" are based on the things I learned by living and speaking with people in and around Lalpur (and to lesser extent Lucknow). A relatively small cohort, those with whom I formed the closest relationships, takes a place at the foreground. Though I have included narratives, stories, observations, and impressions from a range of voices, I find that I come back again and again, in my writing, as in my fond, troubled, embarrassed, angry, and again fond remembrances, to the same set of people. My reflections are most often in terms of their lives, the incidental, chance quality of my research and my life, and the degree to which so much of what I learned, where I went, how I ate, dressed, spoke, and acted, whom I spoke with, was, if not determined, then at least highly informed by them.

Most important was the family with whom I lived, who had been the primary landholders of a large swath of the region for the last two centuries, benefiting from colonial structures of land tenure and taxation and local feudal systems of labor; they were at the top of many heaps. The household was shifting in composition, with people coming and going for long and short stays. Most of the time it consisted of three brothers and their wives—Jawahar, the husband of the woman I knew as "Choti Bhabhi," younger sister-in-law; Sunderlal, husband of "Bari Bhabhi," older sister-in-law; and Raju, then unmarried. Also present was Amma, their elderly mother, and three children—Rohit and Dilip (Jawahar's kids) and Rani, a ten-year-old niece who was staying in the house for a while. Another brother, the eldest, lived in Lucknow with his wife and children. In this account, I continue to refer to the women of the house as Choti Bhabhi and Bari Bhabhi, and to other married women in the village by the ways they were known—as so and so's wife or so and so's mother, with only a few exceptions. Much is often made of the way women's naming practices in rural areas denote their "lack of individuality" or "lack of identity." I refer to them precisely as they were known to me in part to preserve the complexities of how women are known to each other and to counteract with ethnographic detail the assumption that proper names denote consciousness, and a lack of them denotes always and only its lack.

Bari Bhabhi, Sunderlal's wife was, at the time of my fieldwork, thirty-two. Married at sixteen, she had given birth to three sons, two of whom died. The one who survived past infancy, Arjun, was fifteen. He lived in Lucknow with his aunt and uncle and attended the school in which Jawahar taught. He came back to Lalpur several times a year. Like most *bahus* (daughters-in-law) Bari Bhabhi worked extremely hard in the house, and had an amicable but aloof relationship with her husband. She was educated to the sixth grade, and, not unconnected to this, her identity as *dehati* was something she often spoke about. She appreciated "old songs," she said, as evidence of this *dehati*-ness, preferring the long narratives derided by many young women and girls as "old-fashioned" and distasteful. She chastised me for eating food at untouchables' homes, but less so than Choti Bhabhi. When I returned at night from one surreptitious feast or another, she pretended not to notice my poorly hidden belches as she stomped in silent anger at my tardiness and wandering about after dark. She shared a bed with Choti Bhabhi's three-year-old son Rohit, and their bond was close—he called her Mumma, and his mother Mummi. Though our relationship was complex, at times marred by anger, I was closer to her than anyone.

Choti Bhabhi often spoke about the benefits of urban life, and bore longings that could best be termed bourgeois. She was twenty-four, a high school graduate, and loved fine things, dressing up, and displays of wifely virtue urban middle-class women—and less so rural women—demand (regular fasting, rigorous wearing of the *suhag,* the signs of married status). She complained often about how much she worked, how much she detested the uncleanness of untouchables and Muslims, and how different things were in the city, where "everyone is clean and keeps to themselves." She chastised me strongly for my failures to wear, or wear properly, the garb of wifehood—a sari, red bangles, ankle bracelets, toe rings, *sindhur* streaked into the part of my hair, a bindi. She scolded me even more for my transgressions of caste rules, and expressed disgust that I should "let" Dalit women sit on my bed or chair. Her casteism, as I came to see it, and contrary to the views of men in the village who equated more education with less discrimination, was bound up with middle-class longings, visions of morality and urban identity, as well as with her sense of herself as a "more educated" person. It was also, somewhat paradoxically, part of what I came to understand as her intense, almost fearful, desire *not* to offend. Her husband, Jawahar, came from Lucknow every weekend. They had two young sons, and Choti Bhabhi swore up and down that she didn't want any more. Bari Bhabhi and Choti Bhabhi were in strict *purdah,* not permitted, and also not choosing, to leave the house for other homes in the village outside of their kin network (they could and did go to Munniabad to shop, go to the temple, or visit the doctor). They were, in fact, something of a mystery to many other women in the village, some of whom did not know how many *bahus* lived in the household. Because of their status within this prominent family, and their strict maintenance of *purdah* (which had fallen off slightly since the death of Bapu-ji their father-in-law), they were themselves objects of curiosity and fear for other local women.

I spent a great deal of time with people from Lalpur's community of Pasis, an "untouchable" *jati* associated with pig herding but whose primary work was, like most everyone else's, agricultural. Tulsiram, a middle-aged father of five, often lingered into the night in the outer yard of my house, spending long hours with other men discussing politics and agriculture. He appointed himself the task of introducing me to the natural and agricultural worlds of Sitapur, local politics, and the life and perspective of a self-described "small man." Pushpadevi, the wife of a distant cousin of Tulsiram, was also someone I spent many afternoons with. She was probably in her mid thirties, though she could not or would not tell me her age, and scoffed at the idea of knowing so. Her husband was one of several men arrested midyear for a murder and robbery in the nearby *qasbah,* and his departure was a mixed blessing for her. She lacked his presence as an income producer, but she also lacked his beatings, intimidations, and costly demands for sex—costly because they had produced three more children than she wanted, making her tally, as she put it, "a half-dozen." Through Pushpadevi I learned the complexity of the power relations, moral demands, workloads, and institutional failures that impinge on women's lives, most profoundly so for the poor and lowest class and caste.

She admitted that she knew little about history, but talked about "the end of caste" as right-leaning postmodern theorists talk of the "end of history"—as part of a present condition of consciousness containing large and small ironies. At the same time that she spoke of the end of caste, she also demonstrated to me the ways her life was ridden with it. She longed for control of her reproductive life, and, in part because of these thwarted desires, displayed a growing madness, a troubled lack of the upright morality signified by the term *sidha*—straight—in her identity as a Hindu wife. Her sister-in-law, whose husband was more stable, law-abiding, and responsible than Pushpadevi's husband, was truly *sidha,* all that Pushpadevi was not. She covered her mouth and looked away appropriately when talk came around to sex and birth. Pushpadevi brought up the topics repeatedly, and asked for intimate details about life in "my place." If anyone confounded romantic visions of untouchable women defiantly resisting liberal models of modern womanhood, it was Pushpadevi, who desired emancipation in terms at once liberal/political-economic and near mystical, who sought the same things she rejected, and whose body and children's bodies had borne the results of this mix of desire, fear, and resistance. She was, for me, the epitome of the not-straight, demonstrating the often terrible embodiments of conflicting moral logics, conflicting efforts to give care, the way visions of progress converge on reproduction, leaving emotions as crossed and crooked as the lives they make possible and impossible.

There are other figures as well, though I leave them to emerge in the text—Shalini and her mother; two elderly postpartum workers; Chachi, a Muslim birth worker; Pratima, the self-made doctor who lived in a nearby village; and Manjari, a young NGO supervisor who lived in Lalpur. Other key personalities in my fieldwork were the institutions that staked a claim on (or had a stake in) the reproductive lives of rural women. There were several, and their interactions were complex. First and largest was a recent scheme in Uttar Pradesh, described in its own literature as "innovative." I have changed its name to NAFPA, New Approaches to Family Planning Agencies (primarily for symbolic reasons—acronyms are always vague and thus instantly recognizable, even in code), and it was a collaboration of state and nongovernment agents, in which divisions between the public and private good, between national, international, and local were difficult to draw, at least for me. Funded by international donor agencies and the government of India, it was run at the state level from a government office in Lucknow, and at local levels by urban-based NGOs and private hospitals. It consisted of a complex hierarchy of funding, training, master-training, module-producing, implementing, and evaluating agencies, reaching from Sitapur to Lucknow to Delhi to universities, agencies, and governments in foreign countries. At the most local level in Sitapur, NAFPA was implemented by a branch of a Lucknow-based hospital and its workers (aided by next-level-up NGOs) who trained local men and women to serve as on-the-ground agents. Also active in this region was a smaller NGO, based in Lucknow and receiving funds from international donor agencies. I call it Mahila Seva Sansthan (Ladies Service Organization), though, again, its own acronym was far more brilliant and even beautiful than my own clumsy creation. They ran dai trainings, food distributions, educational programs, and other health-related programs in rural communities. Though it predated NAFPA, since NAFPA had come onto the scene (approximately two years before I began my research), Mahila Seva Sansthan worked in communities in which NAFPA did not. There was overlap of personnel between NAFPA and Mahila Seva Sansthan at the upper levels, especially in staffing trainings. In my daily comings and goings I frequently crossed paths with representatives from one or the other agency, one or the other of the many groups involved in NAFPA or Mahila Seva Sansthan, on the road, in Lalpur, in Devia, and in Munniabad, as well as at or near the Primary Health Center (PHC) in the block headquarters about fifteen kilometers from Lalpur.

Though state PHCs and subcenters existed, they were often empty, closed intermittently, staffed irregularly, and severely underequipped. I never saw the subcenter in Devia without a large padlock on its front door, though I was told frequently, "It was open last week," or "It might be open tomorrow." I imagine that my bad luck was not unlike that of many women who came to it in search of a doctor. The PHC was enough of a distance from Lalpur to warrant it being considered difficult to get to, especially at night and in bad weather, and unreliable once reached. Women joked about the infrequent presence of doctors: "Who can tell a baby to be born on a Tuesday or Thursday?" Assistant nurse midwives (ANMs) were more reliable presences, though much of their appeal or lack thereof rested on their own presence, personalities, penchant for work, and attitudes toward minority communities.

Midway through my fieldwork my husband came to visit. Though he spoke little Hindi, his days were as full as mine with visits, journeys, games, and copious amounts of tea and freshly made *gur* (a sugar product made at that time of year). It was not long after he left that I found I was pregnant. From then on things changed for me. After my first month I was doubled over with intense morning sickness, and found myself losing weight I should have been gaining. Nausea ruled my life. I mention it here because this particular way of experiencing pregnancy shifted my subject-position in Lalpur not only to that of pregnant woman, first-time future mother, and even more visibly clueless foreigner, but also to that of sick person. I stayed in Lalpur for the most part, though when things were very bad I returned to Lucknow and, at one point, Delhi. In my fifth month of pregnancy, overcome by summer heat and pregnancy-related sickness, I returned to the United States.

Being pregnant not only, in fairly obvious ways, allowed for new ways of "connecting with" the women I was living with—making me subject to warnings, predictions, new kinds of teasing, unfamiliar idioms, instructions, dream interpretations, and shared fantasies. It also put me in new clinical spaces in the city, to which I returned for check-ups. The process and progress of my pregnancy in terms of *that* experience—dominated by gruff nurses, public disclosures in the crowded clinic, blood tests, ultrasound, ultrasound and more ultrasound (all routine), and tiny yellow antinausea pills (and my own mix of desire, desperation, and fear in relation to them)—were in stark contrast to the contours of my pregnancy in Lalpur. In both spaces I was a novice, sick, foreign, and "alone" (without my husband), but the meanings of these things in each space were different. While being pregnant helped me "connect" with women in Lalpur, in perhaps more telling ways it pushed me further away, making differences between us all the more profound. This experience, even where unspoken, lies underneath much of what I have to say about their lives.

What "care" means

Scene-setting also requires a few comments about health institutions. As R. S. Khare (1996) argues, the broader situation of health care in rural India, its institutional contexts and medical pluralities, make close attention to "practiced medicine" a matter of some importance. This is especially so in an international context in which, given nearly two decades of change in national policy and international flows of funds, policy, ideology, and regulation, at the local level in north India the definition of development is up for grabs, even as it is ever further constrained globally within neoliberal visions and linked historically to structural adjustment (Millen et al. 2000; Qadeer 2001). Recent studies of medical intervention in India, especially those emerging from the south, put notions of "modernity" at center stage. As Lawrence Cohen (2005) and Cecilia Van Hollen (2002) compellingly argue in the case of Tamil Nadu, the body's "availability" to the state (Cohen 2005), demonstrated through extensive use of invasive medical technologies (Van Hollen 2002) and a willingness to subject oneself and one's organs to the cuts of the hospital and circulations of global markets, involves an effort to "remake one's mindful body in accordance with the demands of developmental modernity, to remake one *as if* one were a modern" (Cohen 2005: 87). In Sitapur, perhaps indicative of differences between north and south India along development's various continua, both the association of medical intervention with something like belonging and power (if bioavailability is, at least in part, an index of that kind of affective citizenship) and the ways that the literalized stuff of invasive medicine, namely knives and needles, circulate through everyday talk involve a quite different affective economy. The "health market" means something different here. For one thing, this is a locale in which "participation" is already fraught and in which, more often than not, the "dividuality" (Marriott 1968) of the body tends to settle into matters of moralized consumption as much as, or more than, moralized offerings. As part of consumption logics and their concomitant threat and attraction, things that pierce and cut into the body are treated with a great deal of suspicion, often in evasive terms in which the "group" is perceived as being under threat. Likewise, availability often confounds from the other side of the medical encounter—the availability *of care to people*. With hesitation about introducing another collapse of space and time, another narrative of "developmental modernity," I am tempted to suggest that perhaps, in Sitapur, where care can be enormously unpredictable and difficult to get, the time of bioavailability has not yet come. Though sharing a broadly Indian context in which "family planning" has dominated—in funding, attention, and affective weight—the picture of health care provision, perhaps this is a place where other availabilities, other logics of capital point more to a feeling of being *out of reach* but *in view*—in a very basic way, the sheer difficulties of getting care in the first place. Older conversations about health and development and discourse remain very much relevant in Uttar Pradesh. Or perhaps, given the dynamics of modernity and medicine described by Cohen and Van Hollen in the south, we can hear in a different key the diacritical comments of Ruchi, a doctor who worked in the NAFPA health camps that periodically passed through Lalpur: "Women in the north are lazy and suspicious. In the south they are more interested in their health."

At the same time, recent approaches to reproductive health in India suggest that it is precisely in this domain of affect that "women's reproductive agency" unfolds and people establish relationships—or break them off—with those places that might offer care (Unnithan-Kumar 2001, 2005). Like Cohen, who discusses the way love plays into people's engagement with the global economy by way of their organs and bodies (2005), Maya Unnithan-Kumar, noting connections between emotions and power, finds that among rural women in Rajasthan, relationships with various kinds of medical services and authorities are forged amid "emotions generated by social intimacy," including those between kin and the feelings associated with the burdens of childbearing over the course of a life (2001: 27). Power is involved in crosscutting ways, filtered and mediated by the very emotions that emerge in its points of excess and convergence, as much as in the shape of desire and love so integral to reproduction.

In rural Sitapur, "practiced medicine" and its affective components begin with home births, which constitute the majority of rural births, with circumstances that defy assumptions about how and where medicalization takes place. In Uttar Pradesh, rural home births are often matters of choice and preference. Many women return *from* the city to villages, where they are assisted by family members, local specialists, and uncertified "doctors" summoned to give injections of labor-inducing drugs. Local forms of birth-related work also defy state, international, and feminist fantasies about "traditional midwives," consisting instead of many overlapping practitioners and a basic—and largely ignored—division between baby-delivering and postpartum care (the latter of which is the work of Dalit specialists).

In 2001, the picture of globalization, including structural changes in health care and the ever-increasing emphasis on liberalization and privatization of state services, meant, in India, the "rolling back of the state" (Qadeer et al. 2001: 31) as well as a rolling *over* of much health care to private and not-for-profit organizations, in addition to a reliance on foreign donors and agendas established in distant locales. All of this has meant that health care is dominated by intervention-oriented approaches rather than broad-spectrum care, primary or otherwise, profit-orientation rather than an effort to link health conditions with broader social and infrastructural conditions (Drèze and Sen 2002; Qadeer 2001; Sen 2001). According to Jean Drèze and Amartya Sen, health care in India is marked by low public expenditure, inefficient use of resources, and inequalities in access to health care along lines of class, caste, region, and gender, within a "market system" in which care is a commodity (202). In terms of change, Drèze and Sen note the expansion of health services "in quantitative terms" amid "much evidence that their *quality* has deteriorated" (205; cf. Das 2002, 2003). As has been observed more generally in India is also the case in rural Sitapur: though a skeleton of PHCs and subcenters is technically present, "health centres are dilapidated, medicines are not available, doctors are chronically absent, and patients are routinely charged for services that are meant to be free (when they are treated at all)" (Drèze and Sen 2002: 205–6). In a country that, until recent changes in patent laws, produced cheap generic drugs for the rest of the world, many still cannot afford the "market system where diagnoses and drugs are treated much like any other commodity" (202).

Temporality is key to the health equation in which state facilities and services live (or should) alongside private ones. State hospitals may exist for the long term, but their services, personnel, and reliability come and go. Much depends on the personality and accessibility of ANMs who are often the only people in residence near state health centers, just as much depends on doctors' willingness to spend much—or all—of their week in "rural areas" instead of cities. Likewise, reproductive health programs come and go as priorities shift along with names, agencies, and degrees of association with family planning programs. NGO presence is even more fluctuating; though it aims for "sustainability," its temporary quality is a basic part its structure. Local, national, and international agencies come in, often with fanfare, then recede, maybe to return one day, maybe not. In such a context, painters of signs are often very local; many people create medical roles for themselves, while others are more officially linked with ever-changing development projects. Here, the everyday facts of health care availability mean that the state, in a larger sense, must be thought about in *dehat* as much for how it is evasive and confounding as for the way it can also loom and overarch.

Rural Indian women's bodily practices have been sites of transnational intervention for a long time. While recent efforts are often labeled "innovative," similar programs date back to the 1860s, a trans-

formative period in British colonial rule when ideas about development and "uplift" became central components of a vision of Indian
subjects in relation to state powers. Since then, state and private
health services have arrived as brief, technologically and education-
ally oriented "interventions." Linking pedagogy with performances
of power, "training" is a key praxis—local women are trained to be
institutional agents; "TBAs" (traditional birth attendants) are trained
in "safe delivery;" local men and women are given "skills training" for
"income generation." Though the private health sector is relatively
unmonitored (Drèze and Sen 2002: 206), official programs and the
logics of "training" take advantage of the informal, unregulated quality of medical practice to recruit and to establish local networks.

Where rural women's health is concerned, the state is schizoid,
echoing the longer genealogies of health care in India in which funds
and attention have fallen overwhelmingly on family planning and
vaccination programs to the detriment of other, broader health services. This has involved—and allowed—political framings that have,
over time, "eroded" the very notions of "choice" and democracy from
which they derive their moral weight (Ram 2001). As Kalpana Ram
notes, state family planning efforts demonstrate the collision of two
"imperatives of the Indian state"—liberalism and development (85).
In Sitapur, this situation is firmly in place, along with the lived ironies
of "choice" the policies themselves contain. In Sitapur, the state remains overwhelmingly interested in family planning, with numerous programs encouraging sterilization and contraception, flanks of
local distributors monitoring who buys what, plays, slogans, rallies,
and visits from funders and politicians (local and foreign, of varying
degrees of "VIP" status). But to the coercions, subtle and overt, that
have long shadowed India's family planning efforts (and that make
current efforts advertise prominently their "target-free approach"),
we can add another irony about "eroded choice": for maternal, prenatal, and pediatric care, state health institutions fall into the larger
unreliabilities and absences of care. They are often hard to get to,
hard to pay for (even when services should be free or low-cost), unavailable, involving locked hospitals, absent doctors, dirty conditions, terrible roads, enormous difficulties in transport, little or no
electricity, lousy phone systems, and at times (though of course not
always) threatening and abusive practitioners.

Thus, while this is hardly a place with an "absent state," it is one
in which health care is a patchwork over space and time, and in
which, within global conditions that drain a state already "disinvested
in health" (Drèze and Sen 2002; Rao 1999), affective dilemmas are

part of *both* hegemonic presence and a nearly (if not entirely) averted gaze, and formal health care delivery vacillates between ideals and realities. While in much of rural north India, government and non-government health care institutions are part of the fabric of everyday life, their often uncertain presence means that, for many, institutions exist primarily as points of imagination, a site upon which to lodge affect.

What "power" means

The bond—or bind—between subjects and the state, as between subjects and crosscutting modes of authority that extend well beyond the state, is at the heart of what it takes to care for oneself and one's family in such a context. It is likewise critical to the way childbearing and infant death unfold. Such experiences can unify the "incomparable entities of self and state" (Greenhouse 2001), even as they make what it is to negotiate the promises and failures of institutions essential to survival, such that the state's "*ambiguous* availability [becomes] a pre-condition of human dignity" (Greenhouse 1999: 104, emphasis added). Ambiguity resonates in the longing and fear amid which new life enters and leaves the world. Where infant death is such a shared experience, we must always ask, as Arthur Kleinman (1999) reminds, "what is at stake" in the most everyday of spaces. At the same time, we must take into consideration the ways that the "stakes" for rural poor women (hardly a uniform bunch) are seldom straightforward when it comes to reproduction.

In Sitapur, through women's bodily processes and through their ways of navigating intervention and institutions, utterances deemed furthest from political awareness are often those that express political subjectivity and the conflicted nature of citizenship. In households and the ways births and deaths happen within them, the state becomes mythical, circulating in languages that "[lend] living shape to (and as) coded signs of identity" (Greenhouse 1999: 104). In overlapping forms of suffering and longing, engagement is always at stake. This is so in terms of the ways some actions bespeak a particular orientation toward state power and ideologies of improvement. It also emerges in the ways the tenuous difference between, as women put it, those things God gives (and takes away) and those we bring upon ourselves is experimented on and theorized in this arena.

This is precisely the boundary negotiated, these are the certainties demythologized (and remythologized) in the ways death enters

the time-space of birth and suffering enters the domain of the auspicious and the certain. As Hannah Arendt writes, suffering is the
ever-present other to actions whose consequences in the world can
never be fully known (1998: 190). Suffering, like action, is part of
things in flux, things under debate in reproductive life. Some have
suggested that suffering is compelling to those interested in subjectivity and power because it always "calls into question the real"
(Halpern 2002: 10). Where suffering may be the "hidden opposition
of agency" or the necessary other to action (Halpern 2002: 10, following Arendt), what remains indelibly clear to me in regard to
Sitapur is the way suffering, especially in the case of infant death, can
become an index of multiple forms of agency and accountability,
overlapping (often contradictory) needs, longings, revulsions, and
fears, the way it is often, or always, part of the flow of desires mediated by the very spaces and entities that aim to obviate it. Suffering, in the deeply social form that high rates of infant mortality can
involve, calls agency into question by opening up new ways of imagining connections between subjects and the will, between subjects
and Law, and between capacity and constraint. In many ways, birth
can also do the same. Through everything that new life and childbearing can mean in a context in which so many babies and children
die, suffering can indeed be political (Kleinman et al. 1997). It can
involve expressions of political location, of the delicately sustained
ambiguities between the "I" and the "we" brought to the foreground
in everyday speech. Whether part of a postcolonial state of not-quite-
right-ness (Aretxaga 2000; Bhabha 1994), part of a larger, more
global "necrographic map" (Mbembe 2001) of sovereignty, or part
of the intimate impacts of structural violence and grinding poverty
(Farmer 1999; Scheper-Hughes 1992), grief is part of the ways marginalized (but not marginal) women can express their place in society and in relation to forms of power.

Put in less grand terms, what this means is that in Sitapur, things
like "access," "validity," and modes of othering such as, I argue, contemporary "untouchability" are nestled into one another. This has
everything to do with institutional sites and the convergence of the
market forces of neoliberalization and the battening down of reified
"cultural difference" (Driscoll 2004). Institutions—often global ones,
or local nodes in a global network—produce not only resources (or
the idea of them) *for* rural women, they also produce ideas *about*
rural women. Subjectivities are interlaced with attributed "identities"—renderings and stereotypes which both differ from and, at
times, closely resemble women's own self-reckonings. While features

of the female subject become foci of social change (e.g., an ability to recognize one's own suffering, or to privatize and internalize the relationship between demand and action), subject constitution is, in itself, only as important as the struggles it brings into being. A contemporary form of "untouchability" is not only an encompassing category (incorporating, in rural worlds, poor Muslims and those of lowest class status), it is also one that is increasingly globalized as it takes on the ambiguities associated with class, location, and religion in a world in which so much about equality is now expected to depend upon the individual, the private, and the desocialized.

As part of such global dynamics, childbearing in *dehat* bespeaks the ways lives are located at a convergence of inequalities of gender, caste, and class (Wadley 1994), the ways the management of reproduction and sexuality is part of maintaining social hierarchies (Sangari and Vaid 1997). At the same time, "hierarchy," long the iconic feature of "Indianness," is often described in the ironies of globalization as resurfacing in places where it should not (or no longer) exist, the eruption of caste into spaces of secular democracy, for instance. But as subjects exist in constant tension with power dynamics that both situate and reify their experiences, it becomes critical to consider precisely what kinds of difference might be in play. Let us be more specific about the languages—and language games—of power (hierarchy, if we must). Sometimes social maps involve something different from "hierarchy"; sometimes it is the writing of the self into the world (through talk and interventionist imaginaries, through grief and desire and outrage) according to specific metaphors that do not (or do not quite) suggest "rank" that makes power look and feel the way it does, that makes it have often barely detectable links to the terrible choiceless choices women must make in caring for themselves and their children.

Dehati women's own conversations about these things are located amid rich scholarly debate about how to represent inequality and locate Indian women on global stages and in global(izing) discourses. Specifically, these are debates between critiques seeking distinctly postcolonial, non-Western feminisms, and more positivist, humanist, and Enlightenment-type views—a division once, but no longer, mappable onto the "academic" and the "activist," the "critic" and the "intervener." This division was also once mapped in the other direction, into a distinction between "universalizing" (read: Western) models and particularized local ones. Thanks, on the one hand, to the appropriation of a reified concept of "culture" by large multi-, trans- and extranational health policy sources, and, on the other, to the way, as Anna Tsing remarks, the West can "make no exclusive claim to the doctrine of universals" (2004: 9), such a division is no longer possible. Likewise, in Sitapur, the production of knowledge about "rural women" happens as much within rural communities as beyond them; it is part of the shaping of desire. In a space where the "other" of longing and aversion is not always imagined as residing in "the west," local diacritics employ globalizing elements and strategies of differentiation while also, often, being posited on "non-Western" grounds.

Women's lives in Lalpur force us into considerations of birth and infant death as key nodes of deeply contested political consciousness and citizenship; this involves imagining citizenship broadly, as loaded with affect (Bosniak 2000), as involving the abject, as a condition of desire, as legitimizing, as performative and pedagogical (Bhabha 1994), and as overwhelmingly "empirical" (as opposed to formal)—something more than belonging or its opposites, "an idiom expressive of highly varied, (even crossed) purposes, needs, absences, and desires" (Greenhouse 1999: 105). Likewise, the intervention matrix of medical practice and moral pedagogy make it important to think of citizenship not only as a person's relation *to* civil society (Bosniak 1999), but as a kind of relationship one has *within* civil society. In the way "crossed" purposes may supersede "belonging," or individualizing explanations evoke the straits of group identities, there lies a compelling way to ask what is under threat in the forms of citizenship that emerge at the intersections of what Partha Chatterjee calls the "fragments of the nation" (1993)—the interior coordinates in which citizenship emerges through relationships *beyond* those between self and state.

The primary intersection of diacritics (and their attendant crises of subjectivity) I explore in this book is that of moralities of intervention and something like "untouchability." Writ large, the argument is that through the range of ways that intervention is interwoven with uncertain, ever-receding, temporary, failing structures of care, a figure that looks an awful lot like "the untouchable" has come to haunt the citizen that is the subject of "development." It looms about a postcolonial world expressly concerned with enunciating and enacting equality. This "untouchable" is both an internal other and a threat to progress, emerging not just as a trace or hybrid of "tradition" but as a not-quite-tangible feature of the self-consciously clean, educated, rational female subject. This is especially so in the embodiments of reproduction, in which affective tensions and the dyadic convergence of "I" and "we" demonstrate efforts to grapple with the way "untouchability" has become a crypto-product of discourses and processes explicitly aimed at improving conditions of life *for all*, a silent factor of progress's own rationalities. What I focus on is not the way this marks a bastardization of the global by the local but the way it shows that certain moralities take a formative, generative role in framing globalized ideals. Socialities can reveal convergences discomforting precisely in their easy familiarity (rather than obvious ruptures or ironies of globalization). In logics of legitimization and intervention aimed at the fertile body, citizenship as a mode of disgust becomes the necessary underscript of citizenship expressed as an algorithm of fear and longing.

It has become clear to me, in working through this argument, that it is not always easy—or, in some spaces, appropriate—to talk about "caste" as a contemporary mode of subjectivity or a contemporary practice. How do we turn ethnographic gazes onto such sites of ongoing symbolic and political consolidation, onto the meanings and entities long ago deconstructed as overimagined microcosms of "Indianness"—villages and caste? My own approach has been to sustain a "caste lens," in which "caste," like "the rural," is as good to think with as to think about, and to aim it at the languages, moral symbolics, and practices of those most making a claim on/to "the modern"—not necessarily to "reveal" something latent, remaindered, or even eruptive, but to consider something at once productive and produced. In this sense, if "untouchability" *feels* "eruptive" here— and in many ways it does (to me, at least)—then what should be of interest is precisely the structure of that feeling of wrongness, the very way that "untouchability," like other constructs of disgust (and their objects), has been *made to feel* eruptive in idioms of progress with which it so comfortably sits, the way it—and especially the people associated with it—remain endowed with the ability to cause a shudder of what Freud identified in his essay "The Uncanny" as the eruption of "the primitive," which is also the intrusion of the most messily, bodily, homely feminine (2003). How, in other words, do ruptures in the fabric of reality, be they anthropological or interventionist, allow certain ways of being and doing, speaking and feeling to become at once frightening and necessary?

In ideas about the rural, some modes of power—especially those constituted by the meanings of "untouchability"—are, in academic terms, associated with imagined and constructed pasts, the power/ knowledge of colonialism, and rightly so (Dirks 2001). Likewise, they have been seen as part of the dangerous and desirous imaginaries of we who observe (Inden 1990). This is precisely the mode of inquiry in which and with which I approach "untouchability" in its appear-ance in the flows of intervention—as part of interwoven discourses in which anthropologist, missionary, health care worker, and "rural woman" share certain topographies and maps (that may also, often, appear superficially different, even opposed). At the same time, I would not earn my anthropological stripes if I did not also suggest that accountability must be made for modes of power and diacritics beyond those of "biopower" (as the "explicit calculations," the map-ping, measuring, surveilling mode of power in which, as Michel Fou-cault argued, power over death was replaced by the power to foster or disallow life [1978: 143]). As Partha Chatterjee argues (1994), we may not be able to comprehend contemporary complexities of life without an "immanent critique" of things too often dismissed as "premodern." How can we account, in overdetermined spaces like "villages," for overdetermined modes of othering like "caste" and the ways the very imagination of such entities as bounded is at once part of discursive craftings of modernity and also very real, very em-bodied, very everyday? We begin, I would like to propose, by con-sidering how such clichés and stagnancies play into and through other (and similar) uses and thems. "Untouchability" becomes less about "hierarchy" and more about circulating diacritics that frame the contemporary subject of intervention.

As political, social, and symbolic forms, modes of subjectivity that resemble "untouchability" become facts of life for all rural women, not just those most marginalized—Dalits or Muslims—though the direst consequences of this modern morality fall upon them. If, as Begonia Aretxaga and others have argued, exclusion is often written into the structures of inclusion (2000), how do we find an orienta-tion to justice within such exclusions? I get vertigo from veering back and forth between the idea that "freedom" and "progress" are fetishes (as Wendy Brown [2001] argues) and an appreciation of the stakes marginalized people have in these very concepts. Do these stakes represent a particular (male, Western, elite, etc.) framework in which subaltern women, such as Dalits, amid layers of stigmati-zation become objects in larger discourses on progress? If anything, local stories of birth and loss demand we move beyond the culture wars surrounding relativism—into which these stories could lead us—and beyond the way battles descend on the presence or absence of political consciousness. Conditions of birth in Sitapur demand we approach head-on feminism's ambivalence toward forward mo-tion, its wariness of transitional narratives, and its broad imperatives of change as both subject-producing ideologies and as promises of wellness.

In drafting the Indian constitution, B. R. Ambedkar imagined equality not as a basic attribute, and freedom not something one is inalienably born with, but equality and freedom things the state exists to bring into being to counteract the unequal positions in which people come into the world-as-context (Kaviraj 2000). Equality is, in this view, a matter of reworlding. We must take very seriously, then, efforts to write difference *into* citizenship and the circumstances of those who become targets of ostensibly equality-aimed, difference-ameliorating (or, more often, denying) interventions that, through visions of sovereignty, imagine a constant and threatening "them." The political nature of diacritics and deeply personal identifications underlie this account, as does the sense that *reified* difference (as opposed to socialized and complexified status, a basic condition of social life) in the interest of intervention (or global capital, pace Driscoll 2004) causes enormous harm.

Modes of differing, of locating political and politicized subjects, reflect the crossed purposes of institutions and interventions; they show that there are very real outcomes to language games of intervention: real lives and real deaths. Of course, not everything about birth reiterates "untouchability." Indeed, women's stories about infant death bear a remarkably redemptive quality. Through them, contingencies of daily life and moralities of intervention are critiqued and raged at in terms larger than caste, terms emphasizing the overwhelming quality of conditions of living and trying to survive. In these stories, women outline not only their grief, but also the contours of poverty and their relationships with larger forces. Stories bracketed with fatalistic-sounding phrases describe chains of institutional failure. Rather than absolving blame, they bring mothers, husbands, doctors, the state, ghosts, pharmaceuticals, pathogens, and poverty into the same zone of culpability. Within these tales, the dead baby, like the dying man Michel de Certeau describes, brings to the foreground the "extreme frontier of inaction" (1984: 191) and the ways everyday life amid loud and strident claims to certainty— so often cloaked as "science," "medicine," "development," and so on—can involve negotiating precisely the unbearable boundary between what should be within one's hands but is not.

In the assemblage of actors, discourses, objects, and practices that is health intervention in rural India, so much, for the poor, is considered to hinge on perceptions of what is real: what is real suffer-

ing and what is not, what is the real *cause* of suffering and what obfuscation, what is "knowledge" and what "blind belief," what is a
sense of perspective and what misperception. Education, at the heart
of this apparatus, has as its basic ontological principle the notion
that perception versus misperception of the real demarcates suffering and the way out of it. But rural women's grapplings with birth
and death show that the real *is*, so often, precisely what is being theorized and retheorized and grappled with. In Hindu world(s) we can
add to adamant assertions of the importance of "the real" something
approaching the concept of *lila*—the play or game that is the illusion
of the world we live in, in which consequences are at once tangible
and not quite real. Indeed, the broad, unbearable, and overwhelming causalities of poverty and structural violence do not leave much
room for certainties promised by loud declarations about the real
and its perceptions. In Sitapur, we must account for the fact that the
state may, for some, be the biggest *fakir* around.

Survival, in Sitapur, often seems to be about putting aside categories of real and fake, true and false for the sake of getting through
life, while claims to power, on the other hand, seem to be primarily
about establishing the difference between the real and its others, then
staking a claim on what is established as real. In the flux and flow
of moralities and messages about childbearing, in which women participate as painters and readers of signs, trickery, fakery, performance,
and play, are not in this case the cleverness or desperation of the postmodern or postcolonial, even though as negotiations they are part
of the conceptual frames by which and with which women struggle
with the realities of death amid promises and certainties (if you get
to a doctor your baby will live; if you get an injection you will not
get sick). Of course, this does not obviate what theorists of suffering
such as Kleinman insist is what we should always be after in our
ethnographic endeavors: a sense of what really matters in the ways
people inhabit overlapping cultural, political, and moral structures.

It is through these ideas that we can see the ways that birth and
loss, amid the specific conditions of life and care for the rural poor in
the postcolony, are integral to the way citizenship, or political subjectivity, or where one falls on the map of things, is fundamentally
part of what Michel de Certeau calls "the marvelous and ephemeral
excess of surviving." And so, from that peek at the end, I take you
back to the beginning—to many beginnings, in fact, to pause for a
while on the question of why childbearing brings women, families,
and groups into close contact with the stuff of power: institutional,
global, local, and household. And to ask what can be learned about

power from the terrible intersection of birth and loss in a small part of rural India.

Chapters

But before that, a quick, but necessary, guide to what follows: Chapter 1 situates the account with an outline of the labors involved in home birth. Here I describe the unfolding of birth in the home, the stakes that Dalit women in particular have in this "local" division of labor between baby-delivering and postpartum care, and the ways such work becomes part of Dalit women's reckonings of power and action. Chapter 2 zooms in on the placenta as an object and symbol around which divisions of labor take shape, but also as a site in which meaning games basic to the structure of intervention come into clarity. The abject object here reveals the way thresholds between realms of consciousness, as between life and death, are mediated by structures of care and intervention, broadly speaking. I argue that the placenta, situated at a range of conceptual boundaries, is part of delineating senses of revulsion and labors involving social cordoning-off in both the frames of "caste" and those of biomedically oriented interventions.

Chapter 3 continues to map the shape of care in rural areas, focusing on self-made and uncertified medical practitioners and their complex role in both providing care and sustaining the development myth. Here, too, I address the way socialities that resemble "untouchability" are woven into ethoses of improvement and institutional (and institution-like) programmatics. Chapter 4 is about visuality in pregnancy—dynamics of seeing and being seen and how they form zones of vulnerability in both households and clinics. It is also about how contrasting modes of sight in pregnancy provide material for a critique of the "clinical gaze." It takes us in and out of the clinic—and the many forms this can take in rural prenatal care—and behind and in front of a range of veils to think about what subjectivities emerge through pregnancy. Chapter 5 is about grief. It describes women's narratives of infant death, the ways talk about it creates a soteriology of life and death, action and inaction, and the real and the fake on the margins of institutionality. Chapter 6 returns to the mythical figure of the "dai" and the way imaginaries of the "traditional midwife" inform socialities of intervention and orient them away from "knowledge" and "tradition" so fetishized in policy documents and toward the individualization and privatization of the subject of intervention. Chapter 7 is about "suiting" and gossip, the ways women talk about "other people's" births and babies and care-giving, and the ways they—especially Dalits and Muslims—reconcile these moralities in their own approaches to care. It is also about death and the way it emerges from the moralizing claims of intervention as they circulate through household and neighborhoods. Here I address local fears of medical intervention; this is where I most fully develop the argument that equality- and enfranchisement-oriented discourses of intervention craft an emergent form of "untouchability" around matters such as who takes medicines, who refuses them, who has many kids, who has few, who goes to the doctor, who does not.

Chapter 1

WORK
WHERE THERE IS NO MIDWIFE

Dais who don't deliver

I went to Sitapur to talk to "midwives." An interest in women I had long
known to be called "dais" (something readily translatable as "Indian
traditional midwives"), in their social position, the nature of their work,
their uncertain role in health interventions: these are the things that carried
me through graduate school and readings of historical and ethnographic accounts of birth in South Asia, through interactions with NGOs and advocates in different parts of India, finally to Sitapur, for a "study" of my own.
Dais were something I thought I knew. Now, I find myself beginning stories
about Sitapur with the moment at which the bottom falls out. The inevitability of this framing may come from the force of familiar ethnographic
beginnings, or it may come from what the NGO director in Lucknow tells me
on my first visit to his office to hear about "dai trainings": "Dais here," he
says, "don't do deliveries."

The comment takes me back to my first visit to India when I was already
drawn to the creative and disruptive capacity of this fantasy person—the
midwife. I had wanted to talk to Tibetan women in exile about their birth
experiences, and had thought about locating a "traditional midwife" to talk
to. A friend and I walked into the town in Bihar where we were on a student program, into the "STD" office where patchy, expensive international
calls could be made. His aunt in America had done research with Tibetan
women, and she could tell me where to start. After awkwardly yelled introductions, she said, "The first thing you need to know is that there is no such
thing as a 'traditional midwife' for Tibetans."

Years later, in the Lucknow office of Mahila Seva Sansthan, I try to clarify what "no midwives" means with the director—an American man who has been running dai trainings for several years. He is patient, and seems himself quite taken with the situation. Faced again with "no midwives here," I feel trailed in my obsessions by the predictable (and orientalized) cunning of "the local." But as the clear outline of "the dai" blurs, a specificity emerges that is also about the "global," about a dialectic of ideas about what is "local" that orients much about interventions. I visit Mahila Seva Sansthan field sites with supervisors and field coordinators, talk with women who are and are not quite "dais." I observe complicated hierarchies of trainings with workers from other NGOs in Lucknow—aid organizations and hospitals connected like extended kin through bloodlines of funding, family names of project titles, and complicated myths of origin. I go to villages further and further from Lucknow, talking, still, to women who both are and are not quite "midwives." I visit Varanasi, a half-day's train journey to the east, and have more of the same kinds of conversations with NGO workers and "village women," all in an effort to find a place in Uttar Pradesh where there is something more like "midwives." I plan a trip to Gorakhpur that is thwarted by illness (my own), then decide that maybe it is time to stay put for a while. Dais in Varanasi and Gorakhpur, it seems, also "don't do deliveries," or maybe they aren't quite "dais." I am confused by the language politics: in foregrounding "the dai" I have demoted the women I am meeting (all of whom perform a range of tasks associated with birth, none of whom do everything*) in the same way I have long felt international and Indian agencies demote "dais." How am I to think about the advocacy work I have been moved by in Delhi and Bihar, or the shape of conversations about "traditional knowledge" I have understood to be the central theoretical dilemma of "training"?*

Anthropological beginnings are often marked by the disappearance of the object of inquiry; spaces open up in the places that seem most known, to be filled in again with reckonings of newness. What Lawrence Cohen describes as the search for the missing "it"—the way we chase obsessively after the thing, following nattering old ladies down alleys like paparazzi of the abject, as Cohen so marvelously describes (1999), or the way I spend months in motion around central and eastern Uttar Pradesh in search of the "real dais." My own loss of the cultural object feels somehow right, even as it happens in a place where ethnographic certainty feels indelible. I reread older ethnographies and colonial accounts—some half-memorized by this point— with a different eye. What did it mean that Patricia Jeffery, Roger Jeffery, and Andrew Lyon had noted in their seminal work on birth in western Uttar Pradesh that dais often consider their work to "begin after the baby is born, not before" (1989: 109), or that Doranne Jacobson mentioned that a midwife's arrival may be delayed for hours after the baby is born, but the cord left uncut until her arrival (1989: 64)? I now read the whirl of ghosts, witches, placentas, umbilical cords, and "untouchable women" and their iron blades that populate George Briggs's 1920 account of Chamars as banal, even scientific.

The absence leads to no clear moment of revelation, though at times it is tempting to tell the story that way. Around the time that I begin to see appearing in my notes a structurally appealing map of "birth work," a division of "labor"—the labor of birth workers mapped onto the labor of birthing women, so nicely illustrating P. Jeffery and colleagues' 1989 title (Labour Pains and Labour Power)—I move to a village about eighty kilometers north of Lucknow. I call the village Lalpur now, though its real name is more evocative than any I can come up with (I am stuck with the sense provoked by lal [red], metaphors of redness that drive associations with shakti, women's power, and the stuff of birth). I live there in a room in the outer courtyard of a prominent Srivastav household. Over my room's door, next to the cowshed and threshing machine, hangs a sign saying "Post Office," and just beyond it the brick-paved enclosure is a gathering place of both governmental authority and domestic concern. Long days in the yard with men and in the interior angan (courtyard) with women mean long hours watching comings and goings—visitors, household and agricultural workers, children to "watch" me, and women to chat with the two women I come to call Bari Bhabhi and Choti Bhabhi—elder and younger sister-in-law.

The Bhabhis stay in the inner courtyard most of the time, though Bari Bhabhi comes out every day to milk the cow. Their "seclusion" of purdah is a busy and social one. Amma, their recently widowed mother-in-law, lives out her new social position unfettering the requirements of suhag (the auspiciousness of wifehood) by sitting for hours in the outer yard. There is a mix of relief, fatigue, and uncertainty in the air. Her husband had had a heavy hand with women of the household, and no one knows quite what will happen in his absence. Women, often elderly and low-caste, come and go through outer and inner courtyards. The busyness of the angan has an echo, I sense, in the movements in and out of the space of childbirth. During labor and birth, the sor—the room of childbirth—can be as social, I come to learn, as it is quiet and secluded during postnatal recuperation. My pretty structural map of birth work becomes inhabited. And it becomes temporalized, a matter of movements and rooms and houses and neighbors and changes over a sort of time in which what is "the body" and what is "the social world" are not so easily separated.

Women in Lalpur don't talk much about "dais," but when they do, it has a ring of translation to it. "The state makes you a dai," one woman says to me by way of explaining the term. Others use it as a way of clarifying things for the benefit of someone from "outside." Translation, where birth work is *concerned, is not in the purview of the ethnographer. In other words, with this "division of labor," as I have begun calling it, it is not the case that there is anything new (new old, or new emergent) to be "discovered," nothing to be identified as a basic lacuna in either "local knowledge" or "knowledge about the local." Rather, in the figure of the "dai," certain moralities and assumptions about the world don't so much clash with "local realities" as they flow alongside the lived exuberances, anxieties, and actions of rural birth.*

I begin my stay in Lalpur by trying to hang around with the two women who do the most specialized birth work I can locate—postpartum work. These Dalit sisters-in-law are called by most "the Chamarins." Neither is especially excited about my presence. In different ways, they present my questions and attempts at conversation with evasions, too-short replies, silence, and at times annoyance. I hear detailed, moving birth stories from Bari and Choti Bhabhi, often related on the road to somewhere else—in a bus or the back of a cycle rickshaw—or in the quiet darkness of winter nights while we cook dinner. In other homes, birth stories are harder to come by, hardly the privileged or critical genre recognizable in ethnographic accounts of reproduction, internet blogs, or birth activists' writings in the West. Women don't remember which detail pertains to which child's birth, or who actually delivered which or any baby. "There were so many people there, it is hard to know," one says. Pushpadevi, the Dalit next-door neighbor who becomes one of my most talkative interlocutors, says, "You want to hear stories? What is there to tell? It is like this: there is a lot of pain." Others remember extraordinary cases by recounting less the body's story than the situations surrounding it—"When my daughter-in-law had her baby there was so much rain, rain you can't even imagine, rain coming down constantly for days…"

But with death comes language and narration. I hear death stories on a regular basis. Pushpadevi tells me about her son's death instead of about her other children's births. These stories are detailed and common. They require no elicitation from me and erupt (or flow) into other stories about other things. And then there are other people's birth and death stories—often the same thing—extraordinary tales and plain ones, stories of difficult circumstances, stories circulated, but seldom on demand. A recent difficult delivery, a doctor's failed medicine, a botched hospital delivery, a baby's death four years ago from illness, a birth that would have come out better if one woman or another had been called. Listening to the way stories, such as they are, unfold, to the kinds of actors and actions involved, and even more so, watching the comings and goings through angans, struggling to manage women's frequent references to someone or other in this village or that who "knows a lot" or "has good hands," to someone or other whose daughter or son is "finished," I begin to sense that the idea that "There are no midwives here" offers lack to a situation that is all about abundance. But "No midwives here," or the opposite, "Let's train the dais" (who don't really exist as such), confound the very real lacks that make rural life one of poverty and state failures with a different imaginary of lack. That imaginary is a repository of overlapping fantasies and feelings about the boundedness of reality: "local custom," "tradition," "blind belief," "rural women" "village women," "the village," "the dai." Here, as I will come to see in domains beyond "birth work," is a persistently intertwined sense of abundance and lack around the sor, *the time-space of rural birth.*

This story begins in a familiar place, and with familiar conversations about what might be "local" and what might come from "outside," starting with universal categories ("the traditional midwife") and the many arrivals and transformations that mark the birth of a child. Encompassing these themes is the figure of "the dai."[1] Representing a person and an idea, the term is broad, perhaps even mythical, and points at the same time to the stuff of the household and the shape of institutional visions of the past and future. The term encapsulates histories of intervention, official and local visions of caste, class, and gender, and the very relationship of what we might think of as "local" to what appears at first glance to be "global." But eclipsed by the concept's span and givenness are certain subtleties— the sensations of the *sor,* the nested diacritics of caste and progress. In the question "What is a dai?" lies an inquiry about the emerging (and longstanding) political subjectivities of rural women. And so I begin this account with an attempt to dismantle the category that took me to Sitapur in the first place.

One way to begin to unpack "the dai" would be with state and transnational interventions—and especially the "dai trainings"—that seem to solidify an unstable term, putting development, as Stacey Pigg and others have argued (1997), in terms of relationships based on approved and authoritative knowledge—who has it and who needs to get it. Beyond India, the "traditional midwife" is a trope of knowledge politics across a range of discourses. A standard unit of caregiving, she is, like the dai, romanticized and vilified, symbolic of the timelessness of non-western peoples and "tradition" in general, and axiomatic of where women stand in the ascensions of development. In many public health literatures the "traditional midwife" becomes the "traditional birth attendant," the "TBA," and serves as either a resource for social transformation or the accumulation of all that is dangerous about certain ways of thinking and doing.

From policy documents to training manuals, much can be read about notions of "tradition" and the gendering of progress from the place the TBA holds in what Timothy Mitchell calls the "world-as-picture" of modernity (2000a: xiii). As such, like other categories of transnational feminism and health-related development, most notably the "Third World woman" or "the rural woman," the TBA can be deconstructed for the way, as a category of modernity, it is part of how mappings of time, space, and personhood are put in the service of transnational power (Apffel-Marglin and Simon 1994; Mohanty 1991; Pigg 1997; Trinh 1989). This is especially true in post-colonial times and places in which unique "body politics" unsettle Western "theories of the maternal body" (Ram 1998a). In these sites of intervention, gendered body politics involve overlapping modes of difference that include (alongside household dynamics, patriarchy, and the symbolic frameworks of caste) the position of nations in a global frame, the relationship of states to their citizens, and the tangles of authority that make "governmentality" a "derestricted" mode of accounting and surveillance obsessed with with "population" (Foucault 1991: 99). Likewise, they involve the flows (and blockages) of commodities, ideas, and resources that have come to characterize what we think of as globalization. In such a context, forms of care illegible to international categories of intervention require we question debates pitting "local" against "global," or "traditional" against transnational agents.

The dai is well suited to deromanticizing "the traditional midwife" given the way she is dogged by notions of "pollution" in layers of discourse difficult to parse. Indeed, ways of talking about "pollution" make up a set of moralities that has everything to do with the shape of "progress" and the stakes of its imagined recipients. In a tug of war between representations focusing on pollution and those interested in recuperating "local knowledge," the dai has come to mean something for feminist ethnography as well. Ethnographers have long reminded us that "midwives" in India are in a unique position, of low caste status and performing stigmatized work deemed polluting by association with female bodily fluids (Jacobson 1989; Jacobson and Wadley 1977; P. Jeffery et al. 1989; Rozario 1998; Wadley 1975). Assertions that it is "inappropriate to regard the dai as a 'midwife' in the contemporary Western sense" (R. Jeffery and P. Jeffery 1993: 17) consider the pollutedness of the dai and the stigmatized nature of birth work a challenge to the romance of midwives and other orientalist fantasies of the other, discourses in which non-Western women serve as beacons of "naturalness" in opposition to Western ideas about the modern female self (P. Jeffery et al. 1989; R. Jeffery and P. Jeffery 1993; Ram 1998a; Rozario 1998,

2002; Unnithan-Kumar 2002). The stigma of birth work, according to some, makes South Asia a place where women's subordination rather than their "sources of power and influence" (R. Jeffery and P. Jeffery 1993: 9) determine the way childbirth is handled.

But other accounts note that local forms of knowledge have been forced into accountability to biomedical models, often the very ones that disparage and disqualify them (Ram 1998a: 290). There are charges that the dai has been overassociated with "pollution," that her knowledge, abilities, and religious role have been obscured in descriptions (scholarly and otherwise) emphasizing caste status and a biomedical or public health agenda (a side of the argument to which I have contributed, see Chawla and Pinto 2001). Activists, health workers, scholars, and artists have made efforts to resituate the dai as a skilled practitioner disruptive to a bundled set of institutions— medicine, science, development—as well as to the Brahmanical Hinduisms that can devalue the female body (Chawla 1994).

Where pollution battles local knowledge (to oversimplify) in ethnographic representations, in public health discussions spanning colonial and postcolonial eras, talk about dais equivocates on the matter of value—Are dais good or bad for progress? Are they good or bad representatives of "Indian tradition?" Are they a hindrance to public health or a resource? Are they better resigned to the past or brought into the future? Within debates about how to improve life in rural areas, as within debates over knowledge and stigma, the dai is multiply disruptive and multiply symbolic. But, not unexpectedly, distinctions between ideological camps are difficult to locate in the everyday moral negotiations of the *sor*, clinic, and NGO fieldsite, flooded as they are by currents of meaning. In Sitapur, talk is seldom consistent about what a dai is. Indeed, the term is seldom used at all by rural women except in the context of health interventions. While at a general level the terms "TBA" and "dai" are translations of each other across a local-global spectrum, at the most local level—as in Lalpur—the term "dai" ceases to be useful. In this case, progress' lens on the female body politicizes the spaces considered furthest removed from them (namely, birth at home) as much by the figures they cannot account for as by the subject positions they imagine.

I will return in later chapters to this process, to the cipher of "the dai"—that is, to what "dais" represent. Now I would like to escort "the dai" from the room by taking things out of the register of "knowledge" and into that of "work" or praxis or *kam*, to look at what happens in the first of many concentric circles of what Veena Das calls a "local ecology of care" (2002). Of particular interest here are women

who do bodily work in the time frame of birth but outside the notion of midwifery. While the "dai" as an imaginary is associated with
the moment of "delivery," the socialities of the *sor* require that we
turn our attention *post*natal-wards. Judging by the specialized attention given to "confinement," as my own grandmother might call it,
postnatal female and infant bodies, and their associated embodied
states, can be seen as being situated at an apex of vulnerability to
forces that, with uncanny resonance, breach the gap between the
familiar and the foreign: powers of biomedicine, the state, agents of
authority, jealous gazes, ghosts, pathogens, neighbors, and kin.

Dalit women, those imagined locally as "untouchable," have a
particular stake in the progress politics of the household and in the
transnational politics of new life, notably because of the way that
for many of them, work begins not with birth itself, but during the
time of postnatal recuperation, separation, and reintegration. While
the dai as "village midwife" is often seen in urban accounts as a crea-
ture of stasis, untouchable women who manage postpartum care
manage movement in a range of registers—toward progress, toward
obsolescence, and between the spaces of the margins and the center, the living and the not yet or no longer, alive. Such women are
among the most mobile in their communities, with intimate knowledge of bodies, reproductive lives, and household histories, as well
as a designated, if ambiguous, place in state health schemes. In a
web of work relationships shaped by transformations in the maternal body, forms of "everyday citizenship" (Greenhouse 2001) embedded in the postcolonial modus operandi that is "development"
(Gupta 1998) have bearing on and derive weight from the social dynamics and cosmological proportions of the *sor*. While the *sor* may
appear to some as "raw material" for intervention, it is an already-
engaged zone of action in which and through which forms of belonging and exclusion take shape. It is so as a space of ciphered categories
and broad misunderstandings, in which cosmologies of life and death
impinge on the subject possibilities offered by the stuff of intervention.

Postpartum work

*Shalini and her mother come almost daily to the Bhabhis' angan. Shalini's
Mother (known to the women in my house as such), a lower-caste Lodh (but
not untouchable), helps with agricultural and household work—winnowing grains, sorting pulses and rice—while Shalini does dishes and some
sweeping up. Shalini is the oldest of her mother's three surviving children.*

Her exact age is unknown, as is not uncommon in rural families; she must be somewhere around eleven. But her manner of speaking is grown-up—amused, suspicious, slightly reserved except when the remaining exuberances of childhood overtake her. Together, she, her mother, and her younger sisters gather piles of cow dung and mold them into rounds, slap them onto walls to dry into discs with a symmetry of handprints, then pile them into towers in the garden across the path. Both are paid in objects—blankets, clothes, shoes—and less often, money. One day Shalini, who often hangs around my room, tells me that her mother's baby will be born soon. Like other kids in this region, she refers to her mother as "Bua," Auntie (father's sister)—diverting attention so effectively away from the bodily realities of conjugality and toward other kinds of relatedness that it takes me a moment to figure out who she means. Bari Bhabhi had only mentioned a few days ago that it must be imminent. I had not even noticed the bulge. As the days grow colder and mid winter's dangers come all too quickly after early winter's relief, Shalini and I watch and wait.

*One morning in early January, Shalini comes flying around the corner just as I am unlocking the door to my room. "*Larki hui, larki hui!*"—"It's a girl!" She is smiling, waving her long arms. Once again, I have missed a birth. I only learned minutes earlier that her mother had been having labor pains off and on for three days. I had seen her often in that time but had no idea. Shalini grabs my hand and pulls me back to her house.*

Her younger sisters are sitting in the courtyard. Their father is crouched in the outer doorway, wrapped in the wool blanket I gave Shalini a month ago. He says nothing. I duck and enter the room. At first I cannot tell if the gray haze is mist from outside or smoke. The stinging in my eyes gives me the answer. Shalini's Mother sits on the ground, on a pile of straw, warming her hands and bare legs on a fire she feeds with dried leaves. I reach for her hand and say, "You are shaking." She pulls it away. Behind her is more straw and the telltale winnowing basket. The reed basket, the sup, *flat with edges curved like a shovel, contains an old, browned quilt made from a sari beyond repair. The quilt is folded into a neat square and out from under it snakes a white, rubbery and kinked cord, the blue and red veins wrapping around each other beneath its translucent skin. It leads to the placenta, a fleshy lotus lying wilted on the ground. Uneven pools of purpley brown blood soak into the floor, losing their shiny slickness as they are drunk up by the dirt. "But where is the baby?" I stupidly ask. Shalini's Mother pulls back the quilt, and there she is, at the end of her bodily tether, tiny, naked, new and asleep. "She was born just now. Just before you came." Her voice is shaky with exhaustion, barely audible.*

"Who was with you?" I ask.

"No one. No one was with me."

"Was Shalini here?"

"Yes, Shalini was here." There is a long pause. "The Chamarin has been called," she whispers, "She's on her way."

Rakesh's Mother, known to some as such, to others as "the Chamarin," to others more respectfully as "Chamarin Dadi" (Chamar Grandmother)—arrives. Behind her are some neighbor girls and their mother. They stay in the angan, while Rakesh's Mother comes into the sor, where Shalini's Mother and I are sitting. Shalini has lit a fire in an earthen pot at the doorway. I don't know what kind of herb she has put into it, but it burns with a thick, oily and rich-smelling smoke, heavier and softer than the sharp smoke of the dried leaves. The Chamarin warms her hands and feet. Shalini's Mother, still shaking, stares into the skittish flame. This fire will die fast. It requires constant maintenance while it burns, but its ash will be used to soak up blood from the floor. The Chamarin says to her, "God should have given you a son. You have three girls already. Now look. Another." She reminds us of past losses and the slow fade of grief: "Her son fell in the well and died. Three people have fallen into that well and died. In our well, if someone falls in you can pull him out."

A neighbor woman is standing in the doorway. She says, "Yes, her son died. Some people keep having boys and some people go on having girls. My sister-in-law had four boys and one girl and now she is pregnant and longs for another girl. And look at her." She waves her hand at Shalini's Mother who is busying herself with keeping the fire fed. "Three girls and now one more." Part of me wants them to stop talking like this, in no small part because of the way this talk reinforces some of the more demeaning stereotypes I hear about rural Indian women. Throughout the afternoon, there will be repeated mention of the dead son. Shalini's Mother repeats something I have heard many times, "None of this is in our hands. It is all up to God." She pauses then adds, "And what God gives we must accept."

Shalini brings Rakesh's Mother a clump of dried mud from the pond in the fields. While Rakesh's Mother grinds it to powder, Shalini is sent now for some soap, now for some string. She scrambles into the rafters, on top of earthen grain containers as tall as she is, then tosses the store-bought paper down. When Rakesh's Mother finishes grinding, she takes the blanket off of the baby and looks at it expressionlessly for a moment. She cuts the thread in two with the razor, ties one piece at the navel and ties the other a few inches away. With several sawing strokes she cuts through the rubbery flesh of the cord. The cord falls on the floor; the placenta lies separated from the baby, now something utterly different, something out of place.

The Chamarin rubs in the dirt until the baby is ashen like a sadhu. The dirt is from the large pond about a kilometer out into the fields, I am told. "Paak hai," Rakesh's Mother says, "It is pure." Having never been fatigued *by seed, this is the same mud that is harvested in the spring for patching and rebuilding the walls of houses. Months hence, I will see Shalini, together with her cousins, walk into the pond and bring out heavy mounds of the dense clay in the fold of her* kameez, *then carry it home in enormous bowls. Not all dirt is dirty, I think to myself, not all is "matter out of place." The baby, still in her dusty coating, is put back into the* sup *on top of a few grains of rice. The Chamarin calls for the water that Shalini has been warming on the kitchen hearth. Shalini's Grandmother, her mother's mother-in-law (*sas*), is summoned. We wait. She is required to throw the water onto the baby, I am told by the Chamarin. A woman in the doorway says that the placenta will be thrown away so that it won't be "grabbed" by unhappy spirits of the dead, ghosts that wander in search of vulnerable souls. She tells me, "People who have money ... they burn the placenta. But they will throw it because of poverty."*

Shalini's paternal grandmother (known to many in Lalpur as Shalini's Grandmother) arrives and sits in the doorway. Not quite inside the room, but in reach of Rakesh's Mother and the warmth of the fire, she dips her hand in the pot of warmed water and flicks it in three directions. As Rakesh's Mother holds the baby over a brass cooking vessel, Shalini's Grandmother pours slow streams over the baby. The dirt washes off, leaving stripes of pink and gray skin as the pot below fills with dingy water. The waxy womb-pollution mingles with purifying water and mud. Into this soup the sas *tosses a coin of payment. Rakesh's Mother stops and looks up with bland disbelief. She demands more, holding the steaming baby in one hand. Shalini's mother's* sas *refuses. "We are poor. Poorer than you," she says.*

"Poor, who is poor? What wealth do I have?" Rakesh's Mother replies. Shalini's grandmother continues to refuse. "Look, as you argue your baby gets cold," Rakesh's Mother says. I reach into my own pockets. As I do, Shalini's Grandmother brings out another coin, waves it three times around the baby, then tosses it into the bathwater. A single rupee. I think to myself that bartering (or inflation) can only go so high, dictated by the physicality of money. A coin absorbs malevolent gazes from the baby, and who wants a soggy paper note? Rakesh's Mother rubs the baby with soap, and she gives a sharp, tinny cry. The baby is rinsed, wrapped in a rag, and returned to the basket.

The ash on the floor has absorbed most of the liquidy blood, forming crusty cakes. The Chamarin is given an iron spade with which she scrapes up the bloody muck. She digs divots into the ground beneath the clots that refuse to be absorbed, scraping everything cleanly into an old broken basket lined with a layer of straw. The placenta flops and slips as she picks it up and puts it on top of the collected birth-stuff in the basket. All is covered with a scrap of old fabric that had been lying in the ash.

After she takes the placenta to the edge of the village to throw it away,
Rakesh's Mother returns and cleans the floor of the sor *room with a slick*
layer of cow dung. Someone hands her a bowl of warmed mustard oil, and
she rubs the baby with vigorous strokes. When the baby is wrapped up again
and returned to the sup, *she is laid atop a small pile of rice, which Rakesh's*
Mother will take as payment. Shalini's Mother hikes up her sari. Rakesh's
Mother rubs her legs, her arms, stopping to pull on each hand, giving the
knuckles a resounding crack. Shalini's Mother looks out with apparent ex-
haustion through half-lowered lids, staring blankly at the wall. She lies on
her back in the hay, exposing her now-flaccid stomach. As she rubs, Rakesh's
Mother asks softly where it hurts and how it hurts, and spends time in places
where the pain is greatest. "My legs hurt," *Shalini's Mother says.*

"And your stomach. That will be bad for some days, but you know that,"
Rakesh's Mother says. I ask the purpose of the massage, though I have been
told already by others, and she gives me her usual look of disbelief. "It is for
the pain. Even afterwards there is great pain, and especially for the stomach
you must give massage for many days to break down the hardness that ac-
cumulates and allow the body to heal and the pain to end."

"This thing that accumulates," *I asked,* "What is it?"

"Barhiya." *The* barhiya. *The peregrinating life force that protects and*
accompanies the fetus. "It wanders in the womb," *she says,* "searching for
the baby. The wandering causes the pain." *And the force of the massage*
breaks down this residual, painful bit of life and longing.

After the massage Rakesh's Mother sits for a while in the angan, *teasing*
and shouting back and forth at Shalini's cousins and the neighbor girls. She
eventually leaves, taking the coins and rice. For the next four days she re-
turns in the morning to massage Shalini's Mother. On the second day she
advises her when "the water should fall" *and the initial phase of confine-*
ment should end—this will mark the time when her daily visits will end
and, after a final massage, Shalini's Mother and the new bitiya *(little*
daughter) will bathe and enter the next stage of recuperation and a de-
creased phase of postpartum pollution.

On the fourth day, while Shalini makes food and neighbors chat in the
angan, *her mother bathes next to the well outside. Still dripping, she puts*
on a clean sari. Inside, Rakesh's Mother tosses a few grains of rice into the
sor *room, and then lays the sleeping baby, now clothed for the first time, in*
the sup, *entirely covered by a clean, folded sari. She places Shalini's Mother's*
iron hasiya *on top of this vulnerable bundle of tempered auspiciousness—*
tempered by its femaleness, made at once more and less vulnerable to a
range of forces cosmic, social, and familial. The laden sup *is put in the door-*
way of the sor, *half inside, half in the* angan. *When I ask later what this*
was all about, she says she doesn't know what I am talking about.

Shalini is making food for her mother's first postpartum meal of regular food, and her mother puts the baby to the breast for the first time. Before this she, like many women in this area, gives her droplets of sugar water. The Chamarin sits in the angan amid the goings on and is given a biri *(leaf cigarette). She argues one last time with Shalini and her cousins about payment, pushes the unlit cigarette into her hair, takes a bit of offered cash and walks out the door.*

Postpartum work is one of the few cases in which it might be possible to apply the generalizations of "practice" and "structure" to the lives of women in Sitapur, women who, because they marry out of their *maike* (natal villages), have lives grounded in a gendered sense of diversity—captured in the notion of "household custom" to which many women refer in explaining why they do what they do. For them, variation in language, ritual form, names, myths, and history is part of neighborly bonds. Yet within this diversity, there remains a firm distinction in the time frame of birth: between the work that comes before (and during) delivery and that which comes afterwards; between, respectively, work that can be done by anyone and that which is the purview of "untouchable" specialists. The latter, spread over three to six days' time, includes a matrix of bodily work and cleaning: cutting the umbilical cord, rubbing the baby with ground-up dirt, bathing the infant, massaging infant and mother, removing placenta and trash from the house (or burying or burning the placenta inside the house), and cleaning the *sor.* For a length of time advised either by the Chamarin or a Brahman pandit (depending on a family's financial straits), the postpartum worker returns to massage the *jaccha* (new mother) and baby.

The sociality and labors of birth and managing transition into new life are delineated by the timings of maternal recuperation at once bodily and social. The involvement of various people is determined by the physical, social, and cosmological condition of the *jaccha*—contained in the notion of a gradual fading of pollution, and all that it involves in terms of personal vulnerability and social exclusion. During recuperation, gradual decreases in the pollutedness of the maternal body coincide with the reintegration of the mother into her social world—the family, the household, and the *jati* (caste community). For the baby, the separation period of the *sor* is that of its direst vulnerability, when, like its mother, it is off the social grid, made casteless not only by its untouchable—that is, polluted—status, but by the fact that it has not yet drunk the mother's milk that, through the work of consumption, will give it caste and a place in the world (at least according to some of the women who talked to me about this phase, many of whom were Dalits and described the baby's first days as the time when it was "without caste").

I will explore nuances of pollution in greater detail later. For now, it is adequate to observe in Sitapur what has been noted widely throughout much of India: that childbirth and its substances and processes are considered to pollute both *jaccha* and baby for a period of about one month—as well as those who encounter them. The period of the postpartum worker's labor marks the most severe phase of pollutedness, beginning with the cutting of the umbilical cord and ending after the *jaccha* bathes again about four days later. The secluded time "before the water falls" is, for the *jaccha*, a period of warming milk-tea and special preparations of potatoes, rice, and spices made by others as her hand is forbidden from touching cooking utensils and her body kept away from the cooking hearth. In the language of norms and, according to older women, the idealized era of the past, it is a protected time in which the *jaccha* does not leave the *sor* during the day (she may go to the fields to defecate in the late evening or very early morning, when she is least likely to be seen). "It used to be that in the morning," Amma told me, "the Chamarin came to take away the night-dirt."

The flux of recuperations and the gradual decline of vulnerability, social and physical, continue after "the water falls" when a *naoun*, a woman of the Naai or barber caste is summoned to massage the mother for a time determined by a family's ability to pay. The *naoun* takes on the remaining phase of seclusion, when *jaccha-baccha* are no longer strictly "untouchable" but are also not yet fully reintegrated into household affairs (like cooking, or trips to the bazaar), and as their bodies gain strength. Of low rank (but "higher" than the Chamars, Pasis, Doms, and other "untouchable" *jati*) in Lalpur and surrounding villages, *naouns* were primarily Muslims, putting them in an ambiguous and inconsistent category with regard to "untouchability." Though de facto untouchables for caste-Hindus because of their (imagined) consumption of meat, they were nevertheless in a different and higher order than Rakesh's Mother. "Every village should have a good *naoun*," Choti Bhabhi tells me, as she and Bari Bhabhi laugh about their village's *naoun* who scandalously ran off with a Chamar man. *Naouns*, they tell me, are also within the bounds of *jajmani* exchange, and are everywhere when it comes to marriage and reproduction—especially talented at massage, and often at assisting labor and delivery, alongside their roles of decorating the bride before marriage, delivering dowry gifts from *maike* to *sasural* (marital village for women, home of the in-laws for men), and distributing through the village *prasad* (the auspicious food that is the result of a *puja* or ceremony) from life cycle ceremonies.

For Hindus such as Shalini's family, punctuating the break between the work of postpartum workers and that of *naouns,* "the day the water falls" brings not only a new social and ontological status to the *jaccha-baccha* dyad (and new conditions of consumption and care) but also a ritual called *Chatti puja.* A *diya* (small oil lamp) might be lit and a ceremony of *aarti* (an offering of flame) performed to honor household deities and the Chatti Devi, goddess of *jacchas* and newborns. The white outlines of the Chatti Devi painted on *sor* walls remain for years, marking the auspiciousness and vulnerability, the seclusion, care and fatigue of the new *jaccha.* The square Devi's field of a torso is filled with images of plenty and production—sheaves of grain, lions.

Whether women remain in their *sasural* (marital home) to give birth or return to their *maike* (natal village), with the Chatti come a new set of arrivals marking social integration— the bonds of gifting and shared food that reinforce kin ties. Extended family visits and gifts of clothing arrive from the *jaccha's maike.* Baby and mother put on new (or at least newly cleaned) clothes, and thick, black *kajol* is put around the baby's eyes for the first time by its *bua.* Women and girls gather to sing birth songs late into the night. For Muslims there is no *Chatti* ceremony, though there is a celebration on the twelfth day after the birth; but the postpartum worker's tasks follow a similar trajectory, ending after four to six days.

As in so many celebratory moments in the flow of a life, the dilation of ideals is easily punctured by day-to-day realities. Shalini, her sisters and a few neighbor girls—and I—are the only attendees at the Chatti puja *for this fourth daughter of a poor family. In fact, we are the* puja. *Together we sit under a low straw roof in the post-dinner, post-washing-up darkness. A tiny, plastic oil-powered candle gives off a yellow glow from atop an upside-down metal bucket. Shalini has borrowed a drum from somewhere, and, arguing about the words, the girls sing songs to Maia, the motherly goddess who must be honored before any other singing can be done. The new girl baby, who will not be named for months, and who should have been a boy, as many in the village will say for weeks to come, sleeps with her mother as she is welcomed with out-of-tune girlish delight and a makeshift ceremony by her sisters and cousins in the* angan.

Work from God

"God put the work into my hands? Who would have taught me?" Rakesh's Mother tells me when I ask from whom she learned her skills. She may have followed her mother-in-law to a few house-holds, she says, and watched her attend births in her own home, but for the most part, she didn't *learn* so much as *begin* her work. Hands, as well as Rakesh's Mother's usual rhetorical disdain, evoke the complex valences of caste-based work—obligation and right, coercion and skill, human submission to the divine. Where institutional constructions of the "TBA" envision one whose status as traditional specialist makes her at once open to training and closed to professionalization, postpartum work, though formalized in other regards, does not fit into a pedagogical framework. When I asked others from whom they learned their work, many had difficulty answering; some looked confused, others took the matter out of the idiom of learning, referring to the time when they "began the work"; to a moment, site, or mode of experience, to a punctuation of life's flow, a point of transition such as the death or infirmity of a mother-in-law. "I began when my mother-in-law became too weak to do the work"; "I just started going [to births]"; "God gave me this work"; "I went with my mother-in-law, and then my hands became good."

"The hands" also capture ambiguous sentiments about postpartum labor held by caste-Hindu women—the notion that pollution descends and ascends from its source in action as much as through the contact between self and defilement that hands so often mediate. At the same time, the "dirty hands" of "the dai" represent the site of blame for mortality and morbidity—the "lack of hygiene" and "lack of skill" that make a "dai's" hands vector of a range of ills. The "Five Laws of Cleanliness" (of which clean hands is one) are taught and recalled (by trainers and trainees alike) with the pnemonics of the outspread hand, offering a core image and symbol into which politics of labor (read action), pollution and hygiene (read morality), and identity (read blame) can be collapsed.

And yet, it is via the hands that God moves through both women who deliver babies and those who perform postpartum work (and those who do both). Hands incorporate a multidirectional sense of cause and action, one in which "knowledge" (as *jankari,* "information") is present but secondary. At the same time, hands are part of the way labor relates to the self, part of the way Rakesh's Mother owns her work. Where others may describe her work as "dirty" or "polluting," she refers to it as "ours," sharing the postpartum responsibilities of Lalpur with her elder sister-in-law. Other than them, no one in the village performs the symbolically critical work that begins with the severing of the umbilical cord—not even women from the other Dalit community in this village (Pasi), women whose natal families may do this work in other villages. This is work passed down in the *sasural,* binding *sas* and *bahu* (mother-in-law and daughter-in-law), *jethani* and *devrani* (elder and younger sisters-in-law).

Rakesh's Mother and her sister-in-law have lived next door to each other for decades. As young brides they once shared a large *angan,* but as families grew and fortunes diverged, the courtyard was divided by a sturdy wall erected through the middle. With the wall came growing animosities—over work competition, different boons in money and offspring, and everyday jealousies. As elderly women, their mutual annoyance was palpable. They seldom spoke to each other and both chided me for visiting the other one. In personality and reputation, they could hardly have been more different. The *jethani*—the elder sister-in-law—was known by many as Schoolteacher's Mother. Others called her "Chamarin-Dadi" (as Rakesh's Mother is also known to some). And others referred to her, incorrectly, as "Choti Chamarin"—the younger Chamarin. Though elder, she had more teeth, and was more fleshy and less bent over—signs, perhaps, of her relative prosperity. She was formal and soft-spoken around me. Perhaps out of uncertainty about my own caste position, perhaps out of deference to the status of the household I lived in, or, most likely, wary because of my association with NAFPA, the family planning program that had recently "trained" her, she did not invite me into her courtyard for months. I spoke with her, uncomfortably, in front of an audience of kin from the seat she offered—a rope bed on her veranda, under the NAFPA sign proclaiming her to be a "trained dai"— while she sat on the ground; I felt nudged by this deference into the even more uncomfortable position of formal interviewer. Schoolteacher's Mother answered my questions quietly and simply. Where I wanted stories and conversation, she followed the formulas of social science and public health research interviewers not unfamiliar to the region. But the awkwardness broke down when my own body— rather than the knowledge I seemed to want to harvest—became our point of communication. When I sought her advice in a personal mode, she brought me into her house, urging the discretion and concealment appropriate to the early months of pregnancy. As she felt my stomach for the slip of new pregnancy or the motion of early life, she talked to me about her life beyond the abstractions my earlier questions—and the public way they were situated—prompted.

She had been a widow for many years—at least 25, she reckoned—and claimed to have supported herself and her children off what she earned through her *baccha kam,* baby work. She had borne five sons, all of whom were still alive, now married with children, some with grandchildren. I once asked her, during one of our veranda chats, if the baby often in her lap was a grandchild, and she said, rather wearily, "I am surrounded by grandchildren." Her sons had built houses around her, and she shared her home with one of them, his wife and their small children. While her house was made of mud and thatch, she spoke of her eldest son—the Schoolteacher, a successful and powerful local figure whom even she called Master-ji—as "the one who lives in the brick house."

Where Schoolteacher's Mother was reticent, a point of stillness, perhaps resignation, amid flurries of children, Rakesh's Mother was curt and, I imagined, mistrustful of me. She often responded to my questions about bodies, fetuses, birth, and so on with dismissive responses: "How do I know? God just puts these things there, how do I know why?" and suggestions that I just might be faking my own lack of knowledge: "You're the educated one, you tell me." "Doesn't this happen in your place? Why don't you stay there and find out?" For Rakesh's Mother, my questions, and her rhetorical replies, were all about power. She spoke with a bite to families she served. As well as being known as Rakesh's Mother and, mistakenly, as *"bari-walli"* (the elder), she was also called *"budhi"* (demeaningly, "old lady") and, with more respect, Chamarin-Dadi. My efforts to map their division of clientele were thwarted by the way people in the village identified them incorrectly, did not know which was older or younger, and by the way people knew them only as "Chamarin," and not, as many women are known, by a kinship affiliation—as somebody's wife, somebody's mother.

By many accounts, including her own, Rakesh's Mother had had a difficult life marked by difficulty conceiving, abandonment by her first husband, remarriage, the eventual births of a son and daughter, as well as the daily insults of caste-prejudice. She could often be found trading shouts with the families of her clients. Women described her as *tez*—sharp, and her sister-in-law as *sidha,* or straight. Demand was a common theme in her interactions, an idiom through which she engaged in work, *jajmani* exchanges, and interactions with figures of authority from within and outside the community. She demanded money and goods repeatedly and insistently from her clients, from me, and also from the government, most vividly in an encounter with a supervisor from NAFPA, the recently begun, state/

private sector collaborative family planning "scheme" that had trained her. Her refusals to talk to me or take me with her to clients' homes invoked the authority of the state while revealing its ineffectiveness. If "five hundred rupees" had been "spent on her" (twelve dollars at the time), she reminded me, then our conversations were worth at least that much. She used the same argument in interactions with clients, but to less effect.

Both women's hands performed many labors. They delivered babies in their own households, a not insignificant amount considering the size of Schoolteacher's Mother's family. At the same time, as "dais" trained by the government they were instructed to advertise to the community their ability and training in "safe delivery." Although this training was common knowledge, few outside their own families summoned them to attend deliveries. Schoolteacher's Mother was called by some—the upper-caste family of Meena, a local schoolteacher, some lower-caste households—before the birth and was understood to have "very good hands before and after." But postpartum work was "theirs"—by untouchable status, *jati* affiliation, and ownership. In Sitapur, broadly speaking, a village's postpartum workers come from a single (or several, in the case of bigger villages) *jati* or *upjati* (subcaste) within that village, though not necessarily the same *jati* from village to village. Delineated on several levels—at the dividing point between untouchability and caste-Hinduism, and by *upjati* and kin affiliation at the village level—this "caste-based work" does not ascribe to a vision of caste in which specific *jati* are associated with specific kinds of labor. Yet, as assigned (or owned) labor it is part of visions of rank associated with pollution, part of the cordoning off of tasks associated with death, bodily processes, bodily fluids, and trash. In a context in which "untouchable" *jati* are ranked hierarchically as are those "above" them, postpartum workers come from the lowest ranked untouchable community/-ies within a village.

Where the work of Dalit *jatis* (Pasi, Chamar, Dhanuk, Bakshur, and Dom, in this region) is established—locally, as well as historically—as that which determines "untouchable" status (things related to death, bodies, meat, and bodily fluids), in everyday practice most people from these *jati* were not primarily pig herders (associated with Pasis), leather-workers (Chamars), sweepers and broom-makers (Dhanuks and Bakshurs), or funeral workers (Doms). Daily labors involved agricultural work, on their own or others' land. The overidentification of caste with iconic labor, so familiar from Brahmanical exegesis on the one hand and colonial efforts to categorize, census, and describe their subjects and labor forces (Chatterjee 1993; Dirks 2001; Inden 1990; Prashad 2000) on the other, remains an abstraction that is a facet of contemporary rural life. However, notions of caste as iconic labor, though more foregrounded than notions of caste through birth, live at the level of ideology and imaginary maps, part of projected and imagined moralities formed around praxis and its symbolic weight; origins may be as related to colonial and postcolonial governance as to local identities, but it is the currency of such ideological positions that interest me as much as their genealogies.

For Rakesh's Mother and Schoolteacher's Mother, delineation of clientele and remuneration were part of *jajmani* structures, hereditary patron-client relationships that serve as ritualized sites for enacting local hierarchies. Here, Dalits and pundits, the lowest and highest on the caste spectrum, however defined, fall into parallel positions as those who perform ritual household labors related to the body and life cycle and receive food from patrons on key days in the religious calendar and at moments of celebration in the households of patrons.[2] As well as coins dropped into the baby's bathwater on the day of its birth, a variable amount (from ten to one hundred rupees—twenty-five cents to $2.50 at time of fieldwork—or saris) is paid on the day "the water falls," though payments are often postponed, sometimes indefinitely. In response to NGO encouragement, some postpartum workers described to me their efforts to demand "fixed rates," in which inconsistencies in training schemes and overlapping institutional standards undermined their claims. Some complained that payments diminished after NGO and state schemes began publicizing fixed rates; client families, they said, felt relieved of responsibility to long-standing obligations, or mistakenly believed that "trained dais" get a salary from the government. Because NGO and state campaigns seldom address the difference between peri- and postpartum labor, emphasizing only that "the dai" be compensated, and because families often have less cash available than other kinds of goods, consistent, fixed monetary payments are far from the norm.

Within the *sasural* (marital home), through a line of female affinal kin, the inheritance of clientele and labor weaves into patriarchal structures. Where birth work is concerned, Dalit women's access to clients—and thus income—is part of the emotional tangle of the *sas-bahu* relationship, and, as in the case of Rakesh's Mother and Schoolteacher's Mother, the fraught relationships between female affinal kin. Along with clientele, Dalit women inherit a location in an ongoing relationship of obligation and remuneration from mothers-in-law.

Rakesh's Mother, like her sister-in-law, returns to homes where she or her mother-in-law has worked, coming even in years when there has been no birth to receive goods at festivals, weddings, and at the anguished—and celebrated—departure of young brides to their own marital villages.

"Girlfriends are all around you"

While their kids run around us on the grass between their house and the fields, Pushpadevi and her sister-in-law, women from the "untouchable" Pasi jati, *tell me about the ways their kids were born. They do not remember each birth independently and deflect my questions by joking about pain. Pushpadevi shows me how she prefers to sit to give birth. She pulls her knees up to her shoulders with her hands, and leans back. Her sister-in-law laughs and nods. "Yes, it is like this." In this position, Pushpadevi says, "Having your baby here in* dehat, *it's much better [than in the cities]. There you are alone. Maybe there is a nurse, but you don't know her; she is no one to you. Here, there are so many* sahelis *(girlfriends). Girlfriends are all around you. You are sitting on the ground like this, and one is behind you here, and there is someone in front watching for the baby."*

This is a sentiment I hear again, not much later, when I return to my own household, where a sister-in-law is visiting from Lucknow. She tells me that she returned to Lalpur from the city for all of her births: "In the house you have this one touching you here, that one pressing you there, if there is pain in another place, someone else comes to press on it. In the hospital so many people are coming in and out, doctors, nurses, and still you are all alone. But here in the village you are not alone. Your family is with you."

Against the forward motion of "progress" narratives, whether of national development or birth, I now go backwards from the quiet, restful vulnerabilities of the postpartum phase to the active busyness of birth, where even in "baby delivering" it is not so easy to find "the midwife." In contrast with the bounded quality of postpartum work, the work of delivering babies in Sitapur is flexible and varied, and as I spent more time with women in Lalpur and other villages, it became clear that many, perhaps most deliveries I kept track of and heard about were assisted in homes by family members. Put differently, this means that in rural Sitapur, many women attend a delivery at some point in their lives, usually in their own households. *Jacchas* are often attended by family members—in the *sasural* by mothers-in-law, sisters-in-law, and in the *maike* by aunts, and in some cases, mothers—many of whom possess a great deal of experience and skill in conducting deliveries. Or a *jaccha* may return to her *maike*, where birth may be assisted by sisters, sisters-in-law, mother, or grandmother. Married women with children of their own perform most home deliveries, though the case of Shalini's Mother, described above, is a remarkable exception. Generally, no payment is offered to the member of the household who conducts the delivery.

As Pushpadevi described, having a baby is a matter of comfort in numbers (though for later births, after many previous ones, fewer people assist, and solo births are not unheard of). The pain of birth is, like other kinds of pain, often best managed in the company of others who have known its agony. At the scene of birth, women move in and out of the household and *sor*, participating in different and shifting ways. In the ways women talk about births—of their own and others' children—unless a delivery is particularly difficult, who handles the baby as it emerges does not seem to be of special importance. In stories and descriptions, the person who caught the baby is often neither identified nor made obvious. My efforts to track practitioners and clients were confounded by responses such as "Someone of the house did the delivery," and "There were so many around, it's hard to say." Occasionally, in a group conversation about a particular birth, the woman who had "delivered the baby" announced, "I was there," or "I did it." But more commonly, my questions were dismissed with, "What difference does it make?"

Indeed, even the term "delivery," a Western term emphasizing the task of assisting a birth, is problematic in describing birth work in Sitapur, where delivery is not referred to as a discreet act (J. Chawla, personal communication). "The child happened," (*baccha hua*) or "It's a boy/girl" (*larka hua*) foreground a baby's new presence over the act of getting it out, while the more specific but less common, "The baby's birth happened," (*bacche ka janm hua*) gives a broader household or familial context to the flow of a story or explanation. References to "delivery" use the English term.

Yet not all hands are the same, and skill can be as varied in baby-delivering as in any form of labor. Specialists exist in this frame as well, though not in any bounded or categorized kind of way. Some women, I am told, just have a bit more experience, or a bit more *jankari* (information). Some women's hands are just better.

Only a few days after my arrival in Lalpur, it is clear that word has gotten around that I have been talking to the Chamarins about "baby stuff." One afternoon when I am sitting in the outer yard in the shadows of the veranda, an old woman with eyes that collapse into her head comes into the courtyard. She sits near me and says conspiratorially, "That one who has been coming to see you," and abruptly waves her hand and shakes her head. She is referring to Schoolteacher's Mother.

"She doesn't know anything. I can show you everything." She begins a description, with near-testimonial force, telling me how she positions her hands to catch a baby, what she does if the feet or buttocks come first. Using first my hand and then my arm as a model, she demonstrates how she prevents tearing and shows the kinds of pressure she applies to different parts of the body. "You see? You see?" She points to the house, and says she caught many of the babies born in this household, two generations' worth.

When I ask if she cuts the umbilical cord, she waves her hand abruptly in this manner she has of saying no—emphatically wordless, as if to wipe the stain of the question out of the air. "That is the work of the Chamarins," she whispers. Like many women in her position, she tells me she has no fixed rate for births, nor any leverage from which to make demands—she is happy to take whatever is given, she claims. The Bhabhis later disagree, saying she makes frequent demands on them. I come to learn that her payment is based on her requests and household whimsy. After about twenty minutes she stands up and says, "I have to get back to work. I'll come again tomorrow."

I ask the Bhabhis who she was. "Chachi," they say, Auntie (father's brother's wife). She is something of a household laborer, they tell me, something of an expert on birth, something of a friend and something of a nuisance—all roles collapsed, circumscribed, and defined by her de facto, or practical, "untouchable" status as a low-caste Muslim. "She comes to this house to do deliveries. Or just to help. She used to do the dishes but now she does not," Bari Bhabhi says. Chachi, who had assisted at all of her own babies' births, is from the Julaha jati—weavers. Her husband, Bari Bhabhi tells me, has no land, and is old and infirm. Chachi and her sons work on other people's land and homes. Her eldest son is a laborer in Lucknow. The next in line, Naseem, lives in her home with his wife, son, and two younger brothers. Naseem, like his mother, is frequently in the courtyard of the Bhabhis' household chatting and joking. The Bhabhis say he is especially fun when he puts on a sari and bangles and dances around, something he used to do more often than he does now. Naseem is like his father, Bari Bhabhi says dismissively—he never works anywhere for long.

It takes me several weeks to figure out that Chachi is almost entirely blind. No one mentions it, and she moves easily in and out of the homes she visits and works in—doing dishes here, agricultural work there. She seems to show up almost everywhere, working, hanging out, though other families say they have never heard she is particularly good at delivering babies. I learn she is blind when I show her a picture of my husband and she holds it upside down and says, "He is very handsome," to the amusement of her daughter-in-law, who laughs and grabs the picture; "Why do you try to hide it?" she exclaims. The Bhabhis tell me later that she was blinded by a house fire in this village long ago.

Much later, I visit the nearby village of Devia to see Pratima Srivastav, an upper-caste woman who works as both a self-taught "Ladies Doctor" and a "CBD"—Community-Based Distributor for NAFPA. Pratima takes me to the Chamar mohalla (neighborhood) to talk with a woman she knows to be a postpartum worker. The woman looks nervous, but invites us under her veranda roof. She gives only the briefest answers to questions, and when the conversation comes around to deliveries she says she seldom does any, even in her own family. But her sister-in-law, who lives nearby, is someone I should meet. She calls her over, and she proves to be a gregarious spokeswoman for her baby-delivering skills. She emphasizes stories about difficult births she has performed—"When I arrive, the woman gets relief," and "When I arrive God can take a break." Families throughout Devia, from many different caste communities, call upon her, though most of her work is for those of lower castes.

She seems to be the source of a story that has been going around lately about a baby born with no head. "Do I have a story for your work!" says a neighbor visiting the Bhabhis one day. "A baby was born a few nights ago in a village not far from here. It had no head. None at all!" Though I have had my doubts, this woman claims that not only did it really happen, but she herself performed the delivery. She describes how she pulled out the baby by the shoulders, the protruding veins of the neck stump. How it was "all open" and "terribly red." I still am not sure what to think, though I am later brought back to this moment when, four months pregnant, I go for one of many prescribed ultrasounds in Lucknow and, when I ask the technician what she is looking for with all these early sonograms, am told "Gross anomalies, like no head, for example." Pratima is excited to meet her, and occasionally interrupts the stories about difficult deliveries and turning breech babies to say that such cases should be referred to the hospital. She excitedly takes the woman's name to suggest her for dai training when NAFPA's next round takes place.

Here, closest to "midwifery," we lose a grasp on what might be a "norm." Nothing when it comes to baby-delivering is easily generalized, and categories of task and personnel are malleable; this work is unspecialized, but overlaps with the idea of "midwifery" in other ways. In the case of difficult deliveries, or in families with more money to spend, someone may be called from outside the household to assist, someone who, over the course of a long life of childbearing and child-rearing, has become notably proficient at difficult deliveries. On some occasions such women may not actually catch the baby, but come in and out through the course of labor to give advice, or to help a laboring woman to walk around, or massage her to help ease pain. Some women profess specific skills—like preventing tears, delivering twins, or turning breech babies in the later stages of pregnancy.

Such women, along with those who have conducted "a birth or two" in their own households, represent a broad spectrum of knowledge, skill, and specialization, and come from a range of castes. But one thing that does not vary is that family members and local specialists, unless they are also in the local category of postpartum worker, *do not* openly cut the umbilical cord or perform postpartum work. While some (but not all) with institutional training told me that they will cut the cord if a postpartum worker is not available, others said they only do so *"chup-chap"*—in secrecy. But as baby-deliverers they handle the placenta *before* the cord has been cut and come into contact with the same substances as those who do cord cutting and other postpartum tasks. Yet while postpartum work is delineated by caste, with baby delivering there is no rule of participation. In Lalpur and beyond, while there was much disagreement about how caste influences who attends deliveries *outside* of one's own home, *all* castes in this region deliver babies *within* their own households. Though local experts are primarily from lower or middle-range castes, upper-caste experts are not unheard of, but tend to fall into other self-made categories of specialization, those associated with biomedicine—*daktri* (for such women—who often call themselves "Ladies Doctors"—I have reserved an entire chapter [3]). Because of proximity, many serve primarily in their own *jati* neighborhoods or ones nearby. Some, like Chachi, deliver babies to supplement income, beginning after they have been widowed or when household wage-earners become incapacitated.

Such women are called because, I am told, "they have experience," "their hands are good," and "they have the *jankari*." Usually self-taught, "local experts" (for lack of a better phrase) gave me explanations such as, "I taught myself," "I had ten children of my own, that's how I know," and "I just started going [to houses where a delivery was taking place]." Some women held up their hands or tapped themselves on the chest when asked how they learned; others, like those who do postpartum work, looked at me oddly and said, "God gave me the work." Some, particularly *naouns*, who are the only *jati* group associated with baby-delivering (usually in terms of a predilection for birth work, though local norms and historical shifts are difficult to track—some *naouns* I met said they were remunerated through *jajmani*), said they had learned from a mother or mother-in-law. But inheritance is hardly the rule; many women said they performed work that neither their mothers nor mothers-in-law had done.

Medical anthropologists point out that in many parts of the world "traditional midwives" acquire their trade through apprenticeship, a mode of learning that contrasts sharply with the didactic state programs that "train" them (Jordan 1993). While apprenticeship may involve explicit, "hands-on" tutelage under an "elder," it may also be unshaped, occurring "simply with growing up in a particular environment" (Jordan 1993: 190). It emphasizes the *"ability to do"* rather than the *"ability to talk about* something, and indeed, it may be impossible to verbally elicit from people operating in this mode what they know (how to do)" (Jordan 1993: 192, original emphasis). In Sitapur, where birth skills are not "owned" on the basis of knowledge, embodied or otherwise, it is difficult to know where "wife" ends and "midwife" begins. There is no apprenticeship per se for birth experts in Sitapur. Women seldom absorb birth work in their childhood from mothers or grandmothers, as Jordan described. Rather, it is in the *sasural*, the marital home, where one is surrounded by pregnancies and births, and by bearing children herself, that a woman begins to "do the work." Instead of "learning" from specialists, women "absorb" skills by way of the very nonspecialized nature of birth work, the ways and movements of the *sasural*. They "learn" it because it is all around them. Knowledge of birth does not fall into a local receptacle—the "village midwife." Though women from outside the household might be summoned because labor is prolonged or the birth otherwise "difficult," rather than saying that they possess knowledge restricted from other women, it is more accurate to say they have heightened facility in a base of skill and experience shared by many married women.

Desire, the power of *man*, the heart-soul of volition, is that which many women said had called them to deliver babies, though many also described hardship as pushing them into the field. Indeed, these two narratives of beginning "the work" often served as counterweights of memory, especially among the elderly, lower-caste, and poor women who often become expert baby deliverers. Out of this tension, perhaps, comes a particular relationship to suffering, and many women mentioned to me a special sympathy for the pain of women and to the elementally female suffering of childbirth. According to Chachi, "When a woman has a baby she is in great pain.

How can I see that you are in pain and not come to you?" And as a *naoun* from Devia said, "We do this work in the service of the woman in pain. We do it from our hearts." But the outcome of work done out of sympathy and desire also characterizes the uncertainties of much informal and low-paid work, as meeting work done *man se* (from the heart) is compensation made *khushi se* (out of happiness). Payments may be as flexible as human emotions, matters between persons rather than longstanding ties between families and *jati* groups. Impromptu gifting of saris and cash is a primary means of payment, and gifts depend as much on the baby as on the skill of the practitioner. First children and sons (but also daughters if a family has many sons) bring more happiness and thus more elaborate gifting, and some capitalize on this exuberance because of its sheer unpredictability.

Caste-based work

Well into a dark, new-moon night of a month of gatherings of Kayasth women, late-night circles to sing into auspiciousness a baby born under an inauspicious star-sign, we think we hear a knock at the door. It is difficult to tell, given the cacophony of wind. Someone reaches up to unlatch the door and, as though blown in by a gust, Rakesh's Mother tumbles into the room. Her fall is caught by a girl in the doorway. As we all exclaim about her fall and move aside the drum to make space, two older girls, both upper-caste, exclaim with delight—and respect, "Dadi-ji!" (Grandmother). I am accustomed to the disparaging phrases and grating tones used when the women and girls of my own household speak about Rakesh's Mother and am surprised by the admiration. The two girls rush to touch her feet in respect. At the same time, I catch the face of Rani, the young niece from my household, who rolls her eyes and wrinkles her nose. Lower caste people smell, she later tells me, and the Chamarin's songs are old and boring. Like her younger auntie, she prefers the newer songs, the less dehati ones, with their repetitive and predictable verses—about the stuff of wifehood, the accoutrements of a birth, the relationships between female kin—and their familiar tunes borrowed from the latest film song. That night, Rakesh's Mother sings longer songs, older ones not so often heard anymore, telling longer stories, using terms that the young girls—and I—can barely follow. Some listeners are captivated, straining to follow and maybe even remember her words; others find it yet another reason to think her an old, foolish untouchable. The singing marks another chaos of affection and disgust, admiration and visceral prejudice.

Let us return to the vulnerabilities and negotiations of postpartum workers, for whom, at the level of more Brahmanical exegesis, social relegation incorporates two interlinked frames of pollution. The first considers tasks associated with death, meat, and animal-slaughter polluting according to a karmic principle of nonviolence (*ahimsa*), such that certain communities must shoulder the burden of socially necessary but karmically bad work. The second mode of pollution is based on a body ontology in which certain substances—blood, urine, saliva, mucus, dead flesh, feces, placentas—are, by nature, defiling. While postpartum work brings these tasks into a cosmological register beyond that of pollution (as the next chapter will consider), the association of "cord cutting" and "cleaning up" with untouchable status continues to operate as a caste-Hindu discourse.

It is, however, not patently inaccurate to say that the stuff of birth is considered dirty and polluting in north India. Each term—dirtiness (*gandagi*) and pollution (*pradushin*)—has its own associations, though the two are often used to refer to the same substance, person, or space. The latter refers to symbolic soiling that compromises a person's moral, social, and physical being, impinging on those she comes into contact with. The former refers to substances that can be washed off with water, those things that neither alter the self nor require ritual redress, but are unpleasant nonetheless. As represented in Hindu textual codes, menstrual blood, while dirty and dangerous, is less so than the blood of parturition; the placenta, blood, and feces associated with birth elevate birth fluids to a zenith of pollution in a ranking of bodily substances. However, more ambiguous is the relationship between work and substance; that is, how and in what ways the *work* of birth is polluted and to what extent its delegation is based on such constructs. In Sitapur, upper-caste talk about postpartum work emphasizes the amalgamation of the dirtiness and pollutedness of substance, work, and worker. Pollution binds work to worker in a circular fashion, such that dirty/polluted work is practiced by dirty/polluted people, while the presence of the dirty/polluted people makes the work, the participants and the work space dirty/polluted. Amma told me "the Chamars perform [postpartum] work because it is dirty, but the work is dirty because the Chamars do it," to which her son laughed and added, "It's *chakrivit tark* [circular logic], no? But that's how it works."

Listening to the ways women name postpartum work sheds light on the range of ways it is valued. Even caste-Hindus, generally speaking, describe postpartum work as a set of tasks, not reducible to "cleaning up" or cord cutting. How such workers are viewed often depends on which aspect of their work people see to be most important, and on the way families view *jajmani* exchange (related in no small part to their financial situation)—is giving grain, cooked food, and saris to members of service castes a responsibility or a burden? Like the labels applied to Rakesh's Mother, terminology for "postpartum work" evokes contrasting strains of stigma and reverence. It can be called *dhanuk ka kam* (the work of the *dhanuk*), and the practitioner a *dhanuk* (even if she is a member of another *jati*). Translation of the term *dhanuk* in this region is difficult, as women sometimes use it to refer to birth work (in the sense of *dhanuk ka kam*) and sometimes to trash work and "sweeping," while in western Uttar Pradesh it has been observed that the term refers specifically to those of a "midwife caste" (Wadley 1994).[3] The fact that the term for a trash worker/sweeper can also refer to one who does postpartum work points to a confluence of bodily and social/spatial care in which "housekeeping," including the management of bodies and their offal, has cosmological elements. Women of the Dhanuk and Bakshur *jatis* have particular relevance here; they are both sweepers and the makers of brooms and the winnowing baskets into which are placed (uncasted, according to some) newborn babies, like the unhulled products of the field. In Sitapur, they visit upper caste homes at the inauspicious time of a solar eclipse, receiving food and, in so doing, removing the stain of the eclipse, just as, when acting as postpartum workers, they remove the impurities of birth and threat of jealous gazes when they take away their payments.

The matrix of postpartum tasks can also be referred to synecdochically as "applying the oil," a reference to massage. When asking which workers were summoned to households, I quickly learned it was more appropriate to ask "Who comes to apply the oil?" than "Who comes to cut the cord?" The latter elicits hushed voices and averted eyes, while the former can be said plainly and openly. But equally often, references were specific and contextual, involving the sets of names by which women are identified in their *sasural* (because a postpartum worker works, by definition, only in her marital village), appellations based on caste or family affiliation.

As I shall discuss in greater detail in the next chapter, it is not just the contact with polluting substances or the specialized massage skills (shared, in any case, with *naouns*) that render postpartum labor Dalit women's work. The act of umbilical cord cutting, of severing the new baby from its life-giving (and potentially threatening) placenta lends the weight of labors and ritual acts associated with death, sin, and sacrifice to the intimacies of bodily care. *Pace* the argument that the fact that dais are more "menials" than "midwives" challenges romantic idealizations of specialized or sacred knowledge (P. Jeffery et al. 1989), in the case of postpartum workers, it is trash work that has as much, if not more symbolic and even sacred value (and, in a related way, consequences for health and well-being) as bodily care.

Groups and individuals

We can imagine the political nature of childbirth as situated in the birthing or fertile body, from a perspective in which techniques of governance take a primary interest in sexuality and population while fields of knowledge and power are contested on the grounds of the female body. But there are other ways to think about birth as polit- ical. According to Hannah Arendt, birth is political in its very nature, through the force of newness "natality" represents. She says, "Since action is the political activity par excellence, natality and not mor- tality may be the central category of political ... thought" (1998: 9). At the same time, Arendt says, contained in all action is the fact that it "always establishes relationships and therefore has an inherent tendency to force open all limitations and cut across boundaries." Action's necessary other, suffering, in which "to do" and "to suffer" are "opposite sides of the same coin," makes the political potential of its constant force of newness best represented by birth. If we slant Arendt's meaning somewhat, away from what she calls its "full ap- pearance" and "shining brightness" in "the public realm" (190), but retain her focus on the political weight of action and the bare poten- tiality of new life, this view may contain the germ of recognizability for Dalit women. Their relationship to action (and both its conse- quences and its other side—suffering) gives us insight into their po- litical subjectivity, into possible senses of self amid shifting frames of power and hierarchy. At the same time, we glean from birth and its labors a sense of how action might be understood in terms of "un- touchability" and the female body.

Where knowledge and stigma have places of prominence in dis- cussions of dais (and deliveries), when seen in terms of "work" and "action," birth in Sitapur breaks down into subprocesses that each pertain to different fields of personhood, action, and consequence. In the temporal flow of bringing a baby into the world and healing from birth, contrasting modes of intersubjectivity can be mapped onto a female body transformed and resituated. Writ large, postpartum work is organized according to notions of self and labor based on group identification. Though caste is not uniformly defined by all involved, group identity in terms of caste orchestrates postpartum work. The more flexible work of baby delivering involves meanings that highlight individual identities. Persons attend birth based on their personal relationship to the *jaccha* and her family; work is remunerated on individual, contextual bases, with little sense of formal obligation; women are drawn to the work out of personal desire or history, rather than because of the group they are part of. But the two categories of work, one more "open," the other more "closed," do not represent opposed or alternate "cultural" systems; neither has a greater claim on "modernity" or the categories of "dai," "midwife," or "TBA."

Jonathan Parry, in his work on funeral specialists in Varanasi (1994), describes a division of labor across the time span of death for Hindus, in which different ways of organizing and assigning work according to the phases of death pose a breakdown that "only makes sense in the light of certain ideas about the state of the departed" (1994: 2). Death, he says, is made up of subprocesses, each requiring unique personnel, organization, and care determined by the transition undergone by the deceased. Different workers, Parry says, embody the dead as it changes status, thereby managing the transformation from body to ghost to ancestor. Likewise, different kinds of birth work and the social structures and meanings that situate them are associated with the transformation of the *jaccha* through different phases in the process of having a baby (though birth workers embody neither *jaccha* nor *baccha*). In particular, reproductive work does not engage a single kind of opposition between pollution and purity, but rather, as a set of different kinds of labor, involves kinds and degrees of pollution. Thus the *jaccha* who must be bathed by the postpartum worker immediately after delivery is more polluted during this time than after her second bath, when the postpartum worker leaves and the *naoun* takes over the work of massage. The placenta before it has been severed can be handled by anybody, but after the cord is cut it must only be handled by the postpartum worker. The gradual decrease of pollutedness of the *jaccha* and baby, the transformations that occur in the placenta, and the transition from isolation and castelessness/outcaste status to social integration—all of these movements are mapped onto the healing of the maternal body and the kinds of practitioners that manage and assist it.

Here, we are on familiar ground. Anthropological literatures on childbearing in different cultural and historical contexts suggest that cultural tensions play out on a field of reproduction and the female

body. Some, such as Emily Martin (1987) and Donna Haraway
(1989), have explored the place (and lack thereof) of the female body
in medical and other normative discourses, such that unresolvable
cultural tensions emerge in the ways women negotiate reproduction and the meanings attributed to the female body. Others, such
as Janice Boddy (1989) and Carol Delaney (1992), have taken up
theories of embodiment to address the way cultural dichotomies or-
ganize bodily processes, placing women in at times ambiguous and
at times unambiguously subordinate positions in dominant symbolic frameworks. Unlike many French feminists who have pursued
essentially female bodily conditions or epistemologies, these scholars
argue that it is not due to an inherently or biologically female condition that structural tensions reveal themselves in female bodily
processes, but rather that cultural tensions, upon which various male-
oriented cultural systems are founded, make themselves apparent
in the female body and its inability to live up to normative (male-
oriented, or production-oriented, or individualizing, etc.) ideals.

   There is a correlate—albeit a less embodied one—to these approaches in studies stressing categorical tensions underlying South
Asian cultural and religious forms: renunciation and worldly engagement, king and priest, transcendence and immanence. In particular,
scholars have debated the way a tension between individual and
group identities dominates the landscape of the South Asian self.[4] Let
us embody this contrast, enfold it into birth and recuperation, to see
that the shift from work organized on individual grounds and that
understood as part of group affiliation does not necessarily involve
a *tension* between modes of personhood. If anything, transformations
in the female body involve shifts in social context.[5] As with death
work, tasks are mediated according to the social, cosmological, and
physical context of the *jaccha-baccha* dyad. As systems of action and
engagement rather than specialized knowledge, these social fields
bespeak shifting visions of the gendered, casted self, though they
draw from the same shared font of knowledge about birth, babies,
and the female body. More importantly, they are casted in being
cast upon a duration of reproduction that extends from pregnancy
to birth and into postpartum healing and integration.

Demanding women

For Rakesh's Mother, a "closed" category, like a strategic essentialism
(Spivak 1995: 214) does not mean "closed" to negotiation. Caste, in

particular, is not stable, but is negotiated, contested, performed and counterperformed even where it may seem most stable. It is part of other modes of power that are negotiated in and through birth. In India, it has been noted that the postpartum phase is of concern to state forms of control, a point of insertion of power via family planning measures (quite literally as a site for the often coercive insertion of IUDS) and development discourses (Van Hollen 2002). But beyond institutional settings, the postpartum phase is one in which local politics and visions of social uplift are negotiated alongside meanings of body and identity, stigma and labor. The politics of the postpartum phase are as situated in household and intradomestic intimacies as in institutions. The domestic sphere, as a site of birth, labor, death, and healing, involves negotiations of authority, conflicting symbolics and performances which make for political subjectivities, modes of belonging, and experiences of causation and power. Gender and caste are shaped in the *sor* as both home and place of work. As such, extrainstitutional births are places in which multiple forms of power and authority condense. It should come as no surprise, then, that Dalit women have complex perspectives on their work, views that do not necessarily accord with those of their clients (or their own male kin). "The system" is not uniformly regarded across its spectrum, and Dalit women's sense of ownership does not imply an orientation toward the whole, as Dumont might have it (1980), but rather fragmentation from within.

The first space of negotiation may be "pollution." Dais' status has long been seen as determined by birth pollution, and the low social position of dais an indicator of the status of women in north Indian society (P. Jeffery et al. 1989). This association of birth work (now speaking broadly) with pollution may itself be somewhat overdetermined, notably in its assertion that whole groups are ontologically construed as polluted by direct association with the periodic pollutedness of the female body—at menstruation, birth, and postpartum (P. Jeffery et al. 1989; R. Jeffery and P. Jeffery 1993; Rozario 1998). In this framework, birth pollution and caste pollution merge (Rozario 1998); the pollutedness of the body, the gender (female), the work, the person, and the community (the caste) are part of a single matrix. In some accounts, symbolic stigma is extended to everyday knowledge and ability in an interventionist framework; the low status of birth work is continuous with the "helplessness" of dais presented with difficult situations and with a larger sense of lack—of hygiene, knowledge, medical services, and money (P. Jeffery et al. 1989). While these convergences speak to interconnections between

health care and social status (for practitioners and clients), the con-
flation of potentially different kinds of work and pollution may also
obscure certain understandings of inequality and power. Following
Veena Das (1982) and Jonathan Parry (1994), I suggest that not only
are the pollution of untouchability, birth, and death not the same,
but also that within each of these sites there is room for different
manipulations of pollution ideology and "a degree of indeterminacy"
to symbolic rules (Parry 1994: 111).

In Sitapur, slippages between "dirt" and "pollution," "hygiene" and
"purity" are part of the moralizing mythologies of development. But
it is the semiotic work of untouchable birth workers to hold such
terms *apart*. Postpartum workers do not define themselves or their
work as grounded in the polluting nature of substance or work and
their talk about female bodily fluids downplays "danger" and "pollution" and emphasizes "mere" or practical dirtiness. Likewise, postpartum workers do not consider themselves of an ontologically lower
order *because of* their work, though they may recognize the extent
to which stigma is a social and cultural force and their social status
related to their work in a relative way—that is, in terms of how others view it, rather than in absolute terms. Like the urban low-caste
midwife of Lucknow described by R. S. Khare, Rakesh's Mother,
Schoolteacher's Mother, and others I spoke with, in their dismissals
as much as their explanations, seemed to refuse a vision of themselves, their bodies, and their work as a web of "integrated dirtiness,"
and rejected the "caste-assigned view of 'the sullied (*maila*) body and
immoral soul'" (Khare 1998: 159). Describing their work as "dirty,"
requiring an old sari during and a bath afterwards, they never used
the term *pradushin* (pollution) to describe either substance or work.

Some observers look for evidence of untouchables' acceptance of
the ideologies that subordinate them in the degree to which they
participate in those notions. According to Pauline Kolenda (1978), untouchables do not ascribe to notions of *karma* or *dharma*, constructs
which justify their subordination in a cosmological frame. Gerald
Berreman (1991) argues that untouchables possess a distinct culture
outside of and often in rejection of frameworks of caste, making untouchability a matter of difference in ideology. Others counter this,
arguing that untouchables accept the structures that subordinate
them, demonstrated in the fact that they rank other untouchable
jati according to the same formulae that shape their own status (Moffatt 1979). Putting the debate in the context of representation, Ronald Inden (1990) suggests that, in rendering caste essential to the
imagination of "India," colonial forces and anthropologists have dis-

proportionately focused on pollution (and *jajmani*), denying the singularity of untouchables outside of convergent Brahmanical and colonial visions.

In religious doctrine and everyday life, for better or worse, unified (but not uncontested) visions of pollution exist in Sitapur, defining, on the one hand, the responsibility of women to defend the moral and substantial boundaries of the household and providing, on the other hand, the stage on which "caste" is performed on a daily basis. Such moments and scripts include Choti Bhabhi's anxious explanations for how and why I must refuse to consume food prepared by those ranked lower on a caste spectrum, and the special requirements of exclusionary behavior (primarily, again, through not consuming food) applied to *niche log* (lower people)—"untouchables" and Muslims. Likewise, they include reference *to* such "rules" by Dalit women who fed me in secret—behind closed doors, in darkened back rooms—and said, as one Pasi woman did, "Don't worry. We know who you live with." But like Dalits who recognize the relative, hegemonic quality of caste rules on food consumption, while demanding, as some did, that I consume food as a show of solidarity ("If you don't eat my food, you won't be my friend"), for Dalit postpartum workers, the matter of caste ideology is not necessarily a binary of acceptance or rejection. Nor is it a matter of degree. For many, it seems that pollution remains critically ambiguous, as in the way that Rakesh's Mother rejected outright the notion that such work is "polluting" and foregrounded the fact that it is "hers."

Ambiguity does important work for the subject who makes use of it, even as in institutional frames it can do the work of marginalization (see Chapter 6). Even as she does not embrace it, Rakesh's Mother deployed notions of pollution—and caste-Hindu women's firm assertions of it—and made use of the stigma of cord cutting to demand payment or assert her right to the labor. "As you argue [with me about payment], your baby gets cold," she told Shalini's Dadi. Such bartering points to that fact that, in terms of pollution's relationship to *jajmani* (that other overdetermined trope of north Indian-ness) postpartum workers have an ability for leverage that the less well-defined, less ideologically located baby-deliverers lack. If *jajmani* contains mutual obligations in its abstractions, in its unfolding, certain people are "plainly expected to assert the right to demand or even extort their customary dues" (Parry 1994: 147). Put differently, if Rakesh's Mother or her sister-in-law does not cut the cord, who will?

This is not to underestimate the very real insults and injustices postpartum workers endure on the basis of their caste position. To

be sure they are often underpaid and their demands frequently deferred. But the assertion of "right" to perform caste-based work, and
the sense that all people (perhaps life itself) depends on the work of
untouchables is part of an antagonistic, referentially defined sense
of caste, rather than a sign of agreement across the ranks about how
things should be. Stigma, here, can be a tool of barter, even as it
may also be, in part, that which creates the *need* to barter.

In the *sor* and after it, demands made by postpartum workers can
be thought of as speech acts, less for their results than for what they
enunciate about power dynamics. Rakesh's Mother's demands at
delicate moments—that certainly befuddle efforts to soften the focus or idealize the gentleness of care associated with "midwives"—
and Schoolteacher's Mother's complaints to other members of the
community about various families' underpayments can both be
considered, in Marxian terms, points of revelation. They unmask
the power relations according to which (re)production unfolds, demonstrating the dependence of caste-Hindus on untouchable women
on the basis of fear of pollution and *jajmani* obligation.[6] Or, as part
of an ongoing conversation that keeps open the terms of engagement,
demand can be an act of transformation. It can be seen as asserting
legitimacy, evoking the idiom, if not the actuality, of commensurable
exchange. Indeed, as economic and symbolic hierarchies are revealed
and transformed, at times, into a kind of cultural capital, for Dalit
women, caste-based work becomes a gendered means for limited self-
advancement—as members of a caste, not as individuals. Of course,
Rakesh's Mother doesn't make these enunciations only on symbolic
grounds; she does want to get paid. Still, according to Khare, low-
caste women "neither simply surrender themselves to the dominant
caste order nor [seek] a total separation from it. They use this social
ambiguity to protest, maneuver and negotiate" (Khare 1998: 149).
Untouchable women need not fully "believe" or "not believe" in
pollution in order to utilize it, while their ability to control labor and
maneuver for payment requires that pollution *not* be rendered entirely "unreal." Because of pollution's role in the existence of work
they desire and control, postpartum workers' relationship to "stigmatized" work and ideology is agnostic.

The complex stakes for untouchable women make enunciations
difficult to locate in registers by which caste and gender inequalities
are nationally oriented political concerns, part of party interests and
agendas, requiring loud voices in the key of outrage. Demands for
payment involve the charge that "owned"/"stigmatized" work is not
regarded or compensated highly enough, while at the same time,

paradoxically, resisting the fact of relegation on the basis that such work is devalued, while not resisting the work itself. According to Khare (1984, 1998) untouchable women's perspectives rest at such point of limbo, where ideologies are at the same time put to use, resisted, and reformulated. Even if it is an exaggerated component of ethnographic accounts, pollution is important to gendered definitions of self and labor, and casted (or Dalitized) ways of conceptualizing belief and action. Even where it cannot be said that untouchables "do not believe in untouchability" (Juergensmayer 1980), untouchable birth workers enact a relationship to ideology that is not based on belief (Khare 1998). Instead, they have varied ways of locating themselves and their possibilities for living (and working) on imagined social maps. Postpartum work exemplifies not only the "different views" on caste held by untouchables, but also the ways social structures are part of webs of emotion and everyday strategies for getting by.

Postpartum labor and social change

Schoolteacher's Mother derives her name from the successes of her eldest son, "Master-ji," or "the Schoolteacher," who has, in so many ways, brought his family and jati up in the world. A teacher in a nearby state high school, he owns enough land to make his large family well-off in comparison to much of the rest of Lalpur. His house is large and brick, just beyond the boundary of the village, and his sons' weddings have been lavish. Often I am summoned by a child from his extended family to come watch the Pandit from a nearby village administer wedding-related ceremonies; when I visit him on Diwali, I notice that his religious practice looks very much like that of the upper-caste men in my own household and very little like that of his mother, whose recitations are from memory rather than store-bought religious texts and whose murtis are handmade from mud and clay rather than plastic painted deities and printed posters from the bazaar. At village public singings at festivals—which men and children attend until late into the night, he plays the harmonium rather than the drum, and is a strong voice in the progression of songs. When I speak with him about his mother's labor he cushions his language of jati in the gentle evasions appropriate to such a delicate topic. He explains briefly that his father used to tan hides, but says he knows very little about that. The men, he says, have given up this demeaning labor, but women's advancement is slower, on account of the difficulties of gender and education so recognizable to those concerned with Indian modernization and social change.

"The old women," he says, "do this work because they are not educated to know it is wrong. These are old things, things of the past. But when our people began to become more educated, began to go to school, they learned that such work is dirty. And they gave it up. They were taught not to do certain kinds of work."

The *sor* is not a "new" space of contested political subjectivities. Likewise, Dalit women's carefully sustained ambiguities are not residues of "caste as religious hierarchy" so much as they are continuous with the social implications of "caste as political stance." Contrasting theories of untouchability are reflected in the strategies of Dalit politics, and appear in the range of everyday approaches rights and equality—as they take shape on the backs of Dalit women's labor and lives. At the heart of twentieth century caste uplift movements (and their manifestations in contemporary consciousness) are differences in the ways labor can be related to religious structures and subordination, asking what happens to religious codes when work is politicized as an element of subordination *within* similar moral frameworks (rather than, or as well as, in class-based concepts of labor and exploitation). Different kinds of restricted labor enter identity politics in different ways: consider the refusal by Chamar (men) to perform polluting labor of carcass removal and hide tanning as compared with their unwillingness to reject the work of plowing—work considered sinful within the *varna* system (Mendelsohn and Vicziany 2000: 49). Situated at the junction of the polluting and the sinful, postpartum work suggests politics in which religious and secular frameworks are difficult to disentangle.

Where do Dalit women's labors stand in debates between the revisionist Hinduism of Gandhi that resituated (and pardoned) caste as an abstract system of labor organization, and the radical stance of Ambedkar that involved an orientation toward ideals of secular humanism and outright rejection of Hinduism? Ideas about how labor relates to citizenship and subordination are also situated in visions of national progress: including antipoverty programs, rural development, family planning schemes, and the way state and transnational agencies concern themselves with reproduction. The progress narratives associated with family planning are especially complex in relation to the shaping of Dalit identity; because of connections drawn between overpopulation and poverty, such interventions have often been targeted precisely at the reproductive lives of those in low-caste communities, at times with a strongly eugenic bent (Mendelsohn and Vicziany 2000: 148). Early and mid-century caste mobilization, as well as the contemporary shape of identity politics in more militant organizations such as the Dalit Sena, cannot be separated from (less publicly debated, but no less important) visions of social and cultural mobility, namely the distinction between sanskritization (through shifts in ritual practice, work, and the public role of women) and religious conversion on the one hand and embrace of secular politics on the other. But neither sanskritization nor rejection of Hinduism allows for the complexities of untouchable women's perspectives on power.

Master-Ji's account of his mother's work, of education and caste-awareness as precursors to abandonment of demeaning work, resituates even as it reiterates the long-standing association of caste-status with iconic labor. His view echoes Louis Dumont's argument that caste status and profession are so closely bound that practical changes in bearing or religious practice do less to improve status than giving up the actions that define it: "A caste bearing such a strong religious mark as that of the 'leather people' [Chamars] would gain nothing by introducing refinements into its other customary features: nowadays when it wants to end its infamy, it tries to put an end to the function which justifies this infamy" (1980: 93).[7] For Master-ji, in the context of social uplift, dirtiness (not pollution) is a moral value and dirty work a matter of ignorance. Rather than accounting for women's abandonment of postpartum work through education as a sign that education affords greater opportunity for income generation (and thus no more "need" to do dirty work)—what might be considered part of one standard development story about women in the "Third World"—he associated education with *individual* growth and work with its symbolic value in an idiom of "dirt" in which caste and modernization ideologies are difficult to parse.

The parallel of "old women's" abandonment of "such work" with a wider abandonment of untouchable status puts caste and political consciousness in a gendered framework, one that is not out of line with early and mid-twentieth-century caste movements in which iconic work was fundamentally bound to caste and untouchability, to good or bad effect. Here, as in ethnographic accounts in which stigmatization merges with lack of ability, stigma and knowledge converge, and the failure to abandon stigmatized activities becomes a symptom of a larger state of ill-being, namely, lack of political consciousness, lack of awareness that "this work is dirty." In this view, while "dirtiness" remains absolute (instead of relativized), oppression occurs by participating in caste as an idea *by* performing "dirty" actions—a vision of empowerment based on praxis rather than structure. Slippages in the space of volition are multiple, and, as with the subaltern who cannot speak (Spivak 1988a), the consciousness— visions of caste and power—of Dalit birth workers is given no space to be present except in terms of its absence. While I have argued that anthropological representations of birth as patently polluting follow caste-Hindu frameworks, the stigmatizaton of Dalit women's birth work as "dirty" (rather than devalued) is also present in narratives of uplift. Though such teleologies bespeak a critical *male* consciousness, the ambiguities they employ obscure women as agents and political actors with their own—often strategic—links formed between work, dirtiness, caste, and self.

In early- and mid-twentieth-century Lucknow, Chamars from both urban and rural communities publicly contested their oppression on the grounds of work, specifically the work of hide-tanning (for men), "midwifery"/cord cutting and "menial labor" (for women), and bonded agricultural labor (for both men and women).[8] In this fragment of twentieth century Chamar politics lie crosscutting debates and tensions, a yet-to-be-consolidated movement involving intersecting visions of modernization, equality, nationalism, anti- and procolonial sentiment, and Hinduism (Rawat 2003). Dalits were also engaged by "outsiders" interested in claiming or silencing their cause—British authorities; the Arya Samaj movement; Muslims; Christian missionaries; Sikhs and groups such as the "Nanak Panthers"; Congress and the Muslim League; local landowners and moneylenders; and those identified as "Sanatan Hindus" (orthodox Hindus) (Mendelsohn and Vicziany 2000; Rawat 2003).

Following established patterns of caste mobilization, Chamars sought social and political validity by several means. In the 1920s, '30s, and '40s public discussions debated whether work associated with hide tanning and removal of dead animals, both within and outside the established leather industry, was to be abandoned or whether fair remuneration would be sought for it. According to colonial police and intelligence records, some activists argued that Chamars must abandon labor considered defiling on the grounds that it *was* defiling and had been inflicted on them by both upper-caste Hindu and colonial structures of industry and social control. Others demanded that fellow Chamars abandon coerced, stigmatized, and unpaid labor for landowners. Others called for continuation of such labor, but sought to divorce stigma from market value of labor.[9]

At the same time, there was discussion of means of upward mobility that crossed boundaries between rejection of pollution ideology, liberal humanism, and sanskritization: limiting the movements of Chamar women as part of the advancement of the community, a refusal to carry carcasses, conversion to vegetarianism, insistence on drawing water from all wells and on entry into temples, and insistence that boys be permitted to attend schools.[10] There is also evidence that upward mobility included the refusal to eat or "touch" the food of Muslims.[11] Birth-related work came under similar scrutiny. Some Chamar activists demanded that women give up "work as midwives."[12] Others called for fair remuneration according to standardized rates for the work of cord cutting and "midwifery" (it is unclear to what extent assertions were made by women, as the police record only mentions "resolutions passed"). In the city of Basti, Chamar activists passed a resolution that Chamar women should not accept less than 1.4 rupees when "functioning as midwives."[13] A police account from Benares notes that "as a result of these resolutions a Chamar woman refused to attend the delivery of a child unless she was first paid her fee of Rs 5 and the child died in consequence," casting a familiar taint of failed moral obligation on gendered and casted work.[14] In 1926, reference to a division of labor appears in the police record, as it was reported that at a Chamar group in Benares had passed resolutions that "less than Rs 5 should not be charged for cutting the 'nar' [cord] of a child at the time of delivery."

In this context, women's labor—especially work performed for *zamindars* (landowners) and within the bounds of *jajmani*—like women's mobility, was a pawn in men's activism. Labor forms the link—or the space of slippage and convergence—between sanskritization and rejection of caste ideology, as arguments for limiting women's movements (suggesting *purdah*) overlapped with efforts to curtail women's paid labor. In 1923, Chamar groups in various cities passed resolutions that women should not be permitted to perform agricultural and industrial labor.[15] And in 1946, women's labor was used in retaliation against Chamars: the police record notes "[Chamars] have stopped their womenfolk from doing menial work such as removing dung and grinding and in retaliation Zamindars have disallowed Chamars from cutting grass in their fields and jungles."[16] Where "their womenfolk" stood in relation to these issues is not evident in police records, with the exception of mention that "Chamar women resented [this] interference."[17] But it seems that women did not suggest abandoning work of any kind and insisted, publicly, on adequate remuneration. These accounts demonstrate at once the historical longevity of divisions of labor in birth and a salience of work-based caste identities that extends from the *sor* into the context of citizenship, postcolonial identity, and social change, or rather locates those social and political elements squarely in the *sor*.[18] At the same time, they point to household gender dynamics, in which elderly women exert control over certain forms of work to stave off dependency on male kin. Ultimately, where ability to earn or supplement an income is at stake, stigma is a delicate equation. Work that flows through the patriline as *female* inheritance, work that through its association with pollution and perhaps "shame" stands always to threaten a family (through flows of substance and code) and a community (through the stain of backwardness it brings into family stories of modernization) also stands, in its very genderedness, to reveal the convergence of sanskritization with ideologies of "progress" in a secular frame.

Such fragmentary political moments show that the work of men and women Dalits, and associated views on the meaning of social progress, are felt and organized differently. For women, upward mobility might be envisioned on an economic basis, or gender hierarchies perceived as less negotiable (or perhaps more immediate) than those of caste (so perceived by men). When it comes to everyday survival, the proper valuation of work is at stake, less the act of engaging in it, while socioeconomic upward mobility may, in general, be more available to men. It is not irrelevant that in Sitapur I met few Chamar men engaged in work related to hide tanning or animal removal (though such work had been performed in earlier generations) while women who participated in postpartum work showed little or no conviction that this was work to one day be abandoned.[19] The Schoolteacher's influence on his family's fortunes and outlooks was strong, however, and it remains to be seen whether his daughters-in-law will do birth work one day. While some told me they would, others looked away at the mention of it or said no, they would not.

Where there is no midwife

In Sitapur the romantic figure of the midwife and the progress-bound concept of the "dai" are disappeared on a social stage in which meanings of work do not line up with those that underscore global models of intervention or fantasies about the "traditional" behind-space of the "modern" self. Within the question of who, among many actors, are involved in birth lie layers of subjectivity and negotiation that give belonging its stakes, most vividly so for Dalit women whose perspectives are eclipsed by the dominant concept of "the dai." I have taken as my starting point the assertion that "it is inappropriate to regard the dai as a 'midwife' in the contemporary western sense" (R. Jeffery and P. Jeffery 1993: 17). But I do less on the basis of the "menial" role of local practitioners than on the range of actors and actions involved—and the theories of action and impact under negotiation. I find it important to follow women in Sitapur in understanding postpartum workers on their own terms: as a separate category of practitioner whose work is necessary to bring a baby into the world and manage its vulnerability through *both* body and trash work. In a zone of misapprehended female labor where "the dai" is no longer entirely relevant, they are outside the Western and urban Indian register of birth work. As women with broad mobility and intimate knowledge of bodies, lives, and households, they complicate models of social uplift while challenging, in intimate ways, everyday performances of caste.

The subtleties and dimensions of birth work underscore Partha Chatterjee's statement that "There is not one caste ideology, ... but several, sharing some principles in common, but articulated at variance, and even in opposition to one another" (1993: 179–80). These complexities concur with the idea that the body is a site for articulating and resituating caste identities, particularly for those deemed "untouchable" (Khare 1998). Thinking with Pierre Bourdieu, if social matrices and "political mythology" manifest in "bodily hexis" (1977: 93), female reproductive processes both embody and are capable of revealing inconsistencies and inequalities implicit in social structures. But in the case of postpartum work, the bodily hexes of both childbirth and caste-based work are deployed and reckoned in different ways at different times. For Dalit women, they are perhaps never so fully integrated as to disappear from consciousness.

The work of critical translation illuminates politics of birth by pointing in a different direction than a view that considers the impact of biomedical technology on spaces into which it enters (or intrudes), for example, or the relationship of "traditional practitioners" to institutional interventions. That is, it points us toward praxes and moralities as spaces of convergence rather than contests of knowledge or clashes in ways of being, doing, or thinking. By beginning with the observation that birth work is not organized by knowledge, local or otherwise, but by categorizations of embodied action and associated moralities, we begin to see other ways that birth provides phenomenological grounds for alterities on the one hand and belonging on the other.

Chapter 2

BODIES
THE POISONOUS LOTUS

Abject objects

In Shalini's Mother's sor, in the interim between bathing and cleaning postpartum bodies and rubbing them with warm mustard oil, Rakesh's Mother turns to the part of her work that for many defines it inherently, though not overtly, not in open speech. Where men and women politely refer to her as "she who applies the oil," it is for dealing with the results of "the cut" that "the Chamarin," and no one else, is called.

After scraping the lumps of slick red and brown from the floor, after unceremoniously tossing the placenta—"the purein,*" the lotus—into the broken basket supplied to her, she covers the mess, deemed, literally, unsightly, with an old piece of fabric. She takes the basket outside and washes her hands with water from a bucket placed there specifically for her. Seeing me follow her, she asks what I am doing. Speaking as euphemistically as I can, I say I would like to come with her when she "goes to throw it away." She looks at me, annoyed. I begin my usual explanations. My interest in her work does not flatter. Though I can't put my finger on exactly why, it seems to bother her. On other occasions the reason is clear: "You will take this* jankari *that I give you back to your place and become rich."*

This time there is no jankari *to impart. "Stay here with the baby and the mother," she says, "There is nothing to see."*

"I would like to see what you do with all of this," I motion to the basket.

"I throw it. What else?"

"But where?"

"Where? With the trash." She begins to walk and I go with her. She turns again, says, "This is nothing interesting," but does not insist I stay behind. We wander through the village in an easterly direction, toward the cluster of homes of the Brahman families, between houses, through brambles and fallen mud walls. The Chamarin occasionally stops, looks around and mumbles to herself. In the confusion of age, perhaps, she seems to have lost her way. She stops another old woman walking by and asks how we get to the pond. Directions are given—just beyond the edge of the village, twenty feet or so behind an upper-caste home, through a small patch of wildness of trees and bushes and unkempt growth. I think about what had been said about ghosts eating placentas and possessing babies, about how it is better to burn the placenta, but "Who can afford the wood?" and I ask if placentas are thrown in this place in particular. "There is no special place," she says and dumps out the basket's contents. She does not have much strength in her arms, so the contents roll down the incline, snagging on sticks and roots and bushes on their way to the water. The placenta disappears below the murk. "It's just trash," the Chamarin says and we return to the house where the Chamarin will continue her work. But I have heard enough already about cuts and openings and threats, about winds, witches and churels—ghosts of women dead in childbirth—about the threat of gazes—desiring or malevolent or aspersion-casting—that fall upon things left in the open, enough, that is, to imagine that either something is accomplished by calling this "just trash," or that I must recalibrate my sense of what "trash" might be.

Weeks later, Bari Bhabhi and I pile onto the back of motorcycles. She sits comfortably sidesaddle and is driven by her brother. Unable to balance the way she does, and wearing a selwar-kameez instead of the sari Bari Bhabhi prefers I wear, I sit astride behind Dev, the nephew of Tulsiram (a Pasi man with five kids, his own land, and local political aspirations). We are headed to Bari Bhabhi's maike. Dev and Bari Bhabhi's brother take mostly back roads and dirt tracks through the fields. We pass through villages and I take note of the images painted in white on the outside of houses and molded into the dirt walls—sweeping patterns that look like a well-sown field, auspicious handprints that, in repetition, bloom like plants, swastikas and spirals, and the occasional outline of a lotus—for some a sign of political affiliation, for others, to be sure, something pretty to look at. We pass an overgrown grove where Bari Bhabhi says "some kind of bad work once took place," and numerous small temples—beneath trees, at the edges of fields, in the heart of villages. Just beyond the edge of one small village, I notice something out of place in the road—a lump of flesh connected to a straggling cord and shiny with moisture. I point to it and look over at Bari Bhabhi. She shrugs and says something I can't quite make out over the *growl of the motors, something that sounds like, "A baby must have been born." She turns away.*

Why is postpartum work the provenance of Dalit women? To ask this, we must first ask, what do the thresholds and offal of the body tell us about structures of time, existence, and action that locate a person in the world? Or, why are the things cast off important to those things that are kept? Rakesh's Mother's comments and labors, and the euphemisms, images, and metaphors in women's talk about birth suggested to me that placentas and trash are part of the way new life involves overlapping politics of marginality. In Lalpur, I learned through evasions, whispers, averted eyes, and curt dismissals to focus my questioning gaze, as I averted my everyday, protective one, on the placenta. As the bodily entity that marks the distinction between casted and uncasted labor, the placenta, perhaps more than the womb, seems to explain much about cosmologies and subjectivities attendant to birth. As objects of both disgust and location, placentas are part of maps at once local and institutional. At the same time, in many frames of reference—Hindu, biomedical, Dalit, policy, even academic—the placenta is an object that refuses to be placed, talked about, and at times imagined, though in Sitapur its residue haunts the auspiciousness of birth and the nature of coming into being. The impact of the placenta seems to hinge on the thresholds it crosses—between the visible and invisible, growth and decay, utility and threat, life and memory. Its passages are carefully mediated, demonstrating that as much can be learned about power from the nature of thresholds as from the transitions that things, or people, or groups undergo.

In some ways of speaking common in the metropole, the placenta's topography is distorted by roving Western metaphors that define a human landscape, in which "cutting the cord" signifies the severing of the bond between mother and child, home and the world. Not so in rural Sitapur, except in clinics, spaces where such metaphors have become common, or in "dai training" where it is taught that cords must be cut before placentas emerge because, as one dai trainer told me, "This is what is taught in medical schools." In Sitapur, where women (even "trained dais") adamantly reject the notion that cords should be cut before, not after, delivery of the placenta, the afterbirth becomes an object around which social relations are mapped onto reproductive bodies. Through its disappearance into not only Western metaphors but also bodily maps among among many urban and well educated men and women, and in the *structure* of that disappearance, the placenta becomes an abject object, its capacity to signify as important as its other functions in the world and body.

By way of asking how "untouchability" is shaped in the context of birth, this chapter is a description of the placenta's social meanings. But it is difficult to write with certainty about placentas because it was difficult to get people to talk about them. Men and women responded to my questions with brief answers and pat denials ("The placenta? It doesn't do anything in the body"), statements like "It's just trash." As silence about placentas, like the terms "dirtiness," "sin," "trash," and "pollution," can be multivalent, this account is an effort to approach the implicit and the impasse and is patched together from terminology, observations, bits of described practice, and conversational closures, more than from any exegesis.

Imaginaries of the abject, or the powerful and dangerous, can be a means of expressing "the ambivalent temporality of modernity" (Bhabha 1994: 239) for those for whom it may be precisely "modernity" that is at stake. These are the reverberations across the imagined thresholds of pasts and futures, the ways that "newness enters the world" through the cracks (Bhabha 1994: 212) as well as the seams. As such, this chapter aims to provide some of the cosmological and social ways that disgust is a mode of citizenship and the uncanny shiver becomes a foundational urge for intervention. Through these affective structures, both pedagogical and performative (Bhabha 1994) aspects of citizenship emerge. The fact that this happens on the ground of healing (a ground that can also include vulnerabilities and experiences of loss) situates the possibilities for subjectivity emergent in the time/space of the *sor* and the time/spaces of poverty and intervention in the emotional complexities of untouchability. That it does so in shadowy, *non*institutional spaces, as well as in and through the stuff of governance and governmentality, should come as no surprise.

Even as I approach placentas in their affinities—to lotuses, ghosts, corpses, trash, and so on, affinities, symbolic and otherwise, have their limits. The various uses for and ways of handling placentas demonstrate that here, as elsewhere, little is beyond the reach of poverty. So much—symbols, rituals, and rules for behavior—depends on it. Where the depth of a relative's poverty was best understood, Choti Bhabhi said, by the fact that they had to repeatedly postpone key life cycle rituals such as their youngest son's *mundan* because they could not afford the gifting or festivities required, where life-cycle rituals can be called off "on account of poverty," I am drawn to thinking about qualities of objects and essences within a framework of unfixedness in which lack of means and flaws in infrastructure intrude into existence. They can transform one's relation to the earthly, material plane, and also to the cosmological and ghostly realms of unseen forces.

Lotus

"The purein*?" Bari Bhabhi says, during one of the hot afternoons, after lunch, after the dishes and pots have been cleaned, when we rest under the shade of the room adjacent to the* angan. *It is early in my stay. We have just turned off the handheld radio after one of the afternoon serials about household life and women's struggles that Bari and Choti Bhabhi like to listen to when they can get the station to come in. Bari Bhabhi is lying on the rope* charpai *with Rohit, who does not look very interested in sleep, even as Bari Bhabhi idly rubs his back and plays with his curly hair. Choti Bhabhi, vigorously rubbing mustard oil onto Dilip, who keeps reaching for and trying to overturn the small* kitori *of oil, looks over at us and wrinkles her nose. "What thing?"*

"The purein. *The, what do you call it?" Bari Bhabhi turns to me, "Placenta. It holds the baby's* jivan *[life force] inside the womb. The food comes through it. To the baby."*

I ask if people think of it as something that is the baby's or something that is the mother's. I have asked these questions many times in other settings, but they feel out of place here. Bari Bhabhi says, a bit confused, "It's the baby's thing. What does it have to do with the mother? When it comes out it is attached to the baby. Then it's cut and thrown away. How do they do it in your place?" I say that in America mostly they cut the cord before the purein *comes out. Bari Bhabhi says that she thinks this happens in hospitals here too, but she is not sure, but that at home this would never, ever happen.*

Amma is lying on a bed nearby. She seems to be asleep, but opens her eyes when I mention this. "If it is cut before it comes out, it can rise and strangles the mother. It stops her breath," Amma says.

"How is that?" Choti Bhabhi asks, looking up.

"The jivan *that is there inside has nowhere to go. It blooms and blooms; it suffocates the* jaccha.*"*

Later in the evening, Choti Bhabhi and Bari Bhabhi and I are leafing through my copy of Where There is No Doctor, *a health manual I had been advised to bring into "the field," the "interior," for my own sake—a commentary (and irony—the title, at least) that strikes me on more than one occasion. I use it for its intended purpose exactly twice—once to inspect the rash on a neighbor's arm, and once to decide which antibiotic to give my husband when he picks up giardia in Lucknow. The rest of the time it pro-vides mostly entertainment value. After grossing ourselves out with the pages on various injuries, Bari and Choti Bhabhi and I pore over illustrations of pregnancy and birth. Choti Bhabhi points to a picture of a fetus: "Look at how his hand is over his mouth. They have to cover it like that because that water they are in is so dangerous. If it gets in the mouth the baby will be mute. If it gets in the eyes it will be blind, and in the ears, deaf. That's why sometimes they stick their fingers up their nose. I have seen pictures—of the baby with its fingers up its nose."*

"But look," Bari Bhabhi says, "His ear is totally open, so how can that be?"

"Yes, but it's in that sac, right? But if the sac breaks and it gets that water anywhere it is dangerous."

In Sitapur the placenta is very much "the baby's thing"—source of its life force and also conveying its nurturance. It is called *purein,* an Awadhi term meaning lotus. It can also be referred to as *naal,* a term whose meaning incorporates the stalk of a lotus, the umbilical cord, veins and arteries, and channel more broadly. Associations of the placenta with the lotus can be considered alongside the startling physical resemblance of the two, and evoke a web of meanings link-ing the lotus with fertility. In medieval Hindu iconography and myth, the lotus is a representation of the "manifested universe," signifying forces of creation, abundance, and wealth (Coomeraswamy 1993; Feldhaus 1993; Jayakar 1990; Kinsley 1986; Zimmer 1946). It is as-sociated with both the waters (as a source of fertility and nurtu-rance) and the earth (which rests upon and is supported by the waters, as is the lotus blossom) (Coomeraswamy 1993:155; Jayakar 1990: 129). Linked to the divine and spiritual realms on the one hand, it is also associated with the earthly goddess Laksmi on the other, not Laksmi as consort of Visnu, but Laksmi as universal mother, source of creation, and bestower of wealth and nurturance (food) (Zimmer 1946: 100). In characteristically effusive prose, Heinrich Zimmer de-scribes the eruption of life in Hinduism: "When the divine life sub-stance is about to put forth in the universe, the cosmos waters grow a thousand-petaled lotus of pure gold, radiant as the sun. This is the door or gate, the opening or mouth, of the womb of the universe" (1946: 90).[1] At the same time, the lotus is associated with female genitalia (Jayakar 1990: 129), and with female sexuality and female reproductive organs in art and iconography (Ferro-Luzzi 1980: 48). It can also be seen as a symbol of death and rebirth, and of anything of superior beauty (Ferro-Luzzi 1980: 48).[2]

A number of textual sources make the association of placenta
with lotus (and its associated properties) more explicit. The Vedas
refer to the navel as the seat of the life force. Later, the Puranas bring
together symbolism of the navel with that of the lotus in a manner
strongly evoking the placenta. The *Agni Purana* describes the birth of
Brahma as the emergence of the deity from a lotus springing from
Visnu's navel, with the navel representing the center of energy of
the universe, and the lotus "the material aspect of evolution" (Coomeraswamy 1993: 109). Likewise, in origin myths Puranic and Vedic,
living entities spring directly from the navel in which "The myth of
actual creation takes the form of the origination of a tree from the
navel of a Primal Person, who rests upon the waters and from whose
navel the tree rises up" (1993: 111).

However, as a thing of life and generation, the placenta has its
dangers. With little exception, rural women told me it is exceedingly
dangerous to cut the umbilical cord before the placenta has been
delivered. Many "trained dais" said their trainings were wrong to
insist the cord be cut "immediately"—the life force does not fully
enter the baby's body until both placenta and baby have been pushed
out of the womb, and the placenta itself can rise in the body if it is
untethered from the baby, strangling or smothering the *jaccha*. Others, perhaps offering information gleaned from trainings, said that
after the cord has been cut, the placenta, once beneficial, becomes
"poison." The mandate that the cord be cut after the placenta has
been delivered can also be explained by the use of the placenta as a
device for invigorating the baby. If the baby seems weak, fails to
breathe, or does not cry out, the cord may be milked toward the baby
(this is done in any case), and the placenta itself vigorously massaged.
The placenta might also be heated over a fire or placed in a pit, covered with dirt, and a pile of hot coals placed on top to make a kind
of oven: any kind of warming that may encourage the *jivan* to flow
to a struggling infant. (Most women said that once the cord was cut,
warming or massaging the placenta would no longer have an effect.
Several, however, said that these means could still be taken to bring
life to the baby after the cord was cut, pointing to a retained bond
between placenta and child.)

Like blood and other residue of childbirth, the placenta is spoken
of as "dirty" by those who handle it and by those who refuse to handle it, even as it is also referred to dismissively as "just trash." It is associated with the stuff of birth and menstruation, with other bodily
offal such as excrement, and like the baby and mother, is at once
defiled by birth and one of the elements that makes birth a "dirty"

process. But as with menstrual blood, the dirtiness of the placenta is ambiguous and its power both relates to and surpasses this dirtiness. While most body effluvia (with the exception of semen) is considered polluting in north Indian ontologies, as things that involve "life substance and process" (Orenstein 1968: 115), menstrual blood also has connotations of witchiness. The child who sees his menstruating mother is reminded of stories of the *dakin*, witch, who hides away, "abandon[ing] herself to her hostile desires, drinking the blood of some, eating the livers of others" (Carstairs 1958: 73, cited in O'Flaherty 1980: 279). Indeed, it is in the active powers of the witch and her dangerous and "hostile desires" that bodily fluids threaten. In post-Vedic texts, O'Flaherty questions the assumption that menstrual blood is always polluting, citing ethnographic writing on Australian Aboriginal menstrual practices to suggest that menstrual blood is less polluting than "taboo in the broadest sense," powerful, even dangerous, by reference to "woman's creative power" (1980: 40). In part, this is a matter of perspective. For the *jaccha*, post-partum blood may be bad because it threatens her well-being, not because it threatens the community at large—the idiom of "pollution" expresses something about danger (Chawla 1994).

But "pollution" and "dirtiness," like "trash" and "nothing special" can be thought of as enunciations as much as concepts: things people say for the effect they have, turning the gaze away from one thing or another, concealing what, in the light of day (or dark of night) can threaten, or protecting auspiciousness always under threat—the dangerous power of the physical stuff of generation, on the one hand, and the auspicious goodness of fertility on the other. But then again, sometimes dirt is just dirty, and to say as much demotes the potentially misogynist and casteist elements of ideas about the danger of female bodily substances. Here I approach the impasse of conversational foreclosure and implicit meanings. The women with whom I spoke most often gave the reverse of O'Flaherty's view, saying instead that menstrual blood is "just dirty, not dangerous," thereby evoking a common, everyday quality of defilement, and subverting a Western feminist tendency to transform passive connotations of "dirt" into active concepts of "danger" and "threat." Yet, even as women spoke about menstrual blood and placentas with a dismissive "they're just dirty," they were also able to describe outcomes of contact with these substances and necessary forms of management and redress, strategies for *minimizing* "danger," even as "danger" remains implicit. It is difficult to "read" and distinguish implicit and explicit meanings in this case without imposing a paradigm that

aims to transform seemingly misogynist symbols into more empow-
ering ones.

In the formulations of the women in Sitapur, the womb is both a
dirty pit and a space of life. Life begins at conception according to
some (this is the orthodox view), or at "quickening"—the first sign
of the baby's movement—according to others (that is, according to
most women in Lalpur). But while it contains life, the womb is not
a space of social engagement.[3] The *sor* is not unlike this. When I
asked women if any kind of *puja* (ritual offering) might be done to
help a baby in distress they often looked at me in puzzlement. "This
is what that thing [the placenta] is for," one said. A Dalit woman in
a village outside of Lucknow told me, "That is no place for a *devi*
[goddess]. Why would a *devi* want to come to such a dirty place?"
When I asked her what was dirty about it she said that menstrual
blood is among the dirtiest of substances. I asked if it was dirty or
dangerous, and she said, "Not dangerous. Just dirty." Other observers note that while a *puja* may be done in other parts of the house,
the birth room itself is not a place into which the gods will enter (cf.
Kakar 1981). The invigoration and vitalization of a baby takes place
through worldly means, and the birth room, due to its dirtiness and
association with untouchables, is no temple or household shrine in
the normal sense. Yet cord cutting retains an ambivalent air of the
"sacred"—but the kind of sacred of a place that is "no place for a
devi." Certain components of postpartum work—placing the baby in
the *sup* (winnowing basket) beneath a clean sari and alongside an
iron *hansiya* (sickle) in the doorway of the *sor* on the day the water
falls, casting coins into bathwater and rice into the *sor*, and, especially,
removal of coins and the placenta and other offal—all of these actions
locate postpartum labors at a conjunction of body work, trash work,
and ritual work. As tasks performed by "untouchables," such work
challenges divisions between sacred and profane that seem to characterize statements about the dirtiness of bodily stuff and the clean-
ness of temples. It suggests, if quietly, without the sparkle and rumpus
of the temple, that "no place for a *devi*" might involve specialized movements between states, categories, and realms that are nothing if not,
again quietly, sacred.

Janet Chawla (2002) describes the use of the term *narak* by birth
practitioners to refer to the space of the womb and the time of ges-
tation. *Narak* generally translates as "hell," and the womb, Chawla
observes, is referred to as *nau mahina narak kund* (the nine months'
hell container). Rather than hearing this term as synonymous with
pollution, Chawla understands it to be more complex, loaded with

implicit meanings. While directly referencing the space of filth and malevolent forces, *narak* also refers to the unseen spaces of both body and cosmos, signifying at once dirtiness and fertility (Chawla 2002). Indeed, the lotus itself is often spoken of as a flower that blooms in the dirtiest of places, rising from the muck of still waters and blooming untouched by whatever kinds of dirt inhabit them. Although the placenta may not be considered pure, it is a source of life inhabiting the *gandagi* (dirtiness) of the womb, speaking to the continuous interrelationship of death/decay and birth/growth, even as its ambiguities, like those of the womb, reference a particular vision of generativity. The fetus and the womb can themselves be thought of as ambiguous things and spaces. O'Flaherty notes that in post-Vedic texts, fetuses are "neither demons nor gods, neither dead nor alive; they drink a fluid that is neither blood nor milk [categorically opposed substances], and so their relationship to the mother is ambivalent" (1980: 42). According to Ayurveda, O'Flaherty says, because the fluid of the womb is a "mediating" substance between milk and blood, the pure and the polluting, "it is dangerous and demonic to eat it" (42), likewise for the things that inhabit it as liminal.

It is tempting, then, to turn to Mary Douglas (1975) to understand the symbolic power of the placenta as body part and, perhaps, as object in itself. For Douglas, especially potent entities, those that are objects of ritual attention, derive their force by being located between categories or at a point at which spheres overlap. As collective representations informing both religious and everyday life (1975: 21), the boundaries between categories are, according to Douglas, carefully maintained and policed through ritual activity intended to stem the contagion of one category for another, particularly the contagion of the sacred and profane. Drawing on the Durkheimian notion that the sacred can, in part, be defined by its contagious and susceptible nature, Douglas considers categories from the perspective of danger not unlike the protective ethos that drives caste-Hindu householders (mostly women) to police the boundaries of the household by policing the bodies of those who dwell within and enter from outside. For Douglas, however, the danger that out-of-place objects pose to the symbolic order involves the threat of boundaries blurred by insufficient ritual handling. Thus, any "relation with the sacred" can be seen as a "ritual of separation and demarcation, and ... reinforced with beliefs in the danger of crossing forbidden boundaries" (1975: 48). So, where Douglas gives us the possibility that the placenta can tell us about categories that map onto the body as well as onto groups (at the site of reproduction), at the same time, the fact that birth involves movement and change means that it is not just what the placenta *is* categorically, but how it moves, how it appears and disappears that enables the fraught object to suggest something about power and social life.

Home ground, or "A girl is flowing water"

Connotations of fertility, abundance, and generative forces give the sense that the "lotus" is a shared symbol with relative consistency between people, texts, and art forms. Symbols, while shared, can also be "multi-vocal, susceptible of many meanings" (Turner 1974: 55), "interchangeable" (Ferro-Luzzi 1980), or, to follow Clifford Geertz, can prompt hermeneutics rather than decoding, their meaning at once part of shared texts and enmeshed in historical context. They can, as Gananath Obeyesekere suggests, be at once "public" and "private," both culturally shared and personally significant (1981: 13). Or they may be seen to involve meanings shared only in the broadest sense, coming to life only when people "fill them with meanings drawn from and relevant to their own particular experiences" (Nabokov 2000: 11). Elements of the placenta's precut capacities take on such personal significance. As a lotus, it references a self when life has begun but is prior to worldly social engagement (outside of mother-infant and infant-God dyads).[4] However, as baby becomes child then adult, the placenta as remembered object denotes not only *a* location, but locatedness broadly speaking. In Hindi, to refer to a place as that "where my placenta is buried" (*jaha naal gara hai*) is to evoke kinship, the patriline, and home. This idiom was occasionally repeated to me (often with a chuckle) when I initiated conversations about placentas, though I never heard it used outside of that context, leading me to feel it has an air of old-fashioned folksiness. According to an encyclopedia of idioms, *jahan naal gara hai* or *naal gara hona* (the burial of the placenta/cord) refers to "a place one becomes part of, never to leave behind" (Sharma 1999: 195, my translation). Always a dislocated source, home is not where the heart is; it is where the placenta is.

There are many ways of disposing of the placenta. Burial under the floor of the home, burning in the *sor*. It may be thrown into a river for the purifying quality of running water and its capacity to carry objects away (cf. Eck 1987). It may be buried outside, or thrown into a pond for the invisibility offered by deep water. If buried, the placenta will most likely be put at the edge of fields, outside of the space of cultivation, in the same boundary spaces (*mer*) in which bodies of dead babies and children are buried. The buried placenta may be returned to for ritual purposes (such as at the child's first birthday, when the mother may perform a small *puja* at the site of its burial, as Amma described as having happened "in the old times"). Placentas are never thrown directly into wells or other still sources of drinking water, as to do so would be permanently contaminating. In Lalpur, placentas were not thrown into the large pond in the fields, about a kilometer from the village, from which the "pure" mud (*kurmani*) for cleaning newborns and constructing homes was collected. Rather, they were disposed of in one of several smaller ponds closer to the village, amid patches of brush and bramble, neither village nor field, marginal, unsocial spaces (in contrast with the larger, open pond) from which no drinking or cleaning water was ever drawn, in which no one swam or bathed, and from which no mud was gathered. Most commonly, postpartum workers told me they "just throw" the placenta, using a vague phrase rich in associations with trash and invisibility and suggestions of demoted power.

The invisibility of the discarded placenta is essential. After Pushpadevi told me stories about babies being "grabbed," pointing out women so unlucky as they walk by her house, I found myself, on return to my room, searching in Briggs' colonial monograph *The Chamars* for a particular moment in which the placenta appeared—briefly—in the colonial record: "The cord and placenta are buried in the house near the door to prevent their coming into the possession of an animal, or of an evil spirit, or of a magician; and over this spot in the house a fire is kept burning for six or more days. Some hide the cord in the house. The falling of the scab of the cord is watched with great care, and the particle is disposed of cautiously; most likely it is buried inside the house, lest it come into the possession of a *bhut* [ghost], of a woman or of a wizard" (1920: 64).

Of course, few people spoke with the detailed precision of colonial certainty and its ethnographic representations, except in a few cases—about the strange, ghostlike man who wears a suit and turns up suddenly in women's *angans* and bedrooms, massages their legs then suddenly disappears, the ghost on the road that Jawahar told me Bapu-ji once confronted. In reference to babies, a zone of malevolence invoked by repeated references and tendencies toward silence is deeply personalized, capable of collapsing and containing other powers and gazes—those of neighbors, the state, the downward pull of poverty on the already vulnerable and vulnerability on the already poor. In the way that ponds, burial, and burning are ideal means of disposal, or that "people who see it will think badly of the family," the "shame" of visible signs of reproduction, the body, and, perhaps, sexuality are also part of this matrix of threat. "If it should get pulled into the street by some animal, then everyone will know it is mine," one woman told me.

Lack of means, then, involves a range of heightened vulnerabilities. Though, as with so much else, placenta disposal depends, I was told frequently, on "household custom," as Shalini's mother's postpartum care demonstrates, ideals may be thwarted by poverty. Poverty prevents many from acquiring the dry, hot-burning wood necessary to burn flesh, or requires that available fuel—wood, dung cakes, leaves, scrub—be saved for cooking food. "Due to poverty" is as familiar a phrase in rural Sitapur as "it depends on household custom." In Tulsiram's home the morning after an elderly woman, a distant relation of Tulsiram, had died in her sleep in a nearby home, a neighbor came in and, after a bit of small talk, asked for a bit of money. "Any amount will help," she said. I asked someone what the money was for and the quick answer was, "Wood." Later, Sita, one of Tulsiram's sisters-in-law explained, "If the whole family gives a bit there will be enough for the wood." In the case of a corpse, such collections can be made, but the mention of the placenta carries the burden of embarrassment, and its proper disposal is not critical enough to warrant solicitations.

To return to the phrase "where my placenta is buried," there is a bivalency to this idiom that makes embodiments of location fundamentally gendered. On the one hand, this phrase denotes the place of one's birth and, as such, one's patriline (though first babies are often born in the mother's *maike, her* natal home—the place of the matriline, the idiom refers at once to the patrilineal home, the mother's *sasural,* and to an affective bond with the mother). On the other hand, it describes the resting place of the placenta itself, a place where a piece of one's body and life force resides. But the story is not the same for all. Boys' and girls' placentas are handled differently, and differences in their disposal indicate that while the placenta is home ground for both boys and girls, such locatedness has meanings dependent on the life course entitled by gender—and the emotional complexities thereof, for both mothers and children. Where women talked about, ideally, burying or burning of a son's placenta, either in the home or at the edge of fields, they most often said that girls' placentas are "just thrown" (though boys' placentas may also be said to be "just thrown").[5]

I was told of remembered rituals, things women had heard about or seen in their *maikes* or done once themselves involving the site in which the placenta was buried. Most addressed thwarted fertility or celebrate the birth. *Chatti pujas* are held on the place where the placenta is buried. A woman having difficulty conceiving, or conceiving a son, may bury the placenta of her long-awaited child under a tree just beyond her house, in the family compound, and return to the spot annually on the child's birthday to light a *diya* (butter lamp), and every year tie a knot in a string she keeps for this purpose along with seven *suhagin* (married, unwidowed—and thus auspicious—women). Such ritual moments are not performed for any deity, per se, one woman told me. Rather, they tap into the auspiciousness of successful fertility in order to "distribute *prasad.*" Again to Briggs (who discusses placentas more than any contemporary observer I can locate): when a boy's placenta is buried in the house, he notes, a *diya* or fire may be lit on that spot for several days after the birth (1920).

But women said that the placenta of a girl baby is never treated in this fashion. For many observers the immediate conclusion to be drawn is that this is a reflection of "cultural" or "traditional" undervaluing of girl children and on a continuum of behaviors ranging from placenta disposal to female infanticide. Many interlocutors beyond the realm of rural Sitapur made just such remarks. At one level this has some truth. The reverence given to a boy child's placenta marks a greater desirability, and thus his vulnerability to those with malicious intents, spirit or human. But how is desire structured, and what does it feel like? Unpacking the desirability of male children exposes socioeconomic, ritual, and kinship factors delinked from parental affect (Kakar 1981). Gender differences in placenta disposal are situated in a context in which birth workers may be paid more lavishly at births of boys than girls, in which rifles are fired into the air to announce births of sons, and men and women say things such as "may god bless you with a son" to pregnant women (though often these wishes are met with a reproachful look or comments like, "*Are,* we don't say these things anymore," or "Oh ho, all children are gifts from God"). Such differences are noted extensively in journalistic accounts of rural life, "dais," and so forth. Yet, personal meanings might also suggest that while the different handling of boys' and girls' placentas is part of a continuum of gender discrimination, it also points to the structuring of affect, home, and homesickness in ways that are more about movement than "value."

Normatively, a boy is expected to remain in his natal home for all his days, though the courtyard may be subdivided and new, redivided spaces made out of old walls, or concrete foundations poured onto dirt ones. If he should live elsewhere, his natal home is still "his." His placenta (ideally) grounds him there, staking within its bounds a piece of his body, the matrix linking him to his mother, residue of his life force—and also of his mother's desire for him. Where the locatedness and groundedness of a boy's placenta predicts his future claims to home and place, the disposal of girls' placentas into ambiguous, transitory spaces beyond village boundaries or into spaces of process (sites of decay) and flow (such as rivers) predict her lifetime of to and fro, of movements away from and back to her natal home. Upon marriage (or, more accurately, at her *bidai,* her first ritual departure from the *maike*) a girl/woman's life is one of motion and dual locatedness. In worlds where men often leave for cities for jobs as laborers, a bride can fill a house in a way that is a comfort to a mother whose son is far away. When Dev took me to fetch his sister, Niti, in her new *sasural,* a few days after a *bidai* had sent her off because "the boy's family was calling for her," he told me, when I asked what the boy was like, that the new husband wasn't actually at home these days. "He has a job in Bombay, stitching bags in some kind of workshop." In Niti's future home, after pleasantries, exchanges of *puris,* and snacks and tea, we got ready to go. Niti's *sas* began to weep, "Don't go, my girl," she said petting Niti's face. "She is very lonely," someone explained, "Her house is empty. It will be good when she [pointing to Niti] can stay for a longer time."

The common epithets that "a girl is someone else's child," or that she is a "guest" in her father's house, born to be given in marriage (literally, in *kanya-dan,* the gift of a virgin) to another household are often taken as indicators of girls' low status. Hindu and Muslim religious texts describe (and prescribe) son preference in a way which can leave little room for ambiguity (Kakar 1981: 58). Texts like the Laws of Manu state with little nuance that girls are burdens to their families, bringing responsibility, inauspiciousness, impurity (at menstruation) and the looming threat of sexuality to the household. But the ambiguity of such statements in everyday speech—and the sadness they may conatin and imply—has also been noted (Das 1979: 93). Sudhir Kakar notes, in the most general terms, the "lenient affection and often compassionate attention" which Indian mothers give daughters, suggesting that "in the earliest period of emotional development [infancy] Indian girls are assured of their worth by whom it really matters" (1981: 60). Indeed, Kakar suggests, Indian mothers may be more emotionally bound to their daughters *because of* son preference and feelings of longing for their own mothers (1981: 90). Putting aside textual sources, statements like "a girl is born for

another house" (especially in the way they are often referred *to* in
everyday speech rather than said directly) may signify less the burden of daughters than the sadness the family will endure at her de-
parture(s). For Pushpadevi, this meant that, "A girl is flowing water.
My daughters will leave this house. They'll go to another family. My
son ... someone will come here [to marry] him. But a girl has to listen to the people of her *sasural*. If her brother wants to call her here
[from her *sasural*], then she will come, if he doesn't [call], she won't
[come]. This will bring me great sadness. But, if you want to know
the truth, I care for my daughters more."

The flowing water of a girl's life, echoed in the way her placenta,
as a fragment of her self, is "just thrown," means that movement and
departure is a constant theme in rural women's lives. In the north
Indian context of village outmarriage, women move first from natal
homes and to marital homes, often to return yearly (sometimes more,
sometimes less) to their natal homes as the *sasural* become more
"theirs." In talk the breach may be instant "a girl is born for another
household," and in the *bidai* the language and the outpouring of
grief suggest absolutes. But in practice, the transition is often gradual, spanning years of goodbyes, tears which may be shed even when
a woman is old and returns as a *bua* (father's sister) rather than a
bitiya ("little daughter"), and in which tears may be shed in both
households on both sides of the divide.

Where a girl is flowing water, a boy is a house—not unchanging
over time, but bound to the same location.[6] The permanent location
of a piece of the placenta in the foundation of the home space un-
derlines a boy's claim to that space, making it a claim about bodies
and *jivan*, memory and origins, as much as about floors and walls.
As a girl can stake no such claim, were the stuff of her bodily beginnings there it would complicate that *lack* of claim, perhaps making
her eventual departure all but unbearable (where feminist activism
has promoted a girl's right—especially if she is unmarried—to legally
inherit the property of her parents, this legality has been difficult to
institute and enforce). Even at infancy her "home ground" is difficult
to locate. As Kakar puts it, "[A girl's] 'real' family is her husband's
family. Whatever her future fortunes, when she marries an Indian girl
knows that, in a psychological sense, she can never go home again"
(1981: 73).

In Sitapur, the question of the "real" family is seldom settled for
women, and the fundamental split and its affective impact make
home—and thus, homesickness—an unstable category yet regular
experience. Women, Veena Das says, are "Janus-faced creatures" in

their husband's home, "belonging to the husband's group, and yet being strangers to it" (1979: 94), in much the same way that they have a dual identity in their mother's home—constantly reminded that one day they will have to leave. As such, the intersection of reproduction, sexuality, and space is located beyond the *maike* for women. Both her sexuality and reproductive potential are located "elsewhere" from the place of birth. Meanings of reproduction may be likewise split—as much about future births (in one place) as about a girl's own origins (in another). A girl will make sons and daughters for another household; a boy will eventually make them for the one in which he was born.

Thus, in referencing kinship patterns and outmarriage, placentas and their disposal may convey the gendered complexities of affective claims on "home" and the meaning of "home" as a reproductive space more than being reflections of "son preference." While partaking of shared symbols of an impersonal nature when considered as part of bodily ontologies, the placenta takes on personal significance when seen from the perspective of the infant. Mary Douglas recommends that the "danger" of categorical anomalies not be taken to indicate a "terror" of them, any more than such "anxiety ... inspires the housewife's daily tidying up" (1975: 58). While the placenta may evoke a mix of fear, reverence, and disgust, strong emotions lie less in its dangerous aspects than in its association with home, whatever that may mean. As a "personal symbol" it may not stand alone (I don't recall anyone speaking fondly of their placentas outside of the use of the above idiom), but as part of a web of associations linking body, mother, and home/homesickness, it may be part of some of the most personal and emotionally powerful sets of symbols there are.

The cut

Initially, I am taken aback by the fact that the timing of the Chamarins' postpartum labors, the time "before the water falls," coincides with a phase in which the newborn is fed water or sugar water (or goat's milk in families with such wealth) dripped off the end of a wad of cotton rather than put to its mother's breast. Bari Bhabhi and I talk about this, and she tells me that she fed her babies right away—her father-in-law, who was educated in medical things, she says, insisted that her babies be breast-fed immediately. "Most women around here," she says, "don't do that, though." When, back in Lucknow for a visit, I share this with a friend who has invited me to dinner with a scholar visiting from Delhi, the scholar reacts angrily: "You can't

*say that. It's not true." I am taken aback. I try to defend myself with my ac-
ademic politics and the street cred they might give. I refer to postcolonial theory, to a reticence to make broad claims about "rural women," and to a need
to account for certain things in spite of the discomfort they may cause. My
friend comes to my defense, "India is diverse," he says, "This might not be
true elsewhere, but she has seen this here." The scholar is insistent and angry: "It doesn't matter," she says, "You can't come here and say these things
about Indian women."*

*Falling so easily into uncomfortable (for some) and all too comfortable
(for others) narratives eager to acknowledge rationality or its lacks, knowledge or its absence, in "rural women" or "Indian women" or "Third World
women" or "women" of one kind or another, the timing of breast-feeding,
and the way it maps onto the caste-based delineation of postpartum care, are
at once deeply problematic and too easily reduced to a building block of "custom" and "behavior." Pushpadevi puts the patter of "rationality" and "knowledge" to rest when we talk about the* purein. *After not long in Lalpur, I find
myself spending many afternoons watching the comings and goings between
the Pasi* mohalla *and the fields. Her veranda has an expansive view, in
spite of the low status such exposure might denote. When I mention that
Ayurvedic texts say the placenta brings food to the baby from the mother, she
disagrees.*

*"What food could the mother give it? All that food it gets, all that food
that comes through the purein, that comes from God. The new baby, just like
the baby in the womb—it has no caste."*

*Up to this point, so many of my movements from the Bhabhis' home have
been monitored for what they may mean about what is entering my body—
in other words, the Bhabhis, out of a dire need to protect family and household from foreign and threatening essences, are worried about what I eat. I
make a few mistakes early on that cinch it for me—I mention that Tulsiram
has given me some cooked meat; I accept a frivolous invitation to a meal at
Naseem's house in the presence of Rani, the Bhabhis' young niece. Choti
Bhabhi lectures me again and again. She comes to my room in the evening
when we can talk alone to reiterate what it means for me to eat food prepared by* "niche log" *(lower people)—the way that the defilement of labors
related to shit and death and placentas and trash, the stain of the sins of
killing, meat consumption and, bringing my academic endeavors into my
own corporeality,* naal-*cutting adhere to the bowls, pots, and utensils of such
people. By eating food they cook, by drinking from their well I become "like
them" and transmit that pollutedness into her household. I knew before
this, from the writings of anthropologists like McKim Marriott that food consumption determines status, indeed, "caste," but from Choti Bhabhi I learn
that this is a distinctive feature of* dehat. *"There is a lot of discrimination*

here," she says matter-of-factly. When I mumble something about equality and the oft-repeated ameliorating (and pat) phrase "everyone is the same," she says, "This may be so in your place, or in cities, but this is not the case here"—hinting toward a language of respect and "diversity," she asserts that "discrimination," knowing and preserving difference, is a "local custom," a parampara *I should observe.*

Amma tells me one afternoon, with poetry and logic, "Everything has its category. Look at the clothes hanging on the line, this one is red, and that one is like that. Or the dal. There is moong *and* urad *and names you wouldn't recognize. Or flour: rice flour, wheat flour, dal flour, flour from lotuses that grow in the pond—the flour used during fasts when we can't take grains. All are flour, and each is different. Men are like this, too, all among our own jati. Don't force together things that will stay separate."*

At the same time, women's enforcement of eating restrictions and maintenance of the categories of the world are, for Choti Bhabhi at least, part of middle-class longing, part of a vision of life in which appropriate differences are maintained, things are "kept clean," appearances are upheld. Yet some bedbhav, *she tells me, is not necessary in the cities where, she says, "everyone prepares their food in a hygienic way." Causalities are, for me, difficult to distinguish, but the message is clear enough.*

In some ways of mapping things, in some cosmologies, new life, the placenta that nurtures it, and a morality of protection speak to a frame in which it is possible to imagine what the unlocated self might involve. When Pushpadevi sets me straight on the role of the placenta—a view I do not always find echoed among other women, especially the Bhabhis who say that food comes via the mother—I find myself retranslating notions of flow into my own biological maps. According to Pushpadevi, where consumption is the source of jati *(and moral status and class status—this conversation must wait for Chapter 7), the days immediately after birth but before breast-feeding, the time "before the water falls," the time of heightened vulnerability and pollution, may also be a time of castelessness. So too the time of the womb, when food comes not via another body or hands, but directly from God. The placenta, mediating this flow, is the thing of dislocated,* unjati'd *life. For Pushpadevi, whose own mother does postpartum work in Pushpadevi's* maike, *the placenta and an understanding of its functioning involves an implicit theory of caste as consumption (rather than by birth); likewise, it involves a set of overlapping vulnerabilities and possibilities from which moral frames like* karma *are, if not absent, then pushed to the background.*

What, then, does "the cut" sever?

While before or after the cut the placenta is thought of as "dirty," the cut changes something about its ontological status. Before it, Bari

Bhabhi, or Shalini, or Pushpadevi, or Amma, or the Pandit woman down the road might handle it without threatening self, *jati*, or kin. Afterwards, they do so under threat of denial of food by one's caste-fellows—*hookah-pani bandh*—which means that they do not handle it. From a certain perspective, this involves ritual containment of a categorically compromising object. Questioning the degree to which ambiguity can be "tolerated" by any society (Douglas 1975: 52), Mary Douglas suggests that "dirt"—famously, "matter out of place" (1975: 59)—represents the edges or outside of boundaries, its very presence implying a system, "cherished classifications," organizing its definition and handling (1975: 51). In a later essay Douglas rethinks the notions of conformity and deviance underlying her arguments. The power of such "codes" lies instead, she says, in people's reverence for them (1975: 63). However, as "reverence" is discordant with Dalit identity and relegated/owned work, a more complex situation obtains with those who are at once bound to certain rules and structures (by coercion, poverty, and symbolic hierarchies) but critique and manipulate them in ways that do not overturn the system but allow them to work within it. While the power of the placenta may be more complex for them than for others, we might also ask whether the liminal status and strict management of the postcut placenta (as a mental and physical cordoning-off) are also part of keeping certain persons at "the bottom," referencing a system in which, for some, "belief" has little purchase. It is just as important, then, to consider the *movements* involved in birth and its healing processes as the structures and maps it involves, to observe the ways objects—and ideas about them, languages to speak of them, emotions that attach to them—move and are moved across imagined realms and landscapes. This has everything to do with modes of subjectivity: elements of "disgust," "danger," "pollution," and "just trash" that make up a contemporary set of overlapping meanings, formative of both caste and its contestations.

As I outlined in the previous chapter, castes associated with postpartum work are considered untouchable as a factor of work associated with bodies, bodily effluvia, meat work/butchery, death, and trash. I also mentioned that the social relegation of these tasks involves two frames of pollution, one determined by contact, the other considering certain tasks polluting according to principles of nonviolence. In a grammar of pollution categories outlined in the Dharmashastras, pollution is categorized according to the kinds of encounters that produce it (Orenstein 1968). A division between relational pollution (when a birth or death occurs in one's kin group) and act pollution

("brought about by some form of contact with biological phenom-
ena") relates to a contrast in rules for management and redress (Orenstein 1968: 114). Act pollution is subdivided into internal pollution,
the result of actions performed, and external pollution, the result of
contact (Orenstein 1968: 114). Cord cutting, never described to me
as explicitly sinful, can still be thought of as akin to butchery and
association with the placenta much like association with bodies of
the dead.[7] Without using the term "sin," women told me that it sev-
ers the flow of life force between the placenta and baby. Thus, while
baby delivering may involve external pollution, cord cutting, by its
affinity with killing, transforms the actor internally.

But postpartum work involves not only bodily "operations" but
trash work that is at once material and a matter of essences. Coins
of payment passed around the baby's head and cast into its dirty bathwater are objects of desire that absorb covetous gazes and inauspiciousness. When Rakesh's Mother leaves she takes the coins and their
ill forces with her. Likewise, trash work involves managing risk—
locating the newly transformed object so as to mitigate its potential
threat. At the same time, as the agent of cord cutting, she (and by
extension her kin and *jati*) absorbs and contains the taint of severing life.

In the way it is "trash work" more than "birth work," Rakesh's
Mother's labors contain, in their fleshy corporeality as well as their
cosmological import, the whiff of sacrifice. The term "to cut" (*katna*),
used to refer to the cutting of the umbilical cord, is a common euphe-
mism for sacrifice in Sitapur and elsewhere (Clark-Decès, personal
communication; Fuller 1992: 84). Jonathan Parry notes a parallel in
the work of the cremation specialist and the work of the "midwife,"
such that cremation, he says, could be considered "a branch of obstetrics" (1994: 179). But it seems to me that it is in cord cutting and
placenta management, rather than the birth of the baby, that the
parallel is most vivid. Similar to the "sacrificial violence" of the separation of the soul from the corpse (1994: 178), cord cutting produces
a corporeal object at once polluted and a thing "of great sacredness"
(1994: 180).

The visceral feelings—fear, disgust, disinterest—associated with
the cut placenta may tell us something about what kind of sacrifice
this may be. Perilously at the boundary between sacred and profane
(in a world in which tantric possibilities play on—or blur—the distinction), the placenta becomes a site of excess when severed, a remnant whose effects spill into the realm of the living. As part of the
khuna-kachra of birth, the "blood-trash," as Schoolteacher's Mother

put it, the cut placenta relates to other bodily excess. (It is here that elements of disgust become most apparent as they slide across etiologies of harm and risk, from those in which the placenta must never be severed before it is delivered, to those in which the mere image of an attached placenta bolsters and provides emotional weight to the urgencies of intervention.) To think about "blood-trash" and the forms of power it is capable of containing, I turn to the writings of George Bataille, who twists and flips Marxian frameworks to illuminate elements of disgust, desire, and the marginal in social economies. Thinking about societies and histories in terms of flows of energy, Bataille distinguishes between things with utility, and those which remain as results of "production" but are not "reducible" to their "utility"—things of surplus (1991: 69). There is, he says, "within us, running through the space we inhabit, a movement of energy that we use, but that is not reducible to its utility (which we are impelled by reason to seek)" (69). This energy beyond necessity is the eponymous "accursed share"; the use a society makes of it is "determin[ing]," "the cause of ... the structural changes and of the entire history of society" (1991: 106).

In Sitapur, things almost—but not quite—beyond utility haunt the edges of immanent, social life: ghosts, trash, objects that never altogether disappear, but occupy the edges of consciousness; like the polyethylene bags that get snared in tree branches and flutter as part of the landscape, hardly recognized, but present nonetheless. Utility in this part of the landscape is often transgressive or malevolent, things take on new use *as* trash. The danger of the cut and discarded placenta is that it is *not* beyond utility. The residue of bond between person and placenta offers access to the soul. The overwhelming power of longing for a child characterizes figures imagined as most threatening: infertile women, witches, the *churel*—the ghost of a woman dead in childbirth, whose hands and feet are turned backwards and who roams the margins of villages waiting to "grab" women on their way to the fields to defecate. The *jaccha* is especially susceptible, being weakened, "cool," and "open" from the process of delivery, to ghosts who enter bodies from below and through open channels.

Bhuts of all kinds, but especially *churels*, involve energized desire—the result of "bad deaths," situations in which "the deceased has revealed no intention of sacrificing his body ... or of renouncing his desires" (Parry 1994: 163). Consumed by desire, they are pushed to consume the placenta, itself a place of leftover longing, receptacle of desire fulfilled, by eating or bewitching it, to "grab" the child, sap its life force. Briggs noted that in Awadh magical use of the placenta/cord taps the reproductive potential of the *mother,* her "gift of fertility," (1920: 60), having effect on the child: "If a woman eat [a piece of the cord], the child will die, but she will obtain children. If a wizard or a witch get possession of it, the child will be said to be ruled by their spells. If an evil spirit get it, the child will be possessed" (64).

Here, we must locate ourselves at the margins of presence: with the pre- and postlife self versus its earthly, conscious remainder, with the self before language takes hold, prior (and post) to personal history, prior (and post) to location, with something that "though constituted in the presence of reality, does not belong in any way to this reality, which it transcends" (Bataille 1985: 131). Things cast off— and the ways they are cast off—pertain to the self even in the way they depart from the realm of signification (or utility). Like excrement, the placenta may be "a figure of the body's materiality, of the asymbolic residue that cannot be put dialectically to work" (Pandolfo 1997: 100). There is no discourse that can contain it. Like excrement it points to death (but unlike excrement, to creation as well), to the point of ends and origins at which "[the body] becomes a non-body" (100). And vice versa. For Bataille (1985), excrement is like an unconscious "jewel," "cursed matter that flows from a wound," "part of oneself destined for open sacrifice." Sacrifice, for Bataille, is "the production of sacred things" and "constituted by an operation of loss" (1985: 119).

Likewise, in its resonances with the writings of Jacques Lacan and the near-cosmological (at times near-Hindu) zones Lacan maps into/onto the psyche (idioms of loss and lack, the real and the imaginary), the cut placenta is an arrow to that beyond the symbolic register. As an ungraspable, unbearable fragment of the real, the placenta may be that which the world of locations and (id)entities cannot contain and yet that which is necessary for such a world to exist. "That is clearly the essence of law," Lacan says, "to divide up, distribute, or reattribute everything that counts as *jouissance*." Yet, if *jouissance* is what serves no (earthly) purpose (Lacan 1998: 3), then by reading ourselves further into the shadows, we can imagine that perhaps the danger of the placenta lies in the (frightening) possibility that it is, perhaps, *not* "leftover": "What lies under the [monk's] habit, what we call the body, is perhaps but the remainder.... What holds the image together is the remainder" (6).

In Sitapur, as elsewhere, babies do not enter the social world in a single radical event but progress gradually into it. Because of the eternal movement of selves through death and rebirth, there is no single moment of becoming. The gradual unworlding of the placenta means the worlding of the baby. Like corpses that must be carefully disentangled from relations with the living, the cut and disposal of the placenta involves "movement away from the original ineffable wholeness of Brahman" (Parry 1994: 167). Cremation, performed correctly, separates the body of the deceased from its soul. For the bereaved, this process is a gradual depersonalizing of the departed, a process of erasing their individual life history (Nabokov 2000). Echoing the departure of the dead, the movement of the placenta from utility and embodiment to post- (or transgressive) utility and disembodiment happens at the same time as the transitions made by mother and infant from pollution and segregation to full social engagement. As the placenta enters the realm of death, gradually fading like the swooshes and swells of womb life, the baby becomes viable.

The placenta moves between "incorporation and marginality," a binary formative of caste-related idioms of pollution (Das 1976: 252, in Parry 1994: 215). In the disincorporation of cut and disposal, the placenta is moved toward marginality and the baby away from it (even as the shadow of marginality remains upon the baby). While both newly born and newly dead may be marginal to "ordered categories" (Parry 1994: 225), the placenta, even more than the newborn, becomes a ritual object that bears marginality's ultimate weight. "Sacrifice is the pre-eminently creative act," Parry says, but "produces only ... a flawed creation" (1994: 190). Hindu sacrifice, strictly speaking, merges victim with god, making the sacrificed object mediator between human and god and substitute for the human (Fuller 1992: 84). The sacrificial nature of the cut may lie in the way it is—like the ritualized status of Brahmans—a second birth, or, perhaps, the continuation of a process only begun at birth. This is its sacrificial nature: to come into earthly existence in the "closed circuit" of the "Hindu universe," something must be lost (Shulman 1980: 90). According to Western metaphors, that something is identification with the mother, and that loss's abruptness conveyed with the idiom "cutting the cord." Lacan suggests the loss may be located elsewhere, "the mother" part of a larger set of infantile experiences. In northern India, I suggest, the immense power of the placenta describes that something as a multiple set of identifications: identification with the elemental *atma* embodied in both the feminine generative capacity and in the notion of asocial existence, and identification with the self of the womb—the presymbolic, marginal self that is also the self at death, a self of the shadows, but also a self whole and unsevered.

To enter the social realm the baby must be released from part of itself; the "something" that is lost may be absolute self-incorporation.

Bataille says that the self is the site of a cut, a "laceration" at the
"boundary of death, which constitutes the very nature of the im-
mensely free *me*, transcending 'that which exists,' [and] is revealed
with violence." (1985: 132). The hushed tones, averted eyes, and
barely perceptible sense of shame of those who do postpartum work
point to the cutting of the umbilical cord as a momentary and permanent violence in which the act of bringing into life entails a small
act of death, the death of the placenta and the severing of the bond
between the earthly baby and the not-quite-earthly lotus. To think
about this laceration in terms of categories is to risk assuming the
binary opposition of life and death, jettisoning the idea that in Hindu
frameworks, "life [is] not opposed to death as the positive is to the
negative, but life emerges out of death" (Apffel-Marglin and Mishra
1991: 209). Placentas are not so much "between" categories as they
require we recognize their simultaneity, turn our attention instead
to that space of the threshold between here and there, visible and
invisible, rather than birth and death. As simultaneously things of
preworld and afterworld, womb and trash heap, growth and decay,
placentas are, if marginal to the world, part of a landscape of the self.

We are brought back around to the form of the sacred specific to
the work relegated to and constitutive of "untouchability." It might
be a stretch to say that cord cutting is sacrifice in Hindu terms (its
products are life/baby and excess/placenta rather than identification
with a deity, and its *prasad* a vague sense of auspiciousness). However,
as a sacred act, cord cutting creates "trash," constituting both a loss
and a beginning. It entails a brand of the sacred that encompasses the
sinful in a way that posits alternate visions to Brahmanical modes
in which the pure and the polluted are separate (Apffel-Marglin
1991). Chawla suggests that this sacredness engages the realm of
narak, the dark, internal, female space in which death and life are
necessary elements of each other (2002).

It is therefore insufficient to say that Rakesh's Mother handles
the placenta because it is dirty and she is "untouchable." Rather, her
untouchable status puts her in a position not only to manage bodily offal, but to mediate passages over a set of thresholds. In the cut,
she enacts the transition of the placenta from embodied, useful object (indeed, part of the baby) to a thing in itself, unconnected, excessive, overflow, decay. What was life-giving becomes life-taking,
what was familiar foreign (while remaining in memory precious and
potent). Rather than being "matter out of place" or a static thing on

a map ("where there is dirt there is system") (Douglas 1975: 59), certain kinds of excess *get made* in a process which is not accidental but carefully managed and mediated. While placentas are dirty products of birth, to become "dangerous" they must be converted and actively transported across the threshold from this-world immanence to that of decay and regeneration.[8] And yet this transition is necessary. Postpartum workers don't just manage "trash," they make it, at the same time that they enable life.

As part of work involving a brand of the sacred encompassing the sinful, leftover, and dirty, the placenta is also a theory of "caste," its management threading possible subjectivities to one another. This may be so even as the relegation of postpartum work suggests an ontological field in which, as I discussed earlier, some causalities are challenged even as they are put to use. Oddly, the Chamarin's work may also be the work of caste, and the work of caste may be, troublingly, a bit like the work of healing, reconstituting the self in the image of social order (Kapferer 1979). Through the bodies and cosmological domains it maps and references, the placenta establishes not just distinctions between people, but the very ways *by which* the subject is located: in relation to work, in relation to substance, in relation to cause and effect, and in relation to other people and other bodies. Its movements from immanence to marginality map onto another threshold—that between the located and unlocated self, or, in certain Dalit frames of reference, between casteless and casted identity. If, for some at least, the newborn is truly without *jati*, if the placenta is the thing of castelessness in a *jati'd* world, do those who wield the *hasiya* or *bilade* also do the work of *jati?* Do they sacrifice castelessness to enable caste to be?

Interventions

Before I move to Lalpur, I spend a few months in Lucknow, hanging out with people from different organizations engaging, in one way or another, or planning to engage in dai trainings: Mahila Seva Sansthan, groups associated with the newly formed state project NAFPA, groups associated with other umbrella organizations. On the one hand, on the not-so-subtle maps of authority, my research happens when I chat with "village women," a problematic, but persistently relevant category of intervention. On the other hand, I am well aware of the performative quality of such encounters. I don't need to revisit field notes to know I have learned less from questions asked and (partially) answered in these awkward interviews than from the sensory and affective qualities of the meetings themselves—and from conver-sations in the vans on the way "out" and "back," and in the way the social contexts of intervention and "social science" mesh so comfortably to create distinct and recognizable and repeated affective experiences, the things that say who I am and that establish the "theys" in question, the things that can be revisited to give intervention its own sensory impetus.

In villages that aren't yet supplying trainees, the health workers and I ask around for "Who does the baby work?" We find women to talk to, some reluctant and suspicious, some interested in chatting. I ask questions; often what I am supposed to ask—or the way I am supposed to be asking—feels guided by the insidious and internal power of the scripts of expectation held not only by the NGO workers (many with some kind of social work train-ing) but by the larger apparatus of intervention in which we are situated— the particular vision of social research it allows.

I ride on the back of Mr. Mehra's motorcycle to a village a few kilometers out of Lucknow. Mr. Mehra is one of the "painters of signs;" I have been re-ferred to him by a mutual acquaintance. He runs an NGO involved in a scattered set of "rural uplift" programs—mostly horticultural and income-generation schemes aimed at rural women, and education and empower-ment-oriented workshops. He began a school for girls in one village and has begun mint-growing collectives in others. His organization is affiliated with other, larger ones in a network of umbrella groups, acronyms, and flows of money I have difficulty keeping straight. But he patiently explains the par-ticularities to me, as well as the complex legalities by which groups are in-corporated and establish legitimacy. He has been thinking about expanding into women's health programs, and especially into dai trainings.

We stop in a small bazaar, buy a few onions, and ask around for who does the "baby work," the "dai-vai ka kam"—the something-like-dai-ish work. We are directed, as we often are, to a home at the edge of the village. It is pakka—*solid, cement block—and large. Some children run inside and an old man comes out. Mr. Mehra explains who we are with the delicacy and appropriate reticence I am at this point only beginning to learn—a social grace necessary in talking about tasks associated with the female body and reproduction/sexuality—those that refer always but implicitly to "untouch-ability." A woman comes out, and a small group forms on the veranda. Be-cause of the small crowd, our conversation stays with topics institutional. She does not say, specifically, which "work" she does, and before I can find the appropriate wording to ask in front of so many family members, she tells me about her government training—how it took several months, the details of how she got to the health center, about the "delivery kit" she received. "I can show it to you." She ducks into the house and comes back with a wood box. She pulls out of it a sheet wrapped in plastic, a shiny new stethoscope (such prizes the government once gave!), her certificate, and a fancy watch. Mr. Mehra comments on the watch, and a young man behind him laughs and says it is his—he put it in the box for safe-keeping. Everything is untouched. "Have you used these things?" I ask, and she shakes her head. "I am not called," she says. Mr. Mehra exclaims that this is an enormous tragedy, such a waste of the government's efforts and money. He looks at the certificate and then shows it to me. The date for the training, which we had both, I later learned, assumed had happened a year or two before, was 1968.*

Later that day, we are directed to another house on the edge of another village. In this home, Mr. Mehra does most of the talking. We sit on a veranda with a very old woman and an old man I assume is her husband. There aren't so many people around this time, and the man is working on fixing a small piece of machinery. The woman is cautious. She sits on the brick veranda. Behind her, hanging from the roof, is a wire cage with a parrot. It shakes its wings occasionally, but is mostly still. The sun is heavy, I am relieved to be in the shade. No one offers us water, or sherbet, or tea—something I come to expect in homes such as this—where such an offer might be taken as an affront or might force an awkward refusal that makes "caste" obvious. The woman and I talk. Mr. Mehra translates; for the most part it is not necessary, though some of the Awadhi terms are still unfamiliar to me. We talk in the safe language of generalities. When "the cord is cut," "what is done to help get the baby out ... help alleviate pain ... help the healing ... help a struggling baby." With the topic of cord cutting comes quieter voices and euphemistic (or more euphemistic) language. I use a term for the placenta from another dialect, but she knows what I am talking about and says, "purein." Mr. Mehra keeps translating, but what he says makes no sense. Finally he stops and says, "What is this 'purein-anwal' you are talking about? What is this thing you keep referring to?"

A young man comes by and sits on the platform with the old man. He is dressed as though he has just returned from the city or the bazaar. "The placenta," I say to Mr. Mehra. "We are talking about the placenta and when it is supposed to come out."

"What 'placenta'? What does that mean?" Mr. Mehra says, and I try to explain—not very well or very clearly. He laughs, "You mean there is something else in there with the baby? I had no idea! I have two sons, and I never knew this!"

The men laugh. I write the word, and draw a diagram in my notebook. When it doesn't explain the anatomy well enough, Mr. Mehra says, "But the Ayurvedic shastras say that the cord is connected to the mother's navel on the inside, no?" He explains about his understanding of Ayurvedic concepts of flows of energy and nutritive substances through this channel, and about the critical importance of the navel and its associated chakra.

The younger man laughs, and the older one shakes his head. He says he has seen lots of calvings and explains about the afterbirth, while the younger man says, "In my biology textbook the placenta is described as a matrix [he says matrix in English] that is an interface [in English] between the mother and the baby. The cord goes from the baby's navel to this matrix." He meshes his hands together.

As we explain the anatomy, map bodies and body parts, and assign competing languages and images to bring the disappeared placenta into the gaze of understanding, the woman mumbles something about getting back to work, about making food, and pushes herself up with her hands on her knees. She walks into the cool shadows of the house. That conversation is over.

While placentas' appearances and disappearances in rural Sitapur are the stuff of careful management, their entries and exits are equally important to the apparatus of intervention. Their management is monitored by representatives of institutions, persons who, generally speaking, imagine themselves to operate in the service of rationalization and disenchantment, whose knowledge is established through performance and instruction (Bhabha 1994) as against the localities of "the village." If "operation" (Cohen 2005) is part of the way contemporary subjectivities establish citizenship through the way the scalpel establishes "availability," another series of cuts—this time both universal and necessary—indicate that bodily interventions that bespeak the body withheld, the body unoffered, are integral to the form of citizenship that is "intervention" in the keys of "progress" and "knowledge." Such bodily cuts may map onto semiotic operations equally essential to the moral claims of certain political visions. Like the cut of circumcision, the cut of the cord and the image of its remainder (the placenta, like the foreskin) provide a means of establishing differences between us and them (Boon 1999, Mehta 2000). As talk about circumcision can be characterized by "an unsettled tonality marked by either reticence or overkill" (Boon 1999: 67), diacritical talk about placentas shares this tendency toward scandal. In sensorial and emotional performances of "progress," placentas map moral and epistemological stances onto people in the world. They are both point of entry and a means of establishing moral breaches between the educated and the uneducated, the urban and the rural, the enfranchised and the subaltern. And yet, in the placenta's tendency to disappear, there is an irony to the disenchanting work of intervention.

Alongside "cleanliness," cord cutting and placenta management are central elements of dai training, from casual encounters to the mandates of policy. Clean hands, clean string to tie the cord off, and clean blades for cutting are among the "Five Laws of Cleanliness" that are a staple of training. The timing of the cut—and by extension, the management of the placenta—is also important. It is taught, as I have noted, that cords must be cut immediately—before the placenta is delivered. In Mahila Seva Sansthan, this was described to me as an effort to confront the division of labor; the aim was to either "get dais to cut cords" or to "get dais to attend deliveries," in other words, to merge separate domains of work. More broadly, while such a division is becoming acknowledged, at least in conversations in NGO offices and in a handful of formal documents, the specificity of postpartum labor does not enter open discourse (beyond "dais not cutting cords" or "not doing deliveries"). As "local custom," "not cutting cords" remains part of the idiom of wrongness. It is often understood to be evidence of the persistence of "pollution belief," the persistence of caste in a world that should have no place for it. Epitomizing such a system of "belief," the attached placenta is a core image.[9] As a frightening sign and rhetorical device, the uncanny chill it evokes creates an impetus for action. As part of a moral frame, it references a particular vision of caste on the one side, and association of hygiene and health with equality on the other. Within this framing, modes of citizenship and equality are rendered compromised by bodily engagement.

Yet in conversations with NGO workers and directors, doctors, and trainers, in a range of networked institutions, I seldom felt I was able to receive an answer to the question of why, in itself, the uncut placenta poses a problem When I asked a trainer-of-trainers associated with NAFPA why the umbilical cord must be cut before the placenta is delivered, she said first that it was "unhygienic," and then, when I asked again, said, "she supposed" that an attached placenta poses a problem in putting the baby to the breast immediately, that it might prevent a baby from being wrapped up and warmed, and that it might interfere if the baby must be transported to a hospital—largely secondary concerns that might be remedied in other ways. In most such conversations, the root of the problem of the attached placenta (in biomedical or other terms) was left implicit. Many involved in dai trainings did not know why the cord should be cut immediately, and when pressed, said precisely that. "This is what is taught in medical schools," as one trainer told me. In rereading and rehearing interviews, I find that the uncut placenta enters the world of discourse as an idiom, a moral/political entity within which specific meanings, processes, and causalities are collapsed.

The profanity of a placenta "left attached" to a newborn is left to speak for itself. Postpartum caregiving and caregivers appear momentarily, if at all, only to disappear into a categorical defilement that bespeaks mystification and a defilement of secular equality.

Through the *longue duree* of intervention and outrage about birth practices, Dalit women and their specific labors have appeared and disappeared into the expanse of visceral idioms. The ever-scandalized Katherine Mayo wrote in 1927: "In Benares, sacred among cities, citadel of orthodox Hinduism, the sweepers, all of whom are 'Untouchables,' are divided into seven grades. From the first come the *dhais*; from the last and lowest come the 'cord-cutters.' To cut the umbilical cord is considered a task so degrading that in the Holy City even a sweep will not undertake it, unless she be at the bottom of her kind. Therefore, the unspeakable *dhai* brings with her a still more unspeakable servant to wreak her quality upon the mother and the child in birth" (Mayo 1927: 96).

In her notorious account of the state of women in early twentieth century India (that was, in effect, a deeply problematic theory of suffering and sexuality), Mayo brought the postpartum worker briefly into the light of published day, only to disappear her again into the gloom of "something wrong." Such sensations of wrongness, as Begonia Aretxaga has said (2000), continue to characterize what we sense (rather than "know") about the "Third World." In Mayo's account, it is at the apex of the sacred (Banaras) that the greatest defilements occur. Through a convergence of moments and acts (kitchen knives used to cut cords, lack of care for mother and baby) the "*dhai*" encapsulates all that is wrong with India's "system." When, with Mayo, we meet the so-called *dhai*, this is what we find: "By that [dim] light one saw her Witch-of-Endor face through its vermin infested elf-locks, her hanging rags, her dirty claws, as she peered with festered and almost sightless eyes (1927: 94)."

Recalling that the biblical Witch of Endor raised the prophet Samuel (or his demonic doppelganger) from the dead, perhaps it is in the relationship of midwives to death, in the echoes of the necromancer who moves life backward across the threshold of death, that witchy imagery becomes amenable to the workaday horrors of Indian life of which Mayo writes. Blindness, dirt, and contagion are literal here; witchiness means woman, untouchable, other (to paraphrase Trinh Minh-Ha [1989]) and is a bearer of death in the place of birth. Merging with "untouchability" (the residue of sacred enchantment), "the untouchable woman" is written into the modernization narrative as a specter haunting Indian women's progress toward freedom.

But if some things appear and disappear, others never appear at all. Of the five assistants I engaged to help with transcription, translation, and, earlier on, facilitating interviews, four were, like Mr. Mehra, completely unaware of "such a thing as the placenta." Two were fathers—one had cut the cord at his son's hospital delivery. All were highly educated. These absences suggest to me that this is not a story about authoritative knowledge, or even about the "power/knowledge" by which subject-constitution undermines the "knowledge is power" equation (Foucault 1977b). This is a story about the way disappearances are structured. The creepy feeling evoked by the uncut placenta demands we ask not how knowledge becomes authoritative and consuming, but *"What makes it possible for something not to be known?"* In the sites of intervention (that are also sites of disenchantment and the assurance of knowledge), why are causalities of harm replaced by (unseen) images of placentas?

A series of thresholds (visibility and invisibility, speakability and unspeakability, presence and absence) shimmer atop startlingly similar doorways (between here and there, us and them, life and its beyonds). These are the thresholds that make the placenta part of a theory of untouchability in the "darkest" of the imaginary shadows of the *sor*. What we are to make of this affinity is uncertain. But it is clear that we should consider the "operations" and "cuts" beyond those of clinics—that is, "operations" in language, discourse, image, and upon bodies—by which certain things are swept from view. The placenta suggests theories of marginality that may be less about forms of knowledge than about the thresholds through which things are passed, thresholds that map onto aspects of consciousness verging on the cosmological. In different but uncannily similar idioms, the placenta is a hinge on which swing doors between death and life, touchability and untouchability. It provides material for the aesthetics of intervention, in which "doing something" emerges from a feeling, a shudder of recognition and horror that orients what will come to be the mode of belonging on offer. Here, we encounter modes of power with jarring affinity, in which it becomes possible for some things not to be known, and some people to bear the burdens of marginality.

Pieces of flesh

In everyday talk in Sitapur, imagined boundaries are evoked and crossed constantly. Elements of biomedical models are often known by "uneducated" postpartum workers; practitioners claiming association with biomedical ways of doing send new babies home for the cord to be cut; people on the side of intervention have never heard of a key bodily organ. There is no crisis for rural women who have their babies in hospitals, for boys whose placentas are incinerated in a clinic rather than buried under the hearth, for Dalit women employed as hospital sweepers who take the placenta to the trash without also cutting the cord. While sites of home and institution may be distinct, they do not align with pat ideas about "tradition" or "medicalization." Every space is between home and institution; and if seen in these terms ("tradition," "modernity," etc.) every space appears full of contradictions—the not quite right (Aretxaga 2002) feeling of the postcolony projected into the hinterlands of *dehat*.

In his writing on culture contact and miscommunication, Marshall Sahlins directed our attention to the human mediation of the cultural field and the world, asking how symbols, objects, ideas are constantly reevaluated in the space of human action (1985). We might also ask how, as part of this ongoing work of reevalutation, objects, symbols, or ideas are both swept from view and allowed to reerupt. For, as well as in elaboration, such movements may establish (if quietly), the zones over which subjectivity is fought. The notion of the uncanny—which, as Freud suggests, is "the return of the repressed" that emerges out of a struggle with "our relation to death" (2003: 148)—may resonate with the placenta in its management in Sitapur even as it takes us away from (predominantly) Hindu ontologies in which death is not separate from birth and (re)generation. Here, bodily excess can be located vis-à-vis the unconscious, part of repressions enabling language, social life, and Law, allowing meaning and desire to be structured. In spite of colorful affinities, notions of repression may be more useful for thinking about modes of power and their language games, perhaps because such models represent less a basic psychic reality than a specific "sex-gender system" (Rubin 1975). It may be that in the repression of certain things, ideas, and specificities, social and symbolic realities take on the mantle of "truth."

Doorways can be crossed backwards as well, and what returns is, as Freud said, precisely that which was familiar but has become foreign, that which gives the shudder of both fear and the once known. The uncanny moment may contain, as Mary Weismantel has shown, the production of neoracist realities, and the evocation of longstanding colonial sufferings (2001), or it may involve the careful preservation of animality and abjection as modes of othering (Biehl 2005), or the way the family—and the female—are sites at once threatening and under threat (Cohen 1999; Taussig 1992b). In this case, it is backward movement that the "uncanny" comes to contain; in such motion, *churels* grab babies across the boundary between life and death; the cut placenta is pulled out of the trash by dogs; the uncut placenta obscenely remains where it should no longer be; the unknown "thing you are talking about" erupts into conversation; the "untouchable" brings death with her dirty hands and unspeakability; caste remains in modern consciousnesses. For Pierre Bourdieu, "Psychoanalysis is the disenchanting product of the disenchantment of the world, which leads to a domain of signification that is mythically overdetermined to be constituted *as such*" (1977: 92). In certain modes of power, we find a third moment of disenchantment—one that may, in fact, reenchant the space of intervention. As feelings of disgust settle on certain objects and certain people, sensation becomes part of the semiotic management of bodily idioms, the management of bodies, and the management of persons. This is so in complex ways (in the *sor*, when things like "danger," "dirtiness," and "pollution" involve shifting acts of concealment and skillful manipulation of meaning) and in balder expressions (in boiled-down utterances about "superstition" and "blind belief"). For Obeyesekere, such repression is the "work of culture," the social and individual sublimations by which fundamental motivations are made into "public culture," "open consciousness" (1988: 63). While I can make no claims for the "originary" motivations underlying the figuring of the placenta in cultural processes, such may also be the work of power. Where Obeyesekere observes in Hindu symbolic processes the "extreme proliferation of cultural symbolization in practically every domain of species existence" (1988: 62), we might ask similar questions of those secular domains in which nothing *feels* elaborated—but clearly, excessively is.

In the oppositionally defined moral spaces of rural and urban, the placenta both orients and disturbs. The sense of its impact is part of both healing and harm. With it, we can situate power less in the ways "knowledge" is authorized or embattled than at the moment at which appearance's binary is crossed. In such instants, "untouchability" lies in easy concordance with "intervention," subjectivity bound up with vulnerability. Such a scope shows that the placenta, or at least its troubled relationship to structure, meaning, and existence, lodges and dislodges behind so much about action, even in places where it can hardly be imagined.

Chapter 3

MEDICINE
DEVELOPMENT WITHOUT INSTITUTIONS[1]

That something so preposterous could be happening in modern times at a place barely 100 km from the capital makes it all the more scandalous.

Manjari Mishra, *Times of India: Lucknow*
(5 April 2001)

Sarkar

*W*eekend evenings in the Bhabhis' household are at once expectant and busy. On Saturdays, men begin wandering into the outer yard by late afternoon, looking in the open gate, asking whoever happens to be around, "Bhaia a gaye?" (Has he come?) Choti Bhabi's husband Jawahar comes to the village every Saturday evening, returning from Lucknow where he works as a school principal. He lives with his older brother during the week in a neighborhood at the northern edge of the city, where urban segues into country and new institutional complexes, housing compounds and schools creep into wheat fields and the mango orchards Jawahar tells me are famous. Regularly around 7:30 P.M., the growl of his motorcycle becomes audible as he turns off the main road, passing the pond where Tulsiram and others catch ducks and fish. By this time, three or four men from the village are waiting for him, sitting on chairs under the overhang in the brick building outside the house.

The building is an open room, built in Bapu-ji's lifetime. It was, Bari Bhabhi tells me, put there by sarkar—the government. But it is also part of *the house in an everyday kind of way as in the facts of architecture—the wall surrounding the outer yard and sealed by a metal gate that is locked nightly. The building, standing opposite the entry to the house and the cow-shed, opposite the post office room that I call my own, has three brick walls and a roof made of thatch and blue plastic. Inside are tables, chairs, and a metal cabinet. During the week, Sunderlal sets up a table here for a few hours a day, from which he administers post office business. On inside walls hang posters that bespeak an archeology of government "schemes"—things at once memories and possibilities, pasts and potential futures, presences that are also absences. One announces a training program to teach young men how to fix electric fans, and is next to another with diagrams of machinery and wiring. This program is just coming to its end when I move in. For a few weeks, every Tuesday and Thursday the yard fills with teenage boys just as I am escaping the heat for the shadows and cool mud walls of my room. Another poster declares, in faded blue writing on yellowing heavy paper stock, that this "center" provides oral rehydration fluids.*

Just outside the building, next to one of the walls enclosing the yard in a public/private, indoor/outdoor embrace, is a hand pump. It is a government hand pump, provided some years ago to be accessible to people of all stations in life and society. This is where I wash my dishes and my hands and face in the morning; this, rather than the pump in the angan, *is where Naseem, Tulsiram, and Dev draw their drinking water when they visit.*

When his father arrives, Rohit is sent out of the angan, or off a lap to greet his father. The three-year-old touches his father's feet with urgency and speed that bespeak shyness and fear of paternal authority. He runs into the more comforting lap of his Chacha Raju or a neighbor. If I am around, Jawahar politely lowers his head and touches his right hand to his forehead. "Hello sister, how is your work progressing?" He waves to the men in the yard, then ducks through the low doorway into the darker recesses of the house. There, he touches the feet of his mother and older brother and then, in turn, has his feet touched by his younger brother, wife, nieces, and sister-in-law. Someone brings him a cup of tea and plate of namkin. *Sometimes he lingers for a few moments here with the women and kids; more often, he quickly squats by the angan hand pump, where he washes off the dust from the road. He changes out of his pants and button-down shirt into a lungi and undershirt, and goes into the outer yard to sit with the men, against his sister-in-law's protestations that he eat something.*

He and Raju, and less often Sunderlal, sit with an ever-shifting group of men in the yard until late at night, a hurricane lamp throwing around them a starkly bounded sphere of light. If a newcomer arrives, he announces himself to those within, who peer into the darkness beyond the glow of the lamp. "Who is that?" someone might say, to which he replies with a name or kin-

ship link. It is rare that women join this group, though Raju often invites me over. Sometimes it is because someone has mentioned something he thinks I should know; more often it is because there is a question about life in "America." I get interviewed extensively on these nights, when I am asked detailed and complex questions about politics, history, economics, and families— often things I have never really put into words. Even when the conversation doesn't involve me, the stories that circulate through them establish points of contrast between rural and urban, educated and uneducated, authoritative and subaltern, familiar and foreign.

Sunday, too, will be much like this. As often as not, Sunday morning and afternoon conversations turn didactic. Men come to Jawahar with questions about law, about institutional procedures, about seeds and fertilizers and plows and pumps, about family and neighborly disputes. They come to hear news from Lucknow, to ask and debate about what Jawahar tells them about what is happening in Uttar Pradesh politics, or certain goings-on or ways of doing in the capital. On some occasions he brings material from the city to read—newspaper articles or magazines. One afternoon he brings out a magazine containing gharelu ilaz *(household remedies). Paging through, as he sits on a chair with one leg propped up and a wad of pan in his cheek, he reads to us about "natural" (*prakrtik*) recipes to replace things like fertilizer, pesticide, herbicide, and cleanser. Men listen and joke around and ask for clarification and translation of chemical terms. They laugh when he tells them that the creosote of a certain plant will dye graying hair black, and argue about whether or not a certain plant might really work to keep away crop diseases.*

People come from other villages with legal questions, or looking for advice and mediation. When I ask Bari Bhabhi what this is all about, she laughs and says, "You think this is bad? You should have been here when Bapu-ji was alive! Men came in crowds. They came from other villages day and night, to ask advice on this legal matter, to solve that dispute. And, you know, Amma couldn't eat until after Bapu-ji had eaten. Sometimes she sat up half the night with an empty stomach, waiting for him to come into the angan."

It was not just advice he offered. "Medicine was Bapu-ji's hobby," Bari-Bhabhi tells me. As well as being a source of knowledge, he did a bit of daktri. *"Like what?" I ask. "Like giving medicines, giving the needle—he was very good with the needle. He gave the needle when all of my babies were born." Though her euphemistic ways of talking about labor-associated drugs makes it initially difficult to determine what he injected her with, later it becomes clear that it was oxytocin, a labor inducing synthetic hormone that Bapu-ji gave Bari Bhabhi—who, by her own surprised admission, was perhaps the only woman in the household he treated with gentle kindness.*

In a context of globalization and structural changes in health care, the turn of the millennium and the end of the globalizing, privatizing, outsourcing 1990s meant that in *dehat* flows of health care were channeled by transnational and national processes like privatization, shifts away from "targets" and toward "profit orientation," and an increasing reliance on foreign donors as well as local private organizations for basic health services (Drèze and Sen 2002; Qadeer 2001; Sen 2001). In such a context, many people in Sitapur sought—and seek—health care from *kaccha* doctors, the raw and informal practitioners who are not quite "quacks" but not legitimate doctors, and who invent roles for themselves as medical authorities and representatives of development. Lacking official certification, seemingly ersatz doctors cross the permeable boundaries of institutions. Though some include elements of indigenous medicine in their practice, most work in a biomedical frame, outside the range of systems like Ayurveda and Unani. Self-made medical authority is also common in urban India, part of crises in quality of care amid high levels of use of care (Das 2002). But the blurring of lines between real and fake takes a particular shape in rural areas, where it is imbricated with the structure and ethos of development and the moral mandates of intervention.

In Lalpur in 2001, development and *daktri* were part of visions of institutionality and governance best captured by the Hindi term *sarkar*. Strictly speaking, *sarkar* is translated into English as "government." But its practical usage is more complex and contextual (cf. Guha 1983). It can refer specifically to the government of India and its agencies, to state and nonstate institutions, and to authority itself. In television, films, and cassette tapes of stories both religious and pulpy, the term *sarkar* is a form of address, a trope of submission and obsequious self-deprecation. In *dehat, sarkar* may be the grandest painter of signs. In everyday talk it is a distant source of programs, an origin of slogans on walls and signifiers in circulation. Women with five children talk about the way *sarkar* is said to give money to mothers for first and second children as part of a new scheme. "Uplift" programs bear its stamp: "Every few months a lady comes from *sarkar* to take the completed sewing pieces and bring new thread and material." Recorders of names, of things grown and harvested, bought and sold, born and dead are agents of *sarkar*—like the *lekhpal*, the government employee who periodically sits at Sunderlal's table in the outer room to record life in a large, yellow ledger. *Sarkar*, like ghosts, can come to grab: "the jeep" from the district loan collector careens into Lalpur from time to time, sending whispers flying from *angan* to *angan*, and scattering local men into the fields.

At once capable of describing something concrete, visible, immediate, and human and also something ineffable and just beyond reach, *sarkar* points to the multivalence of institutional authority and power. It is possible to imagine that its authority exemplifies "governmentality"—techniques that "economize" life under a gaze of neutrality and replicate beyond the boundaries of formal institutions; subject-making modalities that are "capillary" rather than tentacular (Foucault 1991). Beyond the self-regulating (and neutralizing) qualities of governmentality, *sarkar* may also involve shifting forms of reverence, fear, and authority that move within people as much as descend from outside with a heavier hand. It may include the way intervention, at once an ethos, aesthetic, performance, and structure, moves in similar circuits, extending governance into something like, perhaps, "interventionality" (an awkward neologism unfortunately lacking the "ment" that gives "governmentality" its interior, subjective feel).

It is possible to sense in *sarkar* a magical power outside the range of technique, an inscrutable yet palpable essence that Michael Taussig says makes God, economy, and the state "abstract entities we credit with Being, species of things awesome with life-force of their own, transcendent over mere mortals" (1997: 1). Or *sarkar* can show the way magic can arise from myth, involving moments of signification that, as Roland Barthes describes, convey in a single phrase a host of taken-for-granted meanings (1972). In myth, Barthes says, a "concept can spread over a very large expanse of signifier;" likewise, *sarkar*—like "development" or "medicine"—extends into other forms of expression and domains of life. Like myth, medical authority provides means for transformation, even "distortion" (1972: 121) of the socialities caught up in *sarkar*, forming a point of communication whose "fundamental character ... is to be appropriated" (1972: 119).

As part of *sarkar*, at the turn of the millennium, formal health care delivery in rural Sitapur wavered between the real and the ideal amid crises of low public expenditure (Drèze and Sen 2002). While PHCs and government health subcenters were often dilapidated, locked, or empty, occasionally they do provide care, channel immunization drives, house ANMs and doctors. And private hospitals, though expensive, were also *there*, even if their services were largely associated with "those who have the money to spend on hospitals." In such a context, few things illustrate the movable, temporary, yet

intensive quality of rural health care more than the "health camp."
While this is especially so with women's health, perhaps the most
iconic "health camps" are the "eye camps" providing cataract surgery in outlying, poor, and underserved areas. Such events, organized
by both NGOs and the state, can be regular (monthly, etc.) or one-
off. "Health camps" bring doctors from the city to provide on-the-
spot care, assess pregnancy, address reproductive health problems,
insert IUDs, and in some cases provide sterilizations or referrals for
sterilizations. (Mahila Seva Sansthan, the private hospital in Munniabad, and the government also ran occasional health camps in
Sitapur). Health camps may include lectures given by "VIPs"—often
directors of local hospitals or doctors from cities), "healthy baby
contests," and booths manned by representatives of condom manu-
facturers, government and private. Some are more low-key affairs
in which women travel from nearby villages to wait in appointed
places for the arrival of "the van" carrying a doctor from the city. Or
they may involve a higher degree of spectacle in which banners fly,
slogans are chanted over scratchy PA systems rigged to noisy gener-
ators, and young women from the city in pressed *selwar-kameez* or
Gandhian *khadi* (homespun fabric) sit surrounded by "village women"
wearing make-up and their best glass bangles, and doctors wearing
sunglasses speechify from platforms in front of small crowds of
mostly women and babies.

A "system" of complicated webs with enormous holes makes it
crucial to pay close attention to both "practiced medicine" (Khare
1996) and practiced *sarkar*, the practiced state. Recent writings emphasizing the everyday, imaginary, and local dimensions of the state
counter frameworks that distinguish governance from culture, subjectivity, and the domestic sphere, representing the state in its immediacy rather than as a set of codes and entities distant from everyday
life (for instance, see contributions to volumes by Fuller and Bénéï
[2001]; Hansen and Stepputat [2001]). In a similar spirit, we might
ask what kinds of socialities are emergent in the building from which
Bapu-ji dispensed government-given rehydration salts along with
illegitimate injections. How is it that some people move back and
forth across the boundaries of formal, legal institutions? By their own
estimations, *kaccha* doctors are part of the grand and messy process
of development. Their practices complicate a view that development
or intervention come from elsewhere, while demonstrating that
their power as ideas lies in the assertion that they do. Their "here"
demands a concurrently imagined "beyond," the idea of externality
in the face of evidence to the contrary.

Pratima and the Mishrein

*"You must meet the Mishrein. She knows so much. She does all the work
you are asking about and can tell you everything you need to know." Women
often frame my efforts as a quest for "*jankari,*" information or data, such
being what researchers do, why they/we come to such places. The authority
of* jankari *is normally referred to as outside of or far from oneself—something I can get elsewhere, though Rakesh's Mother often subverts this paradigm by asserting that the* jankari *she has to give is valuable enough to be
withheld. Pushpadevi tells me that while she herself can tell me a bit about
certain parts of childbearing, she defers many of my generalizing questions
to a local authority—a "doctor" in the next village. Her sister-in-law agrees
with her that the Mishrein will be the one "from whom [I] will get my data."
Others mention her as well. She does "ladies'* ilaz*" (ladies' healing), the
Bhabhis tell me. She delivers babies, another woman says. She gives the needle, Pushpadevi tells me, then adds quietly that there are other things she
can do as well, other kinds of work. Like making babies fall.*

*I visit the Mishrein with Pratima Srivastav, a distant relative by mar-
riage to my own household, and a woman known in Devia to be, herself, a
skilled "ladies doctor," often called to deliver babies. I first met Pratima when
I visited the local field office of NAFPA to observe a training of CBDs—the
"Community Based Distributors" of contraceptives and advice. Mr. Sharma,
the administrator of NAFPA's field office, pulled her aside to talk with me.
"She is really skilled in her village," he tells me, "and she does the kind of
delivery work that you are interested in." She too, he says, will have* jankari
*for me. Later, when I move to Lalpur, I begin to visit Pratima on a regular
basis. It turns out she is distantly related to the family with whom I live.
They send me to her as well. I accompany her on her rounds in the village,
in which her less formal role as a baby deliverer segues into her efforts to sell
contraceptives. I hang out with her on the long afternoons when she fills in
the columns and rows on the ledger supplied by NAFPA with detailed accounts of which households request which contraceptives and in what quantities, of who is pregnant and who has given birth. I marvel at the tedium
of the way, together with her youngest daughter, a local schoolteacher, her
labors of surveillance enable the quantifying, gridifying gaze of the state to
replace the intimate expanse of Dalit women's knowledge of reproductive life
and sexuality. At the same time these rows and columns translate her own
intimate knowledge derived from her more* kaccha *work, tacking down her
movements into blips of* jankari.

*When she takes me to the Mishrein's clinic, it is late afternoon, and the
clinic is empty. The clinic is in the transformed front room of the Mishrein's*

home, in the Brahmin neighborhood of Devia. Her home is pakka—*cooked—made of cinder block and painted prettily. It contains a small wooden desk on which rests a ledger. A platform serves as table, bed, or chair, and there is a shiny red plastic chair. The single window is crossed with bars to keep out thieves and animals, and a cupboard mounted on the wall behind the desk hangs partially open, revealing hypodermic needles, some cloth, and a few bottles of liquid.*

"I have heard about her," the Mishrein says, not unkindly, pointing to me. I say that I have been meaning to come visit for some time. I ask if there have been many births lately, as she pulls some chairs into the angan *for us to sit on and begins to make tea on a small gas stove. "Oh, it's a very slow time...There haven't been any in a while." Pratima asks after her family. Her children are grown. The girls have all married and are in their* sasural, *and the boys have moved to Lucknow with their wives. She tells me her main practice is normally "deliveries," but that has fallen off lately. Women come to her when a birth is slow, or to turn breech babies. She gives some injections for stalled labor, she tells me, something Pratima says she herself does not do. I ask if she has ever been through a "training."*

"No. I have taught myself over the years. Also I watched my husband." Pratima points out that her husband is a doctor. She later explains that he doesn't have "training" either, but that he has built up a solid medical practice over the years. "He taught me a bit," The Mishrein says, "But mostly I learned ladies' ilaz *on my own."*

The Mishrein cannot spend much time with us this afternoon—she has somewhere to go. I say I will come by another day, and Pratima and I return to her mud and brick house on the other side of Devia. Her older daughter is resting on the bed inside. She has come back from her sasural *so that Pratima can deliver the baby when the time comes. Though her bulge is hiding under a "maxi" today—under a nightie-like dress often worn by urban middle-class women in the home—it looks like that time could be soon. Pratima tells me she probably has another couple of weeks to go, "But it is more comfortable for her here."*

On another day, Pratima takes me to meet two sisters-in-law—naouns—who live nearby. "They do this 'delivery' work," she says. We talk on the veranda of their house while Pratima looks on. When we talk about placentas and cord cutting (which they say they do not do), I ask what work the placenta does in the mother's body. One woman pauses, then begins a tentative response—perhaps confused by my clumsy wording. Pratima taps me on the arm. "They don't know this one. It is the thing that feeds the baby." She shifts into a didactic register. "And you have to make sure it comes out right away [after the baby is born] or else it becomes poisonous."

Pratima and the Mishrein became "ladies doctors" in similar ways. Pratima began to do "delivery *aur* ladies' *ilaz*"—delivery and ladies' healing—a decade ago, when her own children were no longer toddlers. She began the work because she had always felt drawn to it, but also at the urging of her husband, a certified doctor of naturopathy, who gave her some textbooks on pregnancy and birth. Her husband, now quite elderly, showed me his certificate from a prestigious school of naturopathy in eastern Uttar Pradesh, and told me about the clinic he once ran in Munniabad. These days, Pratima told me, she sometimes does up to five deliveries in a single week, or she can go for a month or two without being called once.

Though neither women used terms "modern" or "traditional," the scientific, educated, and institutional quality of their work set it apart from the tasks of women they considered "uneducated" and prone to "blind belief" (but "experienced"). Unlike dais and *dhanuks* who said they acquired their skills "from God" and through practice, Pratima described her education as a process of book learning supplemented by practice. Though she denounced the way local baby deliverers refuse to cut umbilical cords, Pratima did not interfere in postpartum work. She generally did not cut cords "unless it was the middle of the night." Over the years, Pratima's renown as a "ladies' doctor" had spread through Devia and beyond. But such work, like fertility, like the reproductive body here, knows only its own timings. These days, she told me, she might attend five deliveries one week and then go through a dry spell with only one in a month. Often I when I arrive she says she spent much of the night before at a delivery. After several years of working in this capacity, she was identified by an NGO-state collaborative project for training as a CBD of contraceptives. This project also identified and trained local TBAs (drawing on women identified as postpartum workers and those who delivered babies outside their own households). Though Pratima was a self-defined expert at deliveries, she was selected for the more authoritative, managerial—and paid—position of CBD. She was the only CBD I met who also worked as a baby deliverer; no designated "dais" were trained to be CBDs because, I was told by organizers, these women are "mostly illiterate." Pratima showed me the books she sometimes refers to; one from a government training showed in vivid cartoons the dangers of difficult deliveries. When speaking about the way she learned this work from books and through practice, Pratima juxtaposed herself to the local women who deliver babies in a different register. "They are illiterate, and they follow some beliefs, like putting an iron sickle in the baby's bed with it." But she was not as outspoken on this matter as her daughter, an unmarried woman working as a schoolteacher in the village, who frequently cut into such conversations to say, "It's all blind belief; they are not educated, you see." Pratima spoke critically of the "refusal" of "these women" to cut the umbilical cord. When asked if she cut cords she said, "When I know someone will come to cut it I leave it for them, but if it's the middle of the night I will do it."

But her relationship with local birth workers, whether baby deliverers, postpartum workers, or both, was not antagonistic. On several occasions Pratima took me to the homes of practitioners she considered "other" to herself, or called them to her house to speak with me. They sat on the bed or on chairs in the front room and talked to me about recent cases, their NAFPA trainings (as "dais"), and the different kinds of work they do. Pratima used no word such as "traditional" to characterize them, but considered them as a group to be "uneducated" though as individuals also "very experienced" and "very skilled." Their work, whether or not they had received institutional "training," was of a different order from her own, but not necessarily deficient. However, in many interactions she played the role of educator, reframing my questions and telling them to tell me what they learned from her or had learned in trainings. She seemed invested in their answers, and coaxed with cues like, "Remember the five laws of cleanliness," or "Tell her how you measure the umbilical cord with three fingers before you tie the string."

In performances of a familiar scene of authority, as well as reframing my questions into the mode of training, she interjected inquiries of her own, mirroring those asked by NGO workers and visiting doctors to assess "local conditions" or lead into comments intended to "educate." Her queries were situated at the points of process and practice which most concern the medical and public health establishment—pushing on the stomach during labor, means of delivering the placenta, cutting the cord, and attending to the stump. She asked postpartum workers how the cord was cut and what substances were used for cleaning (soap or ash). And she asked baby deliverers how they decided to refer a woman to hospital, and whether they massaged the belly to promote delivery of baby or placenta (if they said yes, she told them why this should not be done).

I also accompanied Pratima on some of her weekly visits to clients and homes where she hoped to solicit new ones. Carrying her bag from the NGO, she entered some houses and engaged in conversations about children and family, then remarked that she works for "*sarkar,*" which has a new family planning program. She could make measures available to them; the best one, she frequently said, was "operation." She attempted to dissuade women from a common rejection of birth control pills on the grounds that they are "hot" or "cause heat in the body," not by arguing with their etiology, but by saying "So what's a little heat? Take it at night before you go to bed" (cf. Nichter 1980 on "heat" and medical pluralism, and Cohen 1999 on heat as a feature of health and subjectivity; see also Chapter 7). On these rounds she visited the mothers and new babies she had delivered, and checked women's bellies to tell them how many months pregnant they were, or if they were pregnant at all.

In some of our outings, Pratima introduced me as "an important doctor from outside (*bahar se*)." I protested that I was not, but between houses, Pratima told me I should not contradict her. "It is important that these people think you are a doctor because it will make them listen," she said; it would lend legitimacy to her message. It was not just my (false) identity as a doctor that gave authority to Pratima's mission, but my being from "outside" (*bahar*)—the way that authorizing power comes, by definition, from somewhere else. The term *bahar* is used in rural settings to denote foreignness at different levels—beyond the village, beyond the rural, beyond the region, beyond the nation. More important than where it is located is the kind of authority "outside" signifies. The outsider as reformer or educator is a recognizable figure of progress and change. Full of claims of knowledge, yet ultimately unknowable, the outsider references both threat and possibility: the Gandhian educator of disenfranchised agriculturalists and lower castes in the face of colonial and *zamindari* rule (as in the film *Mirch Masala*); the skeptical hero who rescues villagers from exploitation (as in *Sholay*); the con man who ultimately restitutes local inequalities (*Shri 420*); or, on the darker side, the newcomer at once victim and threat who fills ears with stories about violence and suffering from places not too distant.

In a setting in which the nature of marriage and households makes all married women, to some extent, "outsiders" in immediately perceptible ways—"foreign" accents, unfamiliar terms for one thing or another, differences in religious practice—the use of Pratima's first name in Devia and beyond signified outsiderness in ways at once familial and institutional. In trainings and meetings with NAFPA supervisors (from yet another "outside"), local women were known by first names, a practice which endowed them with an extravillage identity while referencing, perhaps, the familiarity of the *maike*. Such practice, in the eyes of NAFPA, "modernized" them through ruptures in what were assumed to be the "groupness" of female identity—as indicating lack of individual senses of self. For a woman to be known by first name, while it denotes affiliation in the *maike*, marks her as an outsider in the *sasural* in a different way than married women are already outsiders. It can signify—according to local NAFPA workers— refusal of certain forms of sociality and subjectivity, namely the refusal of "superstitions" underlying reticence about first names, often glossed by NGO and NAFPA workers as a concern that a name spoken in anger can bring harm (see Chapter 4).

While it might be possible to imagine Pratima and the Mishrein as "quacks" (a word often used in the urban media and everyday conversation), few described them as such. Some referred to them as *kaccha* (raw, unofficial, unfinished), as opposed to the *pakka* (cooked, official, solid, formal) nature of certified doctors, but few questioned their legitimacy. Practice and self-made authority outweighed (or did not contradict) what might elsewhere appear as falsity. However, the implications of *kaccha* medicine differ across the social hierarchy in rural communities. Where caste-Hindu women did not dwell on the fact that Pratima and the Mishrein were fake (*nakli*), for the most marginalized, the difference between real and fake was crucial—part of the threat of "the real" or legitimate. Dalit and Muslim women, who spoke to me of fears that hospital needles might contain poison, or that they would receive inadequate care or forced sterilizations there, described *kaccha* practitioners as a safer alternative. Abortions and injections outside of institutions, they felt, entailed less risk than those in official spaces.

From the perspective of institutions, Pratima and the Mishrein's self-made authority and quasi-institutional roles segued unproblematically into legitimate institutional membership. Where the state possesses measures to regulate or prosecute such practitioners, in Sitapur the reverse is often true—they are recruited and officialized. Pratima was selected by NGOs because of her role as an "educated" practitioner (though that status was self-made). And others like her were pointed out to me by official institutional figures—doctors at PHCs, NGO workers—as beacons of development. The Mishrein and Pratima began careers by occupying gaps in the fabric of legitimate health care in rural communities. Lacunae in the formal structure, signs of promises always foreclosed—in the shape, in Devia, of a health center with a deadbolt across the door most days, or PHCs staffed with doctors from Lucknow on only certain days of the week, or private hospitals whose fees are too high—allow such persons to institutionalize themselves, to creatively envision work identities in an entrepreneurial fashion. Many large villages and towns in this region have such a person, mustering "training" in whatever form it took and association (especially via kinship) with authorizing forms (political leaders, legitimate hospitals) to offer services in a medical frame. They range from those like the Mishrein, with no institutional links, to retired ANMs who open uncertified clinics in their homes. What makes their practice legitimate and even institution-like, what makes them different from dais, trained or otherwise, is their ability to invoke outside authority and self-positioning in a frame of education and rationality, claims not refuted by legitimizing institutions. (Indeed, a longstanding component of dai training encourages women to establish clinics in their homes.) In this way, imagination becomes social practice (Appadurai 1996) of the most immediate, intimate consequence, and rural women can have babies with doctors even when none are available and medicalized births in their own homes.

Such complexities of *sor* and *kaccha* clinic reiterate Mark Nichter's observation that the broad and varied manifestations of "medicalization" make it "not just the prerogative of the medical (psychological and medico-legal) professions," but very much part of everyday life (1998: 327). At the same time, this context emphasizes the ways social control can emerge through forms of medicalization delinked from formal institutions and the hegemonic structures they are taken to confer. Authorizing forces are as fluid as the practices they endow with meaning, based on something other than official institutional recognition. For Pratima, having a foot in both worlds allowed her to engage the *idea* of institutions by soliciting and performing the ideas her clients had of institutions and the authority they confer. For practitioners and clients, institutions operate as sites of desire and fear, spaces of not only imagined but real and tappable authority. The unquestioned validity of these practitioners demonstrates that, for many rural people, it does not so much matter where your medicine and abortions come from, so long as they come. For the most disenfranchised it matters greatly, making *kaccha* legitimacy preferable to *pakka* power.

Parrots and mynas

I visit a neighbor in Lalpur one afternoon, invited over by Meena, an unmarried schoolteacher who lives in her brother's home. The pradhan *is visiting. We talk about my research and as soon as I mention dais, he says he educates women in his community about cleanliness: "I tell them, 'Don't spread this cow dung. Use Dettol; use bleach.' Now they do this in my village."*

It is not only "tradition" that is fluid, but hygiene too, I think, recalling the way Raju once told me that gobar (cow dung) is the "Hindu Dettol." The pradhan *says he calls together "these women" to tell them they must use a "clean blade" instead of the iron sickle, that they must wash their hands before attending deliveries or cord cuttings. This is his responsibility, he says, part of his desire to serve people, though he has never been officially part of any government or nongovernment health schemes.*

"I was doing my education," he said. "I have a BA. I thought, I will serve the people. So I sat in the company of doctors. I learned compounding and then I got the knowledge for how to do injections. Slowly, slowly I began to do the ilaz *for my own family. After this, when people knew that he practices* daktri, *patients began to come to me.... A relationship with the public was formed. Today, after twenty years I have slowly become experienced."*

Through the interpenetration of medical and political practice, a larger mode of authority is created around a social and moral mandate. The capacity and legitimacy to follow through on those mandates are self-endowed, part of ongoing imaginations of identification with institutional structures. Before the beginning of the formalized *panchayat* system in the early 1990s, before the current *pradhan* formed his "relationship with the public," Bapu-ji was considered *pradhan* of Lalpur. His family had been primary landowners in the region, controlling labor and production in and around Lalpur until land restructuring in the 1970s, and for some time thereafter. But Jawahar's generation enjoyed only the remnants of Bapu-ji's nostalgically described lifestyle. For them, authority was expressed through advice giving (as well as the simultaneous *purdah* and high education of wives), while money and land were in shorter supply. As Bapu-ji sold off much of the acreage that remained after the end of *zamindari* rule, and gambled and drank away much of the family's capital, reeling in personal ways, Jawahar imagined, from the transformations that land reallocation involved, Jawahar said, the family no longer controlled agricultural production and labor patterns in the village. In many respects, he told me, they had come down in the world in staggering ways over the course of a few decades. Though it may not have been obvious to those who sought their advice and referred to them with honorifics, there were struggles to make ends meet, to afford, as Bari Bhabhi put it, meat, nice veggies, and decent cups from which to serve *chai* to guests, and to send the children to private schools on Jawahar and Raju's incomes as teachers and Sun-

derlal's pay as postmaster. But Jawahar's status as "educated," as a
resident of Lucknow, and as the most authoritative (though not the
eldest) son in this historically powerful family left him in the same
position his father once occupied vis-à-vis the dissemination of
knowledge in the community. His aim, he told me, was to dispel
"ignorance" and bring "a little bit of knowledge" to his community
about "science and medicine." In a remarkable circulation of ideas
and cultural currencies, it was not only self-consciously "modern"
knowledge that he shared but also a sense of the "traditions" of the
rural hinterlands and a translation of their validity into scientific
languages.

Consistencies between *daktri* and political power extend into the
performances by which talk becomes education. Such moments, as
displays of authority, are similar in shape and feel to the formal "trainings" so integral to NGO and government schemes. In the ethos of
improvement they take up at once a medical and educational mandate, in which those in positions of authority bear a responsibility to
"serve" by way of transformation of their public. Any place can become an institutional site as the stuff of formal training and of everyday hierarchical relationships slip back and forth into one another.
Everyday conversations are transformed into didactic encounters.
Verandas and front yards are routinized as spaces for transmitting
knowledge and performing self-endowed authority through familiar ways of communicating. While this may involve simply positing
oneself as an authority, it can also involve particular *ways* of communicating—speaking for longer periods of time, shifting into commands and rhetorical questions, or saying that the listener does not
know a certain fact, which the speaker will explain. Where health
is concerned, this shift requires situating talk around the tropes with
which formal institutions are concerned, tropes that converge on
hygiene and reproduction: limiting family size, cleanliness, the use of
gobar, the use of a "clean blade" to cut the cord. In a politics of "talk"
both institutional and everyday, hierarchies are performed through
management of air time and patterns of communication. As sites for
authority overlap, quasi-institutional practitioners can switch back
and forth from institutional to noninstitutional identities with a slip
of language. Patterns of talk allow less structured conversations to
shift into the register of education, even when the conversation has
not been overtly designated a site for learning. The *pradhan* can, in a
chance meeting with an elderly birth worker, mention that she should
use bleach instead of cow dung in her cleaning-up duties. During a
rambling conversation with village men, Jawahar can read from a

magazine brought from the city. Any place can become institutional as the stuff of formal development and everyday hierarchical relationships merge.

In institutions, hierarchies can be more visible and regularized, though they may also claim to offer the absence of extrainstitutional hierarchy as part of the promise of a universalizing way of knowing, the ideal of "health for all" that extends to the idea that anyone can be a practitioner with the right education (as opposed to the "local," where hierarchy is often assumed to reside). Because it relies so heavily on "trainings," the enterprise of rural uplift is all about talk. And talk is the precursor to choice, will, and control. The motto of NAFPA was "Come and talk" (*Ao Bate Karein*), and potential clients were promised—by words emblazoned on posters, banners, bags, and calendars, "Come and have a chat, the decision is in your hands." The mascots of the program were a parrot and myna bird, perched facing each other on a tree branch, apparently talking. These creatures were chosen to represent the program, a local supervisor told me, because they were two different kinds of bird that come together and communicate across obvious (and, I would imagine, ultimate) differences.

Mahila Seva Sansthan has a field office in Munniabad, but its main office is in the heart of Lucknow, not far from the main railway station and down a narrow side road off a busy central artery. The rickshaw lets me off on the opposite side of the road and it takes me nearly fifteen minutes to penetrate the rush of traffic and get across the street. I am here for a "follow-up" meeting for rural women working as local agents of the NGO. Nine of them have made long journeys from their villages to the Mahila Seva Sansthan office where they are to be "retrained." The trainer, Dr. Patel, works for another NGO as a trainer-of-trainers for organizations associated with NAFPA. The women are seated on the sofas in a circle. The electricity is out, so the fans are still and the overhead tube lights do not buzz. The dimness is at once hot and calm. The women talk a bit to one another, but are mostly quiet while they wait for the session to begin.

Dr. Patel gets things started by joking, "We did not bring you here to listen to me talk. This is a place where you can describe your problems in the field and share your experiences with each other." We will go around the room, she says, so that each woman can talk about what she has learned, can ask what she wants to ask. "From others' problems we can learn about our own and from our own we can help one another." We begin with a woman sitting to my left. She says that her work is fine, but sometimes she has trouble getting women to come to her for advice about contraceptives.

They don't really want to approach her, she says. Other women nod their heads. The second woman begins to talk, saying she has come a really long way, and that she had trouble finding the office, but she is happy to be here. Before she says much more, Dr. Patel interrupts. Her responses to the first woman's concerns provide a perfect launchpad for other issues, most of which reiterate the value of the program and its agents and the nature of problems in "rural areas." The women's role in the villages is crucially important, she says. There are many health problems, especially "white water"—leukorrhea or vaginal discharge, something she speaks about for some time. She seldom acknowledges tentatively raised hands, and speaks in an impressive and un- yielding torrent of words. She goes on for an hour or more, though I myself lose track. From time to time she asks a rhetorical question. If there is no re- sponse, she jokes, "Please, you have to speak or else what good is this?" But when women speak she cuts into responses. We never do get to other women's field experiences. Eventually, tea is brought around and it is clear that the meeting is over. Women speak among themselves, mostly about how long it took them to get here, how early they had to leave to arrive on time, and how difficult it was to catch buses. Dr. Patel leans over to talk with me.

I return, in my mind, to the sensations and affects of that meeting, to the jolly and garrulous feeling of obfuscation, to the ironies of the "participatory approach" when six months later I am in the audience at a conference in Delhi. This seminar on maternal mortality is attended by NGO heads, re- searchers, policy makers, doctors, and nurses. For one panel—the one I have been most looking forward to—two women identified as "traditional birth practitioners" are put on a dais for a session on "Extraordinary Individu- als." They are introduced as enthusiastic and active participants in NGO projects in their communities, "successful" trainees yet also vivid embodiments of tradition. As is becoming more common, one of the aims of the conference is not to condemn but to celebrate "beneficial" traditional knowledge and evidence of successful blends of "traditional practice" and "modern science."

The two women are dressed in cheap and colorful saris, with brightly col- ored wool shawls around their shoulders. One wears large, distinctively tribal silver jewelry and bright pink lipstick. We in the audience—mostly women from the health policy world in Delhi, a few researchers, a few "VIPs" from large transnational organizations—are a muted sea of veg- etable dyes, tasteful suits, and stylishly rustic-looking saris and selwar- kameez. (A contingent of nurses occupies a middle ground in the class/ clothes spectrum.) The two women wait to be told when to speak. The first is introduced as Mona. When given the go-ahead by her NGO director, who is sitting to the left of the stage with a microphone of her own to translate into Hindi, she introduces herself again and begins to describe her interactions with the NGO. A woman in the audience stands up as she speaks—some-

thing that has not happened in presentations by researchers and health workers. Mona stops speaking. The woman translating nods.

"What I would like to know, Mona, and we are so glad you are here ... what I would like to know is if you could tell us how you cut the umbilical cord. Do you use a clean blade? Do you tie the string three fingers from the navel? How do you measure where to cut the string?" She smiles and gestures to the podium in encouragement. The NGO director translates and nods at Mona, who looks a bit confused. Mona replies, giving all the right answers.

The woman stands up again. "And do you wash your hands? Do you know the five cleans?"

More questions come. "Tell us what kinds of symptoms you see that make you take a woman to the hospital." We never get to hear the rest of Mona's story, but are urged to applaud the correct answers. "We wholeheartedly support these extraordinary individuals for all the learning they have done," the woman in the audience says in English. There seems to be no space for discourse outside the range of "learning" and "receiving" for the women on the stage—"trainees," lower class, and representatives of "tradition" even as they are also evidence of the effective "respect" of the programs we are here to celebrate.

Near-scripted politics of talk remind those involved of where they stand in relation to others. Unidirectional fulfillment of the educational mandate enunciates authority, reminding subalterns entering the system where power truly lies. Like the frustrated Mahila Seva Sansthan director, there are many trainers, doctors, and administrators who let their interlocutors speak and ask questions, who listen attentively and elicit responses. Such men and women voiced exasperation to me that they or their trainees were silenced by the talk of their superiors. But critical thoughts were not so readily voiced by those in the position of client or trainee; either the familiarity of such dynamics left them unnoteworthy, or there were too many risks to speaking critically.

To return to the *pradhan*, Jawahar, and Bapu-ji, "uplift" unfolds within and outside of institutions as multiple performances of authority through mimetic speech. Familiar modes of talk allow practitioners to tap into the legitimacy of development and health care institutions; they permit people to partake in institutional authority through an economy of legitimizing signs (Taussig 1992a). In these "rehearsals" of power is the Freudian compulsion to repeat: "What happens ... is ... an obsession with the rehearsal itself, as if by such means an abstracted authority or meta-authority could be siphoned off" (Taussig 1997: 77). Roland Barthes says, "For while I don't know whether, as the saying goes, 'things which are repeated are pleasing', my belief is that they are significant" (1973: 12). Undoubtedly in this case, things repeated are both pleasing (for some) and significant. For Jawahar, quasi-institutional authority, while also a burden that kept him from his wife and dinner, was visibly pleasurable as he sat on a small mat warming his feet on a fire of dried leaves, caressing the lump of *pan* in his cheek. Other sites of desire might include the pleasure of talking authoritatively, giving advice, being called upon to administer a treatment, the pleasure of performing a service (*seva*), executing social mandates (Žižek 1997: 51), or being part of something larger than oneself, something that confers legitimacy. This is the pleasure of "becoming an identifiable and legible word in a social language, of being changed into a fragment within an anonymous text, of being inscribed in a symbolic order that has neither owner nor author" (de Certeau 1984: 140).

Mimetic acts conferring recognition bespeak the magical power of institutions to endow authority, to enable those beyond their official realm to draw from a well of legitimacy and become institutional. In the context of childbirth education, it has been suggested that education is the site for the transmission of legitimacy via communication of biomedical knowledge and the transformation of women into "modern pregnant subjects" (Ketler 2000: 142). But in these cases, education does not necessarily confer legitimacy or transform subjects into legitimate modern ones. Rather, it provides a site for enacting authority; the *performance* of education accomplishes a transformation of subjects. The law, in this case the legitimizing rules of intervention, is "grounded only in its own act of enunciation" (Žižek 1997: 78). But who is transformed? Less those who "learn" from figures or become and remain "trainees" than educators themselves, who become agents of authority and participants in development. This transformation cannot come from nowhere. For while mimetic acts bestow legitimacy, they also require that legitimacy already exist. The *pradhan* could best engage the *seva* (service) of *daktri* because he already had authority through the institutions of democracy, land ownership, and high-caste status. At the same time, he said, it was the authority of medical practice that set him on a political path.

Mimesis occurs at another level. When everyday people mimic the patterns of trainings to engage their forms of authority, they pattern themselves on institutions that are themselves inherently mimetic (Langford 1999). Likewise, institutional talk may involve ways of speaking common to the household, the *chai* stall, the bazaar, the temple. The halls of biomedical and development institutions are places of parroting and repetition, and, as medical anthropology has long observed, patterns of talk and performances of authority. And mimesis extends to colonial pasts, to the striking resemblance between the development of missionary medicine in the nineteenth century and contemporary medical practice. For European missionaries, this was a time when interest in medicine grew alongside desires to "open up" previously resistant regions and preserve Europeans' own health in colonial outposts (Fitzgerald 2001). Before qualified medical practitioners became part of missionary groups, missionaries often acquired medical knowledge in a "haphazard, fragmentary" fashion—attending a lecture here, watching patient treatment there; but as medical work became intrinsic to evangelistic activity, they did not limit themselves to "self-treatment" (2001: 104). Their own *kaccha* medicine may have been part of the way missionaries established authority (105).

In agencies most visible in rural Uttar Pradesh, mascots and icons drive this element home and illustrate the mutuality of mimesis: there is no original songbird, but two inherently mimetic birds chirping back and forth, mimicking and transforming and mimicking again, across a divide of essential difference. People mimic formal trainings and institutions like NGOs, and in official sites, in spite of (or enmeshed with) assertions to the contrary ("come and talk," "we have a participatory approach"), NGOs mimic the patterns of talk of everyday people in everyday encounters, in which hierarchy is performed through economies of speech, in which the powerful talk and subordinates listen. "Visiting doctors," trainers brought in for a few days, or NGO workers who live for part of the week in "the field" and the other part at home in the city, appear like iconic outsiders familiar on the Indian educational and political landscape, or, like Pratima, become that way through the performance of authoritative speech. At the same time, the practices of institutional trainings closely resemble the patterns and projects of knowledge control and dissemination characteristic of rural patterns of authority and older systems of governance and power. The way Bapu-ji was sought for information and authority may have predated the presence of institutional trainings in Lalpur. His practice of administering injections remained on a continuum of similar acts which were the perquisites of authority. His household was selected (or offered) as the place for a government hand pump, the post office, and the "schemes" of social uplift. Such a location—neither fully domestic nor institutional—demonstrated that certain kinds of power trump institutional boundaries—even walls and gates—and obscure distinctions between real and ersatz medical practice.

Where there is no source or original, as much as development is about contests of knowledge, it is also about familiar practices and rehearsed acts with immediate recognizability regardless of the knowledge they convey or contest. Stephen Marglin (1990) understands development processes by way of a distinction between *episteme* and *techne*, that is, between universalized, formal knowledge systems and practical knowledge or practice itself. He argues that these categories of knowledge are universal, as are the conflicts they produce. Frederique Apffel-Marglin challenges this view, arguing that epistemic ways of knowing arise from a Western European historical and cultural context (1996a). The suggestion of their universal applicability, she says, is imbricated with contests of power, particularly colonial domination. People like the *pradhan* lead me to suggest that the architecture of "uplift" at once institutes a distinction between *episteme* and *techne*, and at the same time stakes a claim to *episteme*, leaving *techne* for the "others" upon whom the project of conferring epistemic knowledge will be instituted. Thus, the idea that development practices are primarily contests of knowledge is true insofar as knowledge is part of the way development *practices* take shape and part of the way ideologies and structures of "improvement" imagine themselves. But quasi-institutional practitioners and everyday encounters show that development (and development on the grounds of knowledge) is itself a *techne*.

Just as medicine in the postcolonial world is situated at a tension between the universality and particularity of scientific practice, so too does it live in a space between neutrality and power. This is as much as a matter of process—the ways by which science and medicine become authoritative—as it is of *episteme*. Gyan Prakash says of colonial science, "On the one hand, science was projected as a universal sign of modernity and progress, unaffected by its historical and cultural locations; on the other hand, science could establish its universality only in its particular history as imperial knowledge" (1999: 71). While it is through this projection of medicine as a universal sign that medicine is able to command authority, in everyday life the opposite is also true: to gain access to universal realities (and their legitimizing force), one must already be in a position of authority.

Injecting power

When the pradhan *tells me he gives injections I have trouble hiding my surprise. Meena smiles a lot during our conversation, occasionally remarking that the* pradhan *does such good work. She holds out the plate of cookies to offer more, and as I try to refuse and she continues to insist with what becomes near aggression, the* pradhan *says: "There are antibiotics; there is Crocin. Whatever works; like if there is some kind of swelling, then you need acid; if a pill doesn't help, then there is an injection."*

"So do you call the doctor to the house?" I ask. He shakes his head and taps himself on the chest. "People call you?" I ask.

"People call me to say that the pains [of a woman in labor] haven't begun. So to make the pains increase I give an injection. They don't know what kind of thing oxytocin is. What do they know?"

"Isn't this very dangerous?"

"But I [literally, "we people," ham log*] know that if the baby is in the right position ... like if there is light bleeding, or something like water is coming out ... Then an injection can be given." He tells me more about the signs that an injection is warranted, but I am more interested in how he came to practice this.*

"How did you learn?" He holds up his hands—much in the way that Schoolteacher's Mother did when I asked her how she learned her work.

"One woman had a lot of problems.... So I said, come on, let's go see. I arrived and she was in position. I asked the dai if the baby was straight, or in some kind of wrong position. Because if the baby is transverse and you give the oxytocin the womb can rupture. But the baby was in the right position. I gave the injection and the cervix opened."

"Can you see if the baby is in the right position or not?"

"No. These dais, or some woman of the village, they see if the baby is right or transverse. This thing we people ... it's not work for gents."

Back in the Bhabhis' angan, we see the needle administering work of "gents" in another performance. Rohit is a skilled actor who takes on the personalities of others by literally wearing their shoes. He does uncanny and brilliant send-ups of local schoolteachers and visiting babas *and* babus, *and an especially funny imitation of me. He loves to climb onto his father's motorcycle and pretend to ride, and he has his own small "car," a wooden board with wheels that he "drives" through the* angan. *When, I ask, "Rohit, who are you? Where are you going?" he tells me he is the doctor. (Once, he says, rubbing an exaggeratedly "fat" tummy, "I am Master-ji, and I am going to school where I will hit the students who arrive late.") When he arrives at his imagined destination he struts away from his vehicle and approaches Amma, who is sitting on a* charpai *in the* angan. *"Amma, are you sick? Amma is sick. I will give the needle." He screws up his face, as though it hurts as much to give as to receive a shot, and says, "Don't cry. It's okay." He frowns and hands over some imaginary pills. With a curt voice so accurately conveying "doctor" that the Bhabhis and I marvel at his attention to detail, to "the smallest things," he says "Eat these," and goes back to his "car." He repeats the act again and again, until we joke that Amma's arm will be black and blue from all the shots.*

In the rural homes in which men and women practice as "doctors," giving injections demonstrates technical ability, biomedical knowledge, and access to institutions. This is especially true during childbirth, for which the use of injectable oxytocin to stimulate labor is delinked from (official) hospitals and clinics through its widespread availability from rural pharmacists. Called the "happy hormone" in some medical circles, oxytocin in the female body is associated with female sexual response, mother-infant bonding, and even female friendship. In its synthetic forms it has a range of uses. In cows it can, rather painfully, be used to enhance milk secretion and expel retained placentas. It is used in women to stimulate contractions and promote stalled labor, stimulate lactation, curtail postpartum hemorrhage, and in abortion. Its risks include intense pain, ruptured uterus, fetal distress, and placenta abruptia. Oxytocin has a range of illicit uses, rumored and real: as an intoxicant, is said to be used to enhance bootleg liquor; some farmers reputedly inject it into vegetables to increase their growth. Flows of pharmaceuticals (fake and real) within and out of India include oxytocin among their products, and are linked with prostitution; some red-light districts of Delhi are reputedly associated with Russian and Uzbek women who ferry pharmaceuticals, among other products, across borders.

In the Indian media, oxytocin is a chemical of scandal, its uses marking the breach between the urban/rational and the rural/backward, as well as the gray zone between nature and culture, human and animal, real and fake. Oxytocin's use in bovine milk production has been taken up by animal rights activists, those with both secular and Hindu leanings. Use on cows has been banned, pharmacies raided, licenses revoked, doctors and vets arrested. Its use in rural home births is just as disturbing for urbanites as, for rural people, is its distorted usage in clinical settings, in particular, the use of bovine drugs on women. Leading newspapers cite the unexplained presence of bovine oxytocin in medical stores, filling stocks meant to be used in hospitals and birth clinics, and used extensively in respectable medical institutions until the mistake (or something like it) was exposed (Bannerjee 2001).

A newspaper article headlined, *"Daais*-in-hurry inject death to rural women" (Mishra 2001), begins with a "23-year-old illiterate housewife" from "a small hamlet in Sitapur" who required a hysterectomy after being administered an incorrect dose of oxytocin (it does not say yet by whom). The article is written by a Lucknow journalist, Manjari Mishra, who often writes about the profanities and problems of poor and rural women. Even now, through newsgroups and e-lists, her similarly themed articles occasionally pass through my in-box. The headline turns a common critique of biomedical handling of birth (that doctors are too hasty in giving drugs to speed up labor) onto the rural, Dalit, female, and elderly. Denouncing incompetent dais for profaning medical technology using the same tropes of ignorance ("illiteracy") and immorality that describe complicit rural women, it says, "[T]he *daais* in and around Sitapur have obviously evolved their own shortcut to administrate [sic] the drug." But it turns out that the "housewife's" oxytocin was given by an ANM— a government employee—performing a duty beyond the range of sanctioned practice. In fact, the patient "had no complaints against the ANM who messed up her case. 'She was most helpful and the injection she gave me such instant relief [sic],' she told this correspondent, even as the attending gynecologist tried to explain in vain the incalculable harm it had caused her."

The article ends by citing a hospital employee—Dr. Immaculate: "They are too poor and ignorant to lodge a formal complaint." No specific cases involving "dais" are cited, but when ANMs are mentioned, attention shifts elsewhere—to dais and rural women who sustain the practice by not complaining. It is worth pausing at the "relief" the victim describes. The reported conversation points to the ambiguous way rural women refer to "injections" to indicate either pain-reducing or labor-inducing drugs. In most cases involving poorer, lower-class, and rural women, "the needle" refers to labor induction, often in an idiom of relief, though for observers accustomed to the extensive use of pain-*relieving* drugs in other parts of India and the world, the reference is confusing. In the article, such ambiguity allows for an additional layer of moral coding in which "relief" is counterposed with two forms of "suffering": the "false" suffering that prompted the use of "the needle" and the "real" suffering of the hysterectomy which even the sufferer herself cannot grasp. This contrast involves near-Protestant notions of labor, reward, and production: in opting for "relief," the "poor and ignorant" woman brought upon herself "incalculable harm," a harm which doctor and journalist must "struggle in vain" to convey.

Yet while the media and received urban wisdom overwhelmingly blame "dais" and "rural women" for oxytocin injection and its consequences, in rural Sitapur, those who control the informal economy of needles are almost entirely educated people in positions of political, caste-based, and landowning power. Or they are already associated with institutions, either as government employees, by having participated in trainings, or by establishing institutional identities and practices in the key of biomedical rationality. As needles and drugs are available to whoever can pay for them while institutionally sanctioned hands to administer them are notably *un*available, giving injections is a way to establish oneself as a medical practitioner. But the practice channels needles and drugs primarily through the hands of the already powerful—the educated, the elected, the upper caste, the "trained." While some "dais" may give injections, it is important to note that they are not alone. Imputing scandal onto them obscures the shared dynamics of power that ground quasi-institutional and medically mimetic practices. Certain figures must always remain "the problem."

Legalities can mean delicacy in the ways injection giving is talked about. A retired ANM, the upper-caste wife of a political leader, who opened a clinic in her home denied this practice, though she was locally renowned for it. She seemed offended when I mentioned it and said it was dangerous and unscrupulous. But Bapu-ji's family considered this activity part of his service to the community. Going a step further, the *pradhan* turned the scandal back onto institutions: "Doctors take plenty of money. This ANM, she takes five hundred rupees. Hey! What's a needle? Fifty rupees. Meaning, it's her job! I think that [it should be reimbursed] according to one's abilities.... But [it should be from a] good company. Here people give the one for animals. Antocin. To make the buffalo milk come in. This is wrong. But I do the right kind of work. Here people take one hundred rupees for an eighty-rupee injection. Society's well-wishers [sarcastically]."

In crosscutting scandals, moral ideals reiterate boundaries established in the politics of talk, even as they critique the "center" from one of its many imagined peripheries. The *pradhan*'s "right work" is an antidote for corruption and faulty science. Not just mimicking institutional practices, he offers a corrective to what he sees to be corrupt institutional functioning. In ersatz medicine, the greatest categorical confusions involve, on the one hand, praxes of the elite co-opted by the disempowered, and, on the other, technologies of care withheld. As such, both illegitimate and obscene collapse into mutual critiques.

In India vaccination efforts, such as that for smallpox in the nineteenth century, have long and notoriously encountered resistance and fear. In the case of smallpox, this reaction was channeled, David Arnold argues, in part onto a sense that medical and secular challenges to the body of the smallpox goddess Sitala (amid the often painful and traumatic quality of early techniques) involved a larger "site of conflict between malevolent British intent and something Indian, something sacred" (1993: 144). Smallpox vaccination, however, also involved a kind of triage of care via "noncompliance," in which upper castes and classes withheld vaccination from their children on the grounds that it offended religious sensibilities, while lower castes and classes were a more readily available population, a fact of care the British lamented if medicine was ever to be seen as something for more than the lowest and most marginalized elements of society. Vaccination was emblematic of a colonized body, especially in "particularly stubborn regions like Avadh"—precisely where Sitapur sits (1993: 144). In both colonial and postcolonial contexts of globality and power, resistances and fears bear a family resemblance, though they filter through caste identities in slightly different ways. Injections occupy a zone in which the power and fear of biomedicine are linked (Bierlich 2000), forming an especially iconic mode of biomedicine (Whyte and Van der Geest 1994) in which present vaccination campaigns continue to bear the weight of coercions past and present, real and imagined (Greenough 1995). Yet, as things that enter the body can threaten at once religious sensibilities and the body politic, the relationship between health-seeking ideologies, local visions of illness, and acceptance or rejection of vaccines speaks to injections' multivocality (Nichter 1990; 1995). Needles seem to, recurrently, offer "an opportunity for political commentary as well as the articulation of collective anxieties" (Nichter 1995: 618).

Injections can carry dreams of redress as well as the heavy weight of state power; they absorb and challenge anxieties through their circulation *beyond* legitimate use and institutional programs as much as within them. In informal economies, illegitimate economies and fake drugs—as practices offering care to both bodies and society— describe the embodied conditions through which authority and the real are crafted against global conditions in which states and non-state agents at once "disinvest" in basic health needs and aim to offer short-term, pedagogically oriented "interventions." Shifting claims on "real" medical practice break down the "here" and "there" by which authority comes from somewhere "beyond." The needle, like certain kinds of talk, provides entry into legitimizing structures for those who administer it and a social map for those scandalized by it. For those who receive it, it literally injects power into the body— the force of life giving and life taking. It is not through bastardized legitimacy that social hierarchies emerge through medical practice and development, but rather through the very crafting of legitimacy. What remains to be asked is not just how legitimacy is made, but *whom* it is crafted in opposition to, whom its framings exclude. It is here that untouchability whispers to us from the backstages of "modernity." It has, of course, been here all along.

The failure of institutions

Introducing Preeti to the page is difficult. To begin with any descriptive word or phrase invokes the very categories I aim to expose.

Begin with me? Preeti, like Pushpadevi, lives on the other side of the Bhabhis' kitchen wall, her brick and thatched-roof house visible from our roof. Her stepdaughters seek me out early on, when I am walking through the fields. They shout and wave from their rooftop when I sit on the Bhabhis' roof clacking out my notes on the manual Olivetti a professor passed down to me. At my first meeting with Preeti, days after I move in, she hovers in my doorway with her bag from NAFPA hanging from her shoulder. She makes confusing and sparse small talk, communicating her affiliation with the scheme by carefully exposing the green satchel. My research assistant, who will leave soon anyway, dislikes her instantly and says she seems untrustworthy. "You can see it in her eyes."

Begin with jati*? Preeti is from the Pasi community, ranked above other Dalit* jatis*, but arguably the most stigmatized community in Lalpur, mocked for what are imagined to be thieving and promiscuous ways.*

Begin with institutions? When I met her, Preeti was just beginning to serve, like Pratima Srivastav, as a CBD for NAFPA.

Begin with kin and babies? Preeti is on her second marriage. She has three stepdaughters with whom relations are strained, and two young children of her own—a boy and a girl, about six and four. The eldest of her stepdaughters is in her sasural*; the second oldest, somewhere around sixteen, is married, but spends most of her time here in her* maike*, where her alliance with her younger sister is fierce. They are inseparable during the times when the youngest is not at school. Preeti's fights with them are loud and frequent, drawing neighbors onto rooftops to listen and watch with concern and curiosity. "That big one protects the little one from her anger," Bari Bhabhi tells me.*

Begin with gossip? Preeti has a reputation among the women of the village for being immoral, a prostitute, one who "changes husbands the way some women change blouses." The Bhabhis say she is a whore for the police station down the road. "They come to fetch her sometimes, you can see them," Choti Bhabhi says, "Really, it's true!"

Begin with men and the effects of their transgressions? The men in Preeti's husband's family—including Pushpadevi's husband—are arrested in the middle of winter for a robbery and murder of a rickshaw puller in the qasbah down the road. Preeti's husband is not implicated in the crime, but the stain of the crime casts a pall on the entire Pasi community in Lalpur.

The problem in telling stories is that threads are bound together with gossip and the nastiness of neighborly talk. Some things Preeti tells me herself. She took the job of CBD when another woman quit. A twenty-something unmarried daughter of one of Jawahar's cousins had been convinced to back out of the program, though Mr. Sharma and the trainers and supervisors laud her enthusiasm at her training (where I am present) months earlier. Preeti stepped in, got trained, and picked up the satchel and ledger. But as she trained separate from the other women in her group, who were all supervised by Manjari, the woman from eastern Uttar Pradesh—also young, also unmarried—who lives with an elderly couple across the road, Preeti came into the structure already slightly outcast.

She was an outcast in other ways as well. Preeti had a reputation as a prostitute, and the fact that she divorced her first husband and remarried another only verified, for some, the rumors. Her current work required her to "move around" from house to house and village to village, beyond the sphere of *maike* and *sasural*, beyond the home-bazaar-temple movements that make up upper-caste and upwardly mobile women's days. Bari Bhabhi told me, "She should walk with purpose, with intention, from one place directly to a destination, instead, she stops in the road to talk to people, to men, she goes slowly, she lingers here and there on the way." The Bhabhis teased me about "my new friend" and wrinkled their noses when they heard I had been to her house. They got annoyed that I should "let" Preeti into my room, "Her people are thieves. She will be putting her eyes everywhere, on all of your things." Choti Bhabhi says that she is not welcome in the *angan*, "Other of those women know this, and so they don't come in. But 'Madam' comes inside anyway."

A few years earlier, a rural banking program was introduced in Lalpur. The scheme required a local committee of ten. The committee was made up of nine men and Preeti, and met regularly in the outer yard where Jawahar and the men gathered. The talk in the village? "Picture this. She just sat there out in the courtyard with all those men and only her, nine men and 'madam'." Eventually Preeti left the committee, though in her family's Karva Chauth painting marking the fasting of proper Hindu brides seeking auspiciousness and protection for their husbands, alongside the gods and goddesses, flowers, trees, moons, and water jugs, was a man in a suit, carrying a briefcase. I asked Preeti's daughter who the man was. She told me about the scheme, and about the way Preeti was part of it, but eventually quit.

Many people cuttingly called Preeti "Madam," some openly, some quietly. Such teasing made a mockery of her attempts to enter social legitimacy—not to mention financial stability—by engaging in institutional schemes and structures. It precluded any validity she hoped to accrue. Use of this term to her face reminded her that social legitimacy and authority—being called "madam" in seriousness—would remain out of reach. But Preeti persisted. As a CBD she attempted to garner new clients for contraceptives and sterilization operations, and routinely went house to house in neighboring villages (one of which had mostly Muslim inhabitants, which, according to conventional wisdom, meant that few would be interested in contraception due to religious prohibition). With the stigma of sexuality already attached to her name, with the taint of family members whose arrests only seemed to validate stereotypes of Pasis as criminal, it came as no surprise that Preeti had great difficulty acquiring new clients. Most of her clients were from her own neighborhood.

The other CBDs in her group spoke disparagingly of her, as did the local ANM. They agreed with each other: "Who will let her into their house when they know she will be laying her eye on everything?" Pasis are known to be thieves, they said, when she was late for one meeting; they didn't know why NAFPA had trained her in the first place. Manjari, normally ameliorative and vigilant about casteist language, shushed them. But she also agreed, "Yes, her way [literally "work," *kam*] is strange." At a CBD meeting, Mr. Sharma roundly and publicly chastised Preeti for not having enough clients and not working hard enough to get them. He held her up as a negative example, and threatened her with expulsion if she did not have better results by the next meeting. "You should be aggressive, you should go out and search for new clients, you should work to make sure your clients keep coming back for contraceptives. Not like her, back there. Don't be like her."

Preeti comes over to confer with Jawahar after the arrests. She is visibly distressed, with tears barely contained in her eyes, and she grabs my hand and holds it in a painful grip. "People are talking," she says, "and they are saying that it was my husband who did these things, they are sullying our name. I am so worried about this bad name." These accusations are untrue, she says—but the work of brothers impacts the names of their kin. "How am I supposed to carry out my work under these conditions? Where is Bhaia? He will offer relief, he will have something to say." But Jawahar, who is self-professedly less casteist than his older brother, is in Lucknow, so Preeti turns to Sunderlal. "He will give me some relief too," she says, "He is very wise." She tells him what she told me in truncated form. Sunderlal assures that everything will be okay, not to worry. He then turns to me and laughs, "Her whole family are thieves, they are thieves!"

Outside she says that in the evenings she has to take walks because it clears her head. She gets headaches, she says, from all this tension, and sometimes she just needs to leave the atmosphere in her household and wander on the paths through the fields, between villages, for some peace of mind. Not something, I have already learned, that self-respecting women do alone, or at all in the case of the women of my house.

A few days later I come into the outer yard in the evening. A group of men are discussing local politics. Preeti sits in a chair just beyond the edge of the circle. Her head is properly covered with her pallu *and she leans forward on her chair, as though she might be straining to hear from the shadowy boundaries of the lamplight.*

Imagination and institutional authority

As I rewrite and recheck the final versions of this paper a report passes through the electronic ethers and into my email in-box through a newsgroup. It is the report of a public hearing on government food programs in 2005, organized by several groups, National Alliance of People's Movements, People's Union for Human Rights, and Asha Parivar and Sangatan. The report, "Public hearing on right to food in Sitapur (Jan 25, 2006)," lists, in the bare repetitions of testimonial, names, places, villages, districts, tehsils; it lists programs and policies and the way their promises are embodied in signs and acronyms and cards: food rations are not distributed, promised midday meals not available or worm-ridden, anganwadi workers are absent or nonfunctional, animal fodder meant to be distributed ends up on the market. And it tells of suicides due to deep, deep indebtedness, on account of hunger. A flood of places and names I know so well, weighted with enu-

merated and innumerable failings at a most basic level. I search it for famil-
iar villages. Bari Bhabhi's maike is there. Lalpur—a name I have given to
cover over its real one—is not (though another, "real" Lalpur is). The jani-
pahcani *(familiarity) of surnames and place names makes it clear that the*
Dalit and the landless (very often the same) bear the burden of such monu-
mental failures. This, too, is a map.

Amid such absences and losses, in which life can so often hang in
the balance of institutional (government and private) programs,
what do we make of the way medical and development practices—
especially those related to childbearing—can be transmitted outside
formal structures, yet only, it seems, to certain persons? It seems to
involve at once something about the techniques of institutions (their
own mimetic quality), something about development as an ethos (in
which medicine is both pedagogical and technical), and something
about the moral weight of "hygiene" and of things associated with
fertility that allow these praxes to retain validity outside their legit-
imated sites. And it seems to involve an in-place predictability to
loss and refusal, a broad structure of promises made and foreclosed,
a circumstance that situates poverty at the very point at which need
and desire bring one into a relationship with institutions—at its most
basic, in the cases above, in terms of food and hunger, but also in
relation to health and care.

Step back into the ways medical practice has been articulated with
political authority over the course of colonial history, and much has
to do with its interweavings with land ownership: in the colonially
encouraged *zamindari* system of land ownership, patronage, and taxation, the responsibility of indigenous landowners for the well-being
of their subjects was encouraged by colonial authorities and often
took the form of sponsorship of hospitals and other health care institutions (Harrison 2001). Imperial medicine articulated with power
more generally became "integral to colonialism's political concerns,
its economic interests, and its cultural preoccupations" (Arnold 1993:
8). The "self-conscious" notion of medicine as science was a source
of its power, a mechanism by which it authorized colonial intervention and enforced distinctions between colonizers and colonized (18).
Like their predecessors, the *pradhan*, Pratima, and Jawahar partake
in the fluidity of institutional authority as a site of imagination and
practice, structures that both affirm and rebuke the authority of institutions. While they disseminate the ethos of development, their ille-
gitimacy draws attention to failures of state health structures. Ersatz
medicine operates alongside other sites of governance, but rather

than being built into complex structures, it engages surface qualities and tropes; it taps into near-magical authority without the concern for surveillance so characteristic of biopower and government health institutions (especially in rural India, as Gupta points out [2001]). Foucault's concept of governmentality describes a dispersed form of governance, regulation, and surveillance, the means by which state power is extended into everyday life and socialities (2000). With the regulation of life (biopower) a primary modality, governmentality functions by transforming subjects, by opening up an intimate domain for policing the self. In this concept we are taken "within state institutions and outside them, ... in fact cut[ting] across domains that one would regard as separate: the state, civil society, the family, down to the intimate details of what we would regard as personal life" (Gupta 2001: 111). Governmentality takes on particular meaning and urgency in its relationship to the marginality of the rural, a site in which exclusionary elements of health care can emerge from the shape and structure of care, on the one hand, and the places where it recedes from view, on the other.

Kaccha doctors are an integral part of this process, working both within and against marginalization. They may appear quite differently in the rural zones of intervention than in the urban "centers" (or even urban marginalities). In *dehat*, at least, their work appears to be aimed toward service (*seva*) and filling gaps left by legitimate institutions. Borrowing legitimacy through the back door, so to speak, from institutions, quasi-institutional practitioners engage in repeated moments of myth-making in the sense Roland Barthes described as a moment of communication. What lends these acts potency is their "intelligibility," their familiarity (Barthes 1973: 25). But also granting a mythical air is their frozen quality—when speech "turns away and assumes the look of a generality: it stiffens, it makes itself look neutral and innocent" (125). That is, because claims to knowledge and legitimacy are made at seemingly natural points of authorization and on the very grounds of neutrality they are not undermined by their inventedness.

In her description of a spurious Ayurvedic practitioner in New Delhi, Jean M. Langford argues that through a series of legitimizing practices the "fake" practitioner reveals the inherently mimetic qualities of biomedicine, "troubling the binary of truth and falsehood that is a foundation of scientific knowledge" (1999: 24). Following postcolonial critiques, Langford suggests that mimesis enacts a (sometimes subtle) parody of the original, while also engaging "legitimating signs" (33), disrupting colonial projects by emptying them of meaning.

What might be interpreted as hybridity in the case of Ayurvedic quacks is "actually a particular moment in an ongoing intercultural mimetic and countermimetic reverberation" (33). But for all their imitation, the work of Sitapur's quacks is subtly different from that described by Langford in that rather than (or more than) parodying the original, this ersatz medical practice is part of the fabric of legitimacy, integral to the survival of "development" in rural areas—indeed, to survival. While they may at times mock development, such practices also enable it to remain a natural zone in the rural imagination. According to Barthes, it is the *appearance* of neutrality (its falsity) which determines who may and may not partake of a myth. Preeti's failures demonstrate that while the source of legitimacy lies in this neutrality, there are underlying contingencies and partialities. These are, perhaps, the things that are being "turned away" from in mythical speech—long-standing histories and symbolics of "uplift" that designate who may partake of authority and upon whom authority exists to be imposed.

Preeti's story might, to some ears, suggest that the legitimacy of development practice is indeed available to all, provided that " nonmodern" peoples abandon their prejudices (in this case, casteism). But the complex and very *modern* stigmas of caste demonstrate that certain prejudices are integral to the education/health care matrix that is development. The imagination of development itself requires that certain persons remain in the category of recipients, and cannot be purveyors of the magic (Escobar 1995; Pigg 1992, 1997). It is these persons, against whom the educated and rational self is defined, who must present themselves as always in the realm of the uneducated (even if with the occasional wink). While Preeti was undeniably stigmatized by her community, her treatment within institutional structures was also demeaning—on the same, though subtly transformed, basis as her community's prejudices. In such engagements, through the way not only access *to* care, but the very nature of who is entitled to provide it, "untouchability" is effaced as an overt category and replaced with notions of immorality, laziness, criminality, and ignorance (borne of lack of education), or slips into discourse on hygiene, effort, and responsibility. The effect of such institutional practices (and their ersatz correlates) is that caste- and class-based forms of discrimination are performed in a context that erases caste (and at times class) as explicit signifiers.

Medical interventions may depoliticize social problems by offering technical solutions (Ferguson 1994), but their use as point of reference is often in the service of political relations. Rayna Rapp

suggests that "communication" does not always suffice to promote
changes in behavior, especially when there is a difference in power
between the "health care personnel" and clients (Rapp 1988). Likewise, in Tamil Nadu, Cecilia Van Hollen argues that the symbolic
content of health-related messages is less important than the social
hierarchies such messages reassert (2003). In Sitapur, while such
observations apply, we must also ask what the neutrality means; in
other words, what it means that communication (training, talk) also
resituates power relationships (such as those based on caste or land
ownership) on new ground, one ostensibly free of power. This shift
transforms hierarchical relationships into a narrative in which progress is constituted on the basis of ideals of equality and availability
to all.

Should the wrong person try to carry off mimesis, their failures reveal inconsistencies which are, at their strongest, articles of bad faith.
The first are the ideas that the universal knowledge (of medicine
and development) precedes power and legitimacy, and that power
(economic, political, self-mastery) and authority in a modernizing
world come from right understanding instead of being mutually constitutive, a series of relations (Dirks 1994). In these cases, the performance of right understanding as legitimizing and natural truth
constitutes power. The second set of deceits concerns the bundling
of education and equality: that medicine and development embrace
politics separate from the interests of particular groups or individuals, as asserted in global health policy (V. Adams 1998); that the legitimacy of development is available to all who enter into certain
universalized ways of knowing by participation in authorizing structures; that universal knowledge manifests in the same way and is
equally available to all who seek it out. These lies can be seen as
cousins of the bad faith underlying the colonial venture, in which
performance of Enlightenment-based political models in the service
of colonial rule reveals the instability of those models at their source
(Bhabha 1994; Prakash 1999). Or, the matter of hidden contradictions might be inherent to ideologies more generally, such that the
"materialization of ideology" reveals "antagonisms" which "the explicit formulation of ideology can not afford to acknowledge" (Žižek
1997: 4). And all are situated in a deeper set of bad faith acts—the
denial of the core relationship between desire and action/response
embodied in the ration card (useless), the *anganwadi* worker (gone),
the school (on *chutti* today), the acronym, the closing off of the official ways that poverty and hunger might be alleviated just a little
bit. Either way, when models of equality based on education, med-

icine, and "uplift" are put into practice, equality for all is precluded
and what remains is the Orwellian equality for some.

There is a tension particular to public health, between universal
availability and emphasis on a single population (Foucault 1994); we
might consider that it is this tension that is expressed in bad faith.
On the one hand, it might be suggested that references to equality
and universality are ultimately only teleological, as health care development is, like social medicine, *explicitly* (not just from the perspective of its critics) about the welfare of a certain class of people—
the poor—rather than aimed at all classes, a formulation related, as
Foucault suggests, to the origins of social medicine in Europe in which
state efforts were aimed explicitly at maintaining the laboring class
(2000). But on the other hand, missionary medicine in the late nineteenth century created inroads into local communities *because* of its
claims to availability for all (Fitzgerald 2001: 113). The "penetrating
power" of medicine into all levels of society enabled it to be part of
the matrix of colonial hegemony, integral to the assertion of European superiority to indigenous populations (Arnold 1993).

Ultimately, regardless of their general or specific intent, development, health interventions and their "schemes" are always negotiated in terms of local political relations (V. Adams 1998; Ferguson
1994). But the everyday practices of those on the margins of institutions demand that we shift attention away from the separation of
local politics from institutional ones. They suggest, at least for this
part of India, a complicity of institutional forms of legitimacy with
hierarchies of political power, control over resources, and symbolic
stigmatization that characterize so much of rural life. Yet, as these
are the figures to whom many turn for health care, they also show
that it is the familiarity of these practices that makes them all the
more powerful. What disappears is a distinction between center and
the periphery as the breach between a home-ground of modernity
and its points of insertion. Quasi-institutional practitioners like Pratima and the *pradhan* are not "merely" mimetic or even "quasi" to
development. They are, rather, as raw is to cooked, part of the grand,
inspiring, and desire-provoking myth that is social improvement,
mythical in the sense Roland Barthes (1973) intended, not as a falsehood, but as a narrative site of power become naturalized as real and
inevitable. The mimetic performance is part of the original—indeed,
the very part that keeps it going in spaces from which it always threatens to disappear.

Chapter 4

SEEING
VISUALITY IN PREGNANCY

Unseen

*A*t the midpoint of my fieldwork, after my husband's brief visit has come
to an end, I begin to crave achar. *I cannot get enough of the tart mango
pickle Bari Bhabhi made last year. She laughs and rolls her eyes as she brings
down, one more time, the fluorescent yellow stained plastic jug from the top
of the wall in the inner kitchen and spoons a dollop next to my rice and dal.
An older sister-in-law visiting from Lucknow notices my plate. She raises her
eyebrows to Bari Bhabhi. "Isko kuch hai?" Is something up with her?
Earlier, I had laughed off Bari Bhabhi's cryptic—"Now your husband has
left and you will never be alone again," so she says. "No, it's nothing like
that." But a few weeks later, after I sneak the instructionless, for-hospital-
use-only pregnancy kit into the outhouse and watch the telltale double pink
line appear, I think to myself, among other happinesses and worries, about
trash and visibility: Where oh where can I get rid of this piece of plastic that
says so much?*

*I am at a wedding in Bari Bhabhi's sasural when the nausea hits. A
weeklong celebration of events, guests, cooking, banquets, pujas, videos shown
at top volume all night in village public spaces—this is not a good place to
feel this way. Bari Bhabhi and I, with a shifting array of other women, bed
down in a room on the roof on a floor padded with piles of hay. We draw
from a mountain of rented mattresses to soften our sleep, and stay up late
chatting, as gunshots, screams, and tinny music of B-movies infiltrate the
night air from the outdoor VCR and rigged-up speakers. One morning, the
aroma of onion and garlic hits me differently—oily, cloying, it seems to pen-*

etrate; smell becomes substance. It further blanches my face and sends me running to the gutter out back. I have never vomited quite so much.

Bari Bhabhi—whom I have been told I should here call by her given name, Uma—a dignified, grown-woman kind of name—helps me get biscuits and fruits, and manages my concealment even as she manages disclosure of my "condition." Women are understanding. No one says much other than, "The nausea has come, no?" I am humiliated by the way I cannot help but demand assistance. But Bari Bhabhi is not all kindness. She laughs at me publicly for my dehati, *low-class choice of bangles. "What are you wearing?" she demands, when I arrive, wearing the thick glass bracelets in alternating dark and light blue that I had long admired on Pushpadevi's arm. "You look like a village woman," she says, calling over her mother and sister-in-laws to see. She calls more than usual attention to my bad grammar and worse sari choices. Over the week I can't ignore a guilty feeling of betrayal, in small moments where I am left hanging, teasing she seems to take too much pleasure in, a range of insistences, demands, and unwanted disclosures. I think that perhaps this has been a long time coming. I wonder what pregnancy means to her.*

Bari Bhabhi makes a brother and sister-in-law take me into town to buy more appropriate bangles and meet some other relatives. I get through the trip and stock up on bananas and oranges. Back in Bari Bhabhi's maike, *amid the comings and goings, a friend phones for me from Lucknow—miraculously managing to reach me here in a different district from the one where I normally stay. There, phone lines are all but unworkable, and when Rohit plays "phone" he shouts into his hand, "Who is it? Who is it? I can't hear? The line has been cut." But here, the phone rings regularly—calls come in and calls go out. In what feels like a rupture from patterns of quiet disclosure and subtle concealment I do what helps me counteract, for a moment, the betrayals of my body, onions, garlic, and Uma. I tell my friend, in English, my news. He is as happy as I am, and exclaims about being an uncle. But even then, I find myself speaking sideways. I can't quite bring myself to say the word "pregnancy" among so many people. Throughout the week, in this house crowded with people, in these kitchens and roofs bustling with women, through the circulations of people, food, and gifts, among the unfamiliar faces, I struggle to conceal my nausea and also to manage it. Some things I cannot conceal or control, some things I never knew until now that I should. In a way different from that joked about in the songs Bari Bhabhi's aunties sing late into the night, with the physical and sensory intensity of a wedding comes, for me, the physical and sensory intensity of pregnancy, in the sleeplessness and lack of* akelapan *(aloneness/loneliness). In this sociality in which eating, sleeping, dressing, bathing, adorning, peeing, and defecating are shared acts, I begin to learn a new boundary between the*

visible and concealed. I become aware, in my constant failures, of the impor-
tance of staying at precisely this critical space between concealment and dis-
closure, seeing and hiding.

Dialectics of vision shape bodily experience—especially that associated with generativity—in north India in the home and in institutions. They oriented my own experience of being pregnant there, just
as they frame the ways pregnancy is known, kept safe, threatened,
and brought into the glare (or the shadows) of the clinic. As in the
plays of language and meaning and motion around the placenta, so
much about well-being depends on the ways visibility's binary is
crossed, in the constant motion between concealment and revelation.
"Knowledge," universalized or situated, can be collapsed into this *lila,*
as the perceptive qualities of knowing shape models of emancipation
and progress, the broad scope of critique and intervention.

From many angles, visuality's relationship to power comes to a
point of crisis in clinical encounters and in the subjective conflicts
wrought by clinical modes of surveillance, on the one hand, and
spectacle on the other. In biomedical, "technocratic" (Davis-Floyd
1992), and "Fordist" (Martin 1987) births, Foucault's "clinical gaze" is
at once underlying and literalized, a paramount mode of perceiving
the female body, just as the categories solidified by forms of knowledge may also amount to specific modes of seeing, revealing, and
establishing "truth" (Foucault 1975).[1] For Foucault, the clinical gaze
is defined by its roving, rather than penetrative eye, and the "truth"
constituted in its beam one of "the concrete sensibility, a gaze that
travels from body to body, and whose trajectory is situated in the
space of sensible manifestation" (120). This panoptic, scanning sensibility is literalized in medicalized birth—not just via the lines of
sight of the clinician, but by the ways they are extended by technologies of seeing—speculums, ultrasound, imaging; in apparatuses
that attract or disrupt the gaze—fetal and uterine monitors, bodily
positions for birthing; by forms of imagery—photographs, diagrams,
charts, paintings, film. At the confluence of image and epistemology, visuality in childbearing is part of the way cultural, economic,
and political models inform gender and personhood and what it is
to "have" or "inhabit" or "experience" or "be" a body, especially one
that reproduces (or doesn't) (Martin 1987, 1994; Jordanova 1989;
Newman 1996). Images locate female bodies in political and religious
movements (Ginsburg 1989; Newman 1996) and technologies of seeing provide new ground for gender biases (Patel 1989) just as technologies of fertility confer new and old modes of kinship (Rothman

1986; Strathern 1992) and new forms of diagnosis "disambiguate" and offer certainty in some arenas of life while posing new crises, tensions, and moral dilemmas in others (Rapp 2000: 205)

But even as they aim to "disambiguate," gazes of and in clinical spaces can also be astigmatic, imperfect extensions of an idealized lens. Likewise, they do not stand alone, but encounter and entangle with other modes of seeing, other power/knowledge/sight equations. Where the "observing gaze" of/in the (idealized) clinic, as Foucault described it, is purely perceptive, "bound up with a certain silence" (1975: 107), sight can also be communicative and constitutive, as feminist theorists and those with attention to gazes in nonbiomedical frames have been aware. In Sitapur, visuality plays variously stable and unstable roles in pregnancy and in the institutions and interventions that glance at it. It offers material for rethinking the hegemony of the "clinical gaze" over pregnancy, for exploring convergent and divergent processes by which subjectivities are constituted through regulations of sight and disclosure. In considering vision and embodiment in the paradoxical marginality/"interior" of *dehat,* I locate my starting point less in genealogies in which the "ineluctable" quality of visual metaphors (Jay 1993: 1) points back to a stable, if at times unstably situated self, and less in the Foucaultian sense that vision is part of the bag of tricks by which power is shifted from external forces to within the self. I find myself moving between remarkably resonant phenomenologies of vision and those of being seen, different economies of sight, different ideas about how seeing *works.*

In one such vision, gender inhabits precisely that space between seeing and being seen, and gendered subjectivities are part of the way "knowledge" is constituted in this gap. For instance, French feminist Luce Irigaray asks how shadows and gazes fall around sight and subjectivity for "woman." For Irigaray, gaze is a mode of gendering the subject. The "specular" gaze involves a male self projecting his image onto the feminine, effacing it and rendering it sightless and voiceless except in his own terms. Ontologically at odds with the feminine it at once observes and denies, the objectifying gaze determines the nature of knowing. Knowledge is predicated on a subject-object divide that makes all "self-knowledge" false, such that all "theory of the subject" is "appropriated by the masculine" (Irigaray 1985: 133). "Woman certainly does not know everything (about herself)," Irigaray writes, "She doesn't know (herself to be) anything" (231). Indeed, by succumbing to a "theory of the subject," woman renounces "the specificity of her own relationship to the imaginary"—her ability to be a subject in terms of her own perceptive and creative stance (133). In a way, the constitution of identities of resistance that Partha Chatterjee, speaking of anticolonial nationalism, posits as occurring in the private realm gendered female, at a remove from the colonial gaze (1993), is not dissimilar to Irigaray's sense of the female imaginary. The female self, she says, is constituted elsewhere than where the male gaze falls, expressed on the basis of its own "otherness" (Irigaray 1985: 143). To "fully know" is, then, to fail to know, as full disclosure is a particular (male) encounter with the other.

There is, here, ambiguity on the matter of essences, one that troubles (even as it inspires) conversations about "modernity" in settings imagined as "nonmodern" in a range of idioms. Translated into the context of postcolonial (and anthropological) "encounters," "essences" pose a dilemma of the other. Irigaray's language is similar to other French feminist responses to psychoanalysis, in which female selfhood exists as a site of fundamental difference. It has been suggested that the female "essence" posited by Irigaray is less a monolithic category than a strategy for exposing a contradiction within Aristotelian metaphysics—that woman is considered to have an essence *as* woman, but is relegated to object status and thus denied absolute "Essence." Irigaray may, indeed, explore female access to one's own "essence" without describing of what it might consist or foreclosing the possibility of "multiple" and "contradictory" selves (Fuss 1992: 109).

In terms of the body, it is not only symptoms or etiologies, but sensation and perception that can take different forms, meaning that the body, to paraphrase Shigehisa Kuriyama, is known differently because it is felt differently (1999: 55) in forms not quite "essential," but also broadly "divergent." In this sense, those concerned, like Irigaray, Frantz Fanon (1967), and others, with the gendering and racializing of "gaze" might be thought of standing on a slippery ground between metaphor and phenomenology. In Sitapur, gaze is not only about perception, not merely about establishing "subjects" and "objects," and gazes are at once gendered and gendering. In this setting, gaze can be as much a transmutable substance and communicative act as a mode of perception and knowledge. Seeing can transform, threaten, and makes divine an always-fluid self (Eck 1985). In a broadly Hindu frame, while textual and orthodox visions do not necessarily align with the way things are "on the ground," it can be said that sight involves palpable and transmuting essences of different kind and different effect. Among them are *darsan*, divine seeing that constitutes a relationship between devotee and divine, and *nazar*, the so-called "evil eye." In both, seeing is about more than "knowledge" of the other—it entails transfer of emotion and effects both gazer and gazed-upon (Eck 1985). Such "visual and visionary culture" (Eck 1985: 10) involves acts of worship oriented around ocular communion in which the divine becomes "present in the visible world," knowable by seeing. The fact that, "In India's own terms, seeing is knowing," arises from, Diana Eck says, Hinduism's insistence on the tangible experience of both truth and divinity (1985: 11). Religious seekers, pilgrims, and "sacred sightseers" travel vast distances for the *darsan* of deities embodied in images and statues, as well as of temples, teachers, natural sites, and divine places (1985: 5).

Beyond idealized relationship with the divine, Eck says, in all aspects of life, seeing is a means of "reaching for" or "touching" tangible truth or the beloved: "Whenever Hindus affirm the meaning of life, death and suffering, they affirm with their eyes wide open" (1985: 11). Sight communicates earthly love as well, sending desire in channels proper and improper. In descriptions of their weddings, men and women often emphasize seeing their bride or groom for the first time, and the moment of first gaze climactic for those who gaze upon it as much as for those caught in its bind. In the cinematic flairs of love-marriage, it is through visual union that sparks of love are first ignited. In Indian films too numerous to mention, love begins with the eyes, at accidental meeting of glances, conveyed to we who watch and swoon as the screen goes soft and the sitar or mandolin or sarangi or synthesizer ripples.

The way that gendered, tangible, communicative, and objectifying gazes force us to consider a range of ways of locating "knowledge" in relation to sight suggests a range of ways of experiencing longing and threat, of thinking about what seeing and being seen *do*. The clinic is not the only place where power and vision converge. Rather than locating subjectivity at the juncture between gaze and gazed-upon, I would like to think about gazes—of different kinds, different mechanisms and in ever-shifting levels of meaning (metaphoric, symbolic, literal)—in circulation and encounter with each other. Where it is easy to imagine gazing as active, it may be more difficult to consider the engaged quality of being gazed upon, though this too is part of the interplay of power and knowledge. For rural women, a range of gazes—converging and diverging—mean that seeing and being seen are integral to relationships forged with each other, with kin, with institutions, in all their shady unreliability, and institutional imaginaries.

Seeing (and) the bride

Preparations for Preeti's stepdaughter's bidai *have been going on since last night. Men from Chhaya's* sasural *arrived yesterday and were given food by her family. The men sat out until late in the night playing cards and listening to a loud cassette tape of* bidai git*—songs celebrating marriage, hinting at sexuality, and telling happy stories about the young bride's departure for her husband's village. One song casts this as new kind of event—"Oh how times have changed," the singer tells us, "the bride used to leave in an ox-cart, now she rides off on a motorcycle. Her sister used to visit wearing* selwar-kameez*, now her girlfriend comes wearing pants and a blouse." The men finally sleep in the ox-cart that brought them—the motorcycle's presence in song enough to cast a sheen of affluence on their dreams.*

In the morning I pass the men on my way to Preeti's house. They do not look up from their cards. I step over a beak, talons, and bloody feathers. There will be meat for Chhaya's feast. In the outer room Chhaya is standing with her dewar*, her husband's younger brother. They laugh and joke and she keeps her head covered with her* pallu*. The groom has not come, but it doesn't matter—his brother will bring Chhaya back. The men will all leave after another meal, before Chhaya's own departure in a tempo (auto-rickshaw). This is not her first* bidai*, I have been told—she had the first one, the big one, nearly a year ago. She must have been about sixteen at the time, though she cannot tell me her exact age. At that time she went for two days, then came back, as seems to be the norm. Her husband, still spoken of as "the groom," and his family have summoned her again. This time it will be for longer, she says. Maybe a month, she doesn't know.*

The morning is filled largely with cooking—Preeti and Kulu's Mother fry puris *to be sent among the gifts. I ask Kulu's Mother if Preeti is keeping track of the number. She taps her chest and says quietly, "I count them." The bangle seller comes, and a small crowd of neighbor girls and boys amasses to watch her choose. Chhaya folds her hands in reverence and prayer and touches the bangles, then touches her head. She asks me to photograph her as she does this.*

More cooking, more feeding, the afternoon wears on, and talk about the men's impatience begins to rumble. Something is happening, confusion about the transport. The tempo that had been called did not arrive. Someone has been sent back to the crossroad. In the meantime, Chhaya is a center of activity—the reverse of the eye of a storm. She is watched by a growing crowd of children and teenage girls, her cousins, neighbors, girls from the other side of the village whom she barely knows, as she bathes at the hand pump, soaping through her clothes, scrubbing for ages. She moves from an old blouse and petticoat into newer ones without exposing anything. People peek through the grass wall separating angans. *Sitting in the corner, Chhaya calls for her younger sister, Vinita, to bring nail polish and red coloring for her feet. Around herself, on the ground, Chhaya arranges a mirror, a comb, stalks of dried grass to apply the color. As she brushes her hair, oils her arms, puts on makeup, colors her feet and puts polish on fingernails and toenails, the crowd grows and I marvel—in my own aversion to being stared at—that she can seem so oblivious, display so little sign of either loving or hating being on stage.*

She asks someone to bring a bag from the back room—this one containing lipstick, bindis, *and* sindhur. *A few well-placed strokes of red, and the "girl of the village" becomes "bride." Preeti stops cooking to help put on necklaces and earrings. Chhaya pulls out her nose ring and replaces the small flower with a large gold hoop. She moves to the middle room, on the other side of the* angan. *The crowd eddies and swirls around her.*

By now it is late afternoon. The men have left, taking baskets of goods. Chhaya opens a suitcase and takes out a sari. She stands and begins to wrap it. After laboriously folding the pleats (she is still new at this) it becomes clear that she has not left enough material for the anchal. *She unfolds it and starts again. Observers whisper, "She has to do it again." "Why? What's wrong?" "There's not enough for the* anchal." *She does this three times, wrapping, letting pleats unfurl, refolding, measuring the remainder, letting it all unfurl again. Women from the crowd offer advice—"Measure it." "Count the pleats." "Hold the fabric like this." But they do not step forward. On the fourth go she succeeds, folds the* anchal *over her shoulder and pulls the front down to cover her stomach, putting a large pin at the pleats in the shoulder. She reaches into a polyethylene bag suspended from a nail in the wall and pulls out a little pill. She asks me for some water. I get her some, and she swallows the pill. I am perplexed—I don't know what it is, and no one can tell me.*

This process has taken hours. Through all of it Chhaya barely communicates—asking only for the occasional object. Slowly, she closes the suitcase and wipes it with a rag. While everyone is talking about the tempo that has not come, Chhaya is a picture of equanimity. I feel such deliberation in her actions, wonder if she knows something we do not—as though she will finish getting ready, stand up, walk out just as the tempo arrives.

But there is more work to be done.

She sits on the floor and puts her head down on her knees. Slowly, with what feels like the same precision she used to put on her makeup, she begins to cry. First small gasps, then larger shaking ones. Everyone watches. "She is crying now." When it is clear that a tempo has finally arrived, Preeti pulls Chhaya by the arm. Stepmother and stepdaughter lean onto each other's shoulder and start to wail. The cry is high pitched, specific to the bidai, *rec-*

ognizable in tone and form. They move through the now-large crowd of
women and children. This is the climax, the moment everyone has come to
see, and many eyes, including mine, well with tears. Chhaya is passed from
her stepmother to her aunt, they embrace and cry. They stop in front of me,
and I think Chhaya is going to embrace me to, so I lean in. She holds me
and sobs, but briefly. As she pulls back Preeti signals that they want me to
take a picture. She and Chhaya stand facing me, holding very still, their
grief well composed on their faces. I take two pictures; they move on. I notice
that Chhaya does not embrace her sister, from whom she is usually insepa-
rable, for whom she is protector from Preeti's rages. Vinita is not crying, not
silently, not loudly.

Chhaya is now wrapped in a shawl and her head is entirely covered. As
Preeti guides her, Chhaya's father steps out of the crowd. He hugs her; his
sobs are not loud and womanly, but they shake his body. He pulls away.
"Don't cry, don't cry," he says to Chhaya through his own tears, "You have
been sick. Be careful and take care of your health." Chhaya gets into the
tempo. Vinita gets in with her, holding the suitcase on her lap. The driver
revs the engine. With a shudder it pulls away. Chhaya's dewar, *who will*
accompany her to his village, walks behind and throws candy to the crowd.
The children's faces lurch from grief to glee—if expressions could get whip-
lash these would. Kids lunge for the candy. People disperse. Preeti and her
husband go in the house. I see that Kulu's Mother is standing further down
the road, by herself, watching the tempo drive away. We can almost hear
Chhaya's loud sobs over the engine. Or even if we can't, we imagine we do.

In South Asia, gaze—and its regulation—have been considered extensively for the way they relate to the female life cycle and, notably,
the modes of subordination contained therein. Representations of
Indian women emphasize the place of concealment in relationships
between men and women and in restrictions on women's movements
under a male gaze. These accounts fall, roughly, into two camps,
both of which place veiling, or *purdah*, as a sign of women's status,
strategies, and condition. First are more popular and intervention-
oriented accounts, rendering *purdah* a counterpoint to modernity, a
perplexing persistence of "tradition" in a country showing "other"
signs of more "modern" forms of women's emancipation. Countless
book covers and titles of volumes such as *Indian Women: From Pur-*
dah to Modernity attest to this (B. Nanda 1976). As a trope of travel
literature and journalism both Western and Indian, and as integral
to both colonial and nationalist accounts of women's "role" in Indian society, concealment (and, by association, constricted vision)
involves concepts of subordination in which being seen entails full

sovereignty, full participation as a rights-bearing subject. Here, the image is a potent part of narratives of personhood and citizenship. In colonial accounts, this preclusion of sovereignty, paradoxically, helps to justify the colonial venture (cf. Mani 1985), just as in anti-colonial reforms "the image of womanhood was more important than the reality" (Chakravarti 1997: 78).

Second, and often in response to accounts in which visuality is rendered part of control over women, is the long history of ethnographic engagement with layerings of subordination and subtleties of resistance, challenges to what appears, "under Western eyes" (Mohanty 1991), as patent oppression. (Of course, in this context, "Western eyes" are as much an abstract mode of critique as literal, localized gaze—the critical gaze is not always "Western," just as "the West" has been effectively relocated as a shifting mode of being.) Self-protection, religious modalities, expressions of sexuality, and critique are, in these accounts, the less-overt aims of veiling and seclusion, integral to protection and expression, and taken up by women as much as they are taken on critically by them, as much as they are imposed by others (Raheja and Gold 1994). Doranne Jacobson's 1977 account of an abstracted, idealized rural north Indian woman is exemplary in this regard, describing the bivalency of female sexuality (at once feared and necessary for reproduction) and women's roles as mother (life-giving and potentially life-taking), and the complementary nature of gender roles (Jacobson 1977: 60). Jacobson describes *purdah* as a mark of high status that offers a measure of protection from a male gaze while contributing to women's subordination (1977: 63-64). Both Jacobson (1977) and Susan Wadley (1975) note that while textual sources of orthodoxy such as the Laws of Manu render veiling and seclusion matters of control (of women's movements, sexuality, and capacity to pollute), women's daily lives are at a far remove from these formulations. Prohibitions involving both self-protection and control speak to the complex force of *shakti,* women's power, and its presence in lives both everyday and divine (Wadley 1975). Other accounts emphasize the ways women's seclusion, as control of sexuality, is a sign of male honor and prestige and *purdah* inseparable from the honor of kin networks and the patriline (Mandelbaum 1988).

In Sitapur, the tension between these two (loosely grouped) gazes on gazes is diffused into broader moral, spatial, and temporal concepts. Modes of seeing and being seen, moral imperatives to regulate gazes and deflect glances (one's own and others) locate gaze—as mode of perception and action—into the power(s) that flow through the gendered life cycle and the changing, changeable social world. Within the movements constituting love, marriage, sexuality, and reproduction (not necessarily in that order), what has been thought of as "restriction" on visibility and gazes also constitutes modes of protection, the shaping of affect, the stirrings of political conviction—in other words, the things that implant "modes of personhood" in the world. Beginning at marriage, just as a (rural) woman's emotional life is likely to be divided between worlds of affinal and consanguineal kin, reproduction and sexuality involve a play of tensions between things told and kept secret, displays of concealment and concealment of display. Sociality, identity, and morality, the ways a person becomes *suhagin* (an auspicious married woman), can be largely shaped by successes and failures in navigating disclosure—the *ghungat* pulled over all but a quarter-moon of the face, held firmly in place by the teeth in the presence of some, or pulled over the back of the head, only suggesting veiling, preserving modesty while displaying a sensibility more urban and enlightened.

Veiling signifies location as well, providing a way of knowing and mapping the unfamiliar, just as it is a means of recognizing power in its complex gradations. Carefully arranged scenes I was asked to photograph—of women lined up in the middle of blossoming mustard fields, or in front of the house, or against the most prettily decorated *angan* wall—become, long after the fact, keys for my memory to local identity and kinship. Women married into the village have veils pulled over head and face, women born to the house have uncovered heads. Pushapdevi told me, as her eldest daughter prepared greens for their meal and we talked about the way daughters become wives, that while she gets annoyed by the rules of *ghungat* or *purdah*, its imperative means that the bride stands for not only the honor of the family, but its appropriate display of location in broader maps: "If a new bride comes, if the father-in-law is there, or the elder brother-in-law, and people of the village, the community … then you should hide your face so no one can see. If someone big comes to our house, then I have to keep *purdah* in front of him. The people of the house make [the bride] do it … It's only like this in the village."

Choti Bhabhi puts the visual economy in slightly different terms: "In the cities all the houses are closed, so you cannot see what is happening in the house next door, you don't know even if a guest has come. Everyone does everything closed up. You never know anything because you can't see it."

The geopolitico-moral topographies that locate "village" and "city" also locate modesty and emancipation as possible and necessary ways of being. Such diacritical imaginaries are situated in the already-fluid space of "the village," in which interlopers are a regular feature and "the local" itself is an imaginary of boiled-down realities. Anjali, a schoolteacher from Agra placed in a nearby elementary school, lived with her young son in a rented a room near the central temple. She was teased, "This one never covers her head. If you don't cover your head, how will people know you are married?"

"I wear a sari," she laughed. "Everyone is obsessed with veiling," she said turning to me. "You must veil, you must veil. But look at these women—their stomachs are exposed up to here, their breasts are hanging out, but they have their heads covered." Concealment as modesty and concealment as display converge and collide with visions of bourgeois modesty and emancipation, mapped onto the ever-circulating locatedness of "these women."

As Pratima's training and naming showed, versions of disclosure converge in women's use of their names—on the use of given or "household" names in the *maike,* and kin terms in the *sasural,* where her name must not be spoken by or around her affinal kin, even as children refer to their mothers by a term for paternal kin. For some, the "absence" of a name signifies the undervaluing of women, the subsuming of personhood into kin and reproductive capacity, the relational identity of women (Kakar 1981; Khare 1992). "A woman is never herself, she is always somebody's mother, somebody's wife," said Bari Bhabhi. But in another register the withholding of names is not imposed upon women but is demanded *by* them as a means of protection from other women, based less on lack of identity than on concern for the closeness of names to the *heart* of identity, for the uses to which names can be put. "If someone knows your name," Pushpadevi said, "and you get into a fight, they will use your name to bring you to harm" (cf. Woodburne 1981: 58)—an item of "blind belief" often referred to in urban locales and intervention-oriented spaces.[2] Men tease wives and elders about this concern, skirting the edges of their sexuality. They may teasingly reveal older women's names (or give outrageous-sounding false names) to provoke anger or embarrassment, or ask a child to say her mother's name. Women's concern about use of their names can extend to a refusal to give names in official contexts. Raju, who kept local polling records, said, "They might say, 'I'm Madhuri Dixit' [a popular film star], or 'I'm Indira Gandhi' and I have to find their names another way." Where women's names evoke an immediacy that conveys a tinge of sexuality and a nearness to the self, and where women fear revealing their names to the state, it is through state and institutional agencies that women gain social permission to use them—as in the case of NAFPA or other settings where women are "local agents" of one scheme or another.

Economies of exposure orient living spaces as well. Courtyards are the partially concealed domain of women, open to the sky but invisible to outsiders (except the rooftops of immediate neighbors); verandas are more arguably male (though less so for lower-caste women who are less likely to be bound by or adhere to such spatializations of concealment). Inside rooms are dark and private spaces of closed cupboards and closed eyes, of storage, sex, and sleep. Rooftops are in between, affording a glimpse down at the world, but with limited exposure to its gazes. Women, in their management of the bodily and sensory boundaries of household (through gaze as much as through food consumption), protect interiors, often within moral idioms involving the eyes and gendered idioms of power and threat. As Bari Bhabhi reminded me often when I returned from the Pasi neighborhood: "We don't want them in here. We know they will look at all the stuff and say, 'This is kept here, that is kept there,' and go and tell their husbands so they can come and steal it. Those people are dangerous. What men will go and sit inside a house? But women go inside the house, they look around [literally "apply their gaze"]. This looking around, seeing what people have? This is woman's work."

Where seeing threatens, it also involves shared emotion. It acknowledges the new—newcomers, those with a new status—and punctuates change. I was frequently visited by groups of people coming "to see," or called to houses so that a guest might "see" me. People advised me, on different occasions, that I should go to the home of a person (often people I had never met) recently returned from hospital because "everyone will be going to see," or to a home where someone had died in order to "see" the corpse. Such acknowledgment is also part of the socialities of emotion, a way to "share" or "divide" grief. Mandates and desires to "see"—the new, the visitor, the transformed, the resplendent, the bride, the groom, the sick, the injured, the dead—are based in a mode of communion in which visual witnessing does not objectify or efface the subject, but rather shares an essence or emotion and facilitates transformation. Such things become replicable with the aid of the camera lens, as experience, emotion, and communion remain as traces in the image. Photography may solidify the object of gaze into a static image, may "capture" beauty and tragedy, but more importantly, it enables continued socialities, ongoing participation in the weight—or levity—of the moment. Susan Sontag suggests that photography allows for the appropriation, replication, and redefinition of reality, constituting a consumption-oriented way of being/knowing (1976). But in rural India, photographs are not just images to be consumed. They are points and objects of communication. Photographs of the bride are more than shows of beauty, just as images of the dead are more than memorials.

After the festival of Holi, I return from a brief stay in Delhi, where I have mostly been sleeping off nausea and trying to keep food down. I ride out to Devia to see Pratima Srivastav. When I arrive, she says, "Oh, we haven't seen you for a while."

"I wanted to come by for Holi, but I was unwell and away."

She nods her head to the side. "Bhaiya [Sunderlal] came by and said you weren't well."

"Do you know the reason why?" I ask.

She nods her head, then looks away quietly. Though I know better, I push the matter—I have been eager to hear what she has to say. "I have had many problems." She looks up and says, now in her normal tone of voice, "Yes, I was so sick too during that time. For five months I couldn't take any food, I couldn't tolerate the smell of anything. I wrapped my pallu *around my head like this, see?" She pulls the fabric tightly around her mouth and looks to me like a bandit from a western. "You must eat lots of iron. Are you taking the pills?"*

"I try, but it's difficult."

"One way to keep from vomiting—find a dirt wall, a kaccha *one. Spit on it. Then smell the dirt until you begin to feel better."*

Her youngest daughter brings out tea and biscuits. I struggle to eat them, though the sweet chai is satisfying as is the damp coolness of the room, a respite from what feels like an onslaught of sensations, of sounds, smells, and sunlight, that I have never experienced this way before. Pratima pulls out a photo album. I think, a wedding, another bride. But the page shows a baby, no, more like a toddler, its eyes half open, its body dressed in a clean, pressed frock. It is held to the camera by the arms of someone whose face is not in the frame.

"My oldest daughter ... this is her baby. She passed away." [Literally, "is finished."]

"Oh ho. How sad. How big was she?"

"About seven months." The baby looks much older to me, though the angle of her body makes its size difficult to discern.

"What happened?"

"She died. Bari dukh se. *With great sadness. It was very sudden—she*

got sick and within an hour and a half she was dead. Nobody knows what happened."

I look again. I now realize that she is not showing me a picture of the child in life, but in death.

"This is at that time?" I ask.

Pratima nods, then turns the page. Another picture, again a close-up of the child, its head at an awkward angle against the elbow of the male arms that hold it, its legs on someone's lap. The dress is frilly and black and pink. Pratima turns the page again. The father now, next to the child in someone else's lap; a crowd of faces, mostly young ones—children, teenagers—surrounds him. His mouth is open in what I can only imagine to be a wail of grief, its frozen activity jarring against the passive composure of the child. The faces around him look as though they have been struck. Pratima turns the page again. In this one her daughter sits on the charpai *holding the child in her lap. Her other children—four boys—are around her, their faces wet with tears, and her own expression unreachable.*

I struggle to figure out what I am supposed to say, and to contain and conceal the welling up of my own cultural bounds of sensation … the sense of wrongness, that I should not see "reproduced to infinity," as Roland Barthes said, "what could never be repeated existentially" (1981: 4). But, I realize, rather than objectifying and depersonalizing in a slip from the real to the less real, in the repetition of the image what has been reproduced is intensely personal, the emotion contained in the continued enfolding of the real. Grief has been further distributed, further divided, as Bari Bhabhi tells me happens when people come to a home to see the newly dead, to see the mother who has lost a child. Even if we cannot, as Bari Bhabhi tells me, communicate, "This too happened to me," we do so implicitly with our eyes. For me, however, it is not the image but its casing that moves me most, though I feel uneasy about this the moment I am aware of it. But at the same time, something about this way of seeing and sharing experience points to the very immanence of death—that way by which, as Barthes, again, says, a photograph "is wholly ballasted by the contingency of which it is the weightless, transparent envelope" (1981: 5). What are we capable of doing with our eyes and their surrogates?

Pregnancy and disclosure

"Did you tell that woman?"

"Who?"

"That one you go see."

"Rambal ki Dulhan?" (Rambal's wife—i.e., Pushpadevi.)

"Yes. Did you tell her?"

"Yes, they know. But they figured it out on their own."

"Don't tell anyone else. Absolutely don't tell anyone else. It would be very bad if the whole village knows."

Kamlesh's Grandmother comes by when I am writing in the outer yard. She sits down near me and says, "I heard you are not feeling well."

I say I have been vomiting a lot. "I have medicine, but I don't want to take it."

She shakes her head. "And your husband so far away. He doesn't even know."

"No, he knows. I told him by phone from Munniabad."

She nods slowly, carefully. "Good."

Sitting on the veranda of Pushpadevi's house with the usual crew. Pushpadevi's devrani *(sister-in-law) says I should have a* taviz *(protective amulet) made for me to protect the baby and help me feel better. Perhaps my illness is from too much "showing," too much "talking." I ask where I can get one and she says, "My husband can get one for you." She holds up a* taviz *tied around her neck. "He got this one in Devia."*

I say, "So does this mean?" She smiles, pulling her pallu *over her mouth until only her eyes are showing.*

I ask how many months. She stays behind her pallu *and holds up two fingers. Pushpadevi, always concerned with my comprehension, laughs and holds out her hand as if to slap me. "You have understood," she says. Then we talk about nausea, about the things one wants to eat and the things one cannot stomach. The* pallu *comes down, her face is exposed and we speak openly and freely, never having said a word about "pregnancy."*

Again in my spot on Pushpadevi's veranda, talking with Shalini's Dadi who is, Pushpadevi swears, close to 100. A precious moment, a gem of a conversation. She is sharing stories, telling me about babies she delivered in her long, long lifetime. A young woman walks by on the path from the fields that goes by the doorstep. She is one of a group of women who tease and make fun of me, mocking my misunderstandings, making sexual jokes to see if I can comprehend their innuendos. ("Do you like eggplants? The long, long ones and the round, round ones? When your husband visits, will he bring eggplants?") She ducks under the low roof and shouts, laughing, "Hey, Didi-ji, So your condition is not good!"

"I am speaking with Dadi at the moment," I say with unintentional primness. But she keeps joking around about "my condition" and the results of men's disastrous "work."

Suddenly she turns serious. She jerks her head upward and lowers her voice, "So you will stay here?"

"How can I stay here?" I unconsciously adopt the angry rhetorical tone the Bhabhis use. "My family is over there."

"You will go into a hospital, no?" For the birth, she means.

"No. I want to be at home." I am enjoying being contrary, even though I do not lie. Then, abruptly, while I am explaining why most people, but certainly not everyone in America goes to a hospital, her louder, joking voice interrupts,

"Hey, Didi-ji, your husband came here and ruined you, didn't he?"

Shalini's Dadi gets up to leave. I am about to say, "No, but you ruined my conversation with Dadi," but she cuts in again with a loud laugh, "Hey, you are really stuck in a bind, aren't you?"

I say, "I really want to talk to Dadi."

She turns serious again, "Yes, you should talk to her. She can give you a lot of information." Then she says, "You should go see the Mishrein. She knows a lot too. And she gives injections."

I nod and say, "Hey, don't tell anyone."

She says, softer now, "No, no, I won't tell anyone. No one should know." After all the raucous joking I am not sure how to take this.

Amma says to me, in a low voice, after I have just vomited in the gutter by the hand pump in the outer yard, "Bitiya (little daughter), don't vomit out there, vomit back here in the gutter in the angan *or behind the house."*

"But that one is closer to my room," I protest.

"Yes, but there are so many people sitting out there. God knows who. Do it back here where no one can see you. It's better."

How to locate these instances of reticence and concealment, hidden faces and mouths, strategically lowered voices, things said and left out, with the scene of my revelation to the Bhabhis—who proceed to count the days from my last period, discuss whether things are only "possible" or "certain," and debate intimate things like fertile days and whether one can bleed and still be pregnant. They joke, "We know everything about each other. Even our periods. I know when yours is and you know about mine." And I am aware of the way they pride themselves on their educated and scientific knowledge—their ability to "count the days and months" in contrast with "those people" who "don't even know in which month a baby will arrive." They tell me not to tell anyone else, but everything, it seems, is fair game among us— at least as far as my revelations go.

Nowhere, perhaps, are reaching, touching, and longing so elemental to visuality in India than during pregnancy, when the effects

of gazes, auspicious and inauspicious, are heightened and their impact part of everyday experience for women and their families. During pregnancy, acts of disclosure and concealment become crucial to
bodily and moral praxes, situated in a context in which life processes unfold through and are affirmed by "eyes wide open." In this
context, sight is less a mode of what Rapp, in the context of the lab-
oratory, refers to as learning how to distinguish by learning how to
see (2000). It involves managing, rather than overcoming, the ambiguities of knowledge. At the same time, disclosure engages a tension between visibilities literal and metaphoric (the ways sight can
be a metaphor for knowledge), and a tension between things known
by seeing and known through words.

As women told me, when a woman becomes pregnant there is
seldom spoken announcement to husband and family. Life goes on as
usual, until some signs are impossible to "not see," or are recognized,
often by a female family member: The signs of a missed period—when
a woman does not refrain from cooking (though in many households
menstruation is no bar to cooking in spite of general prohibitions),
when she does not "wash her hair" (the sign that menstruation has
ended, and thus occurred). Vomiting, weakness, sallow complexion,
desire for certain foods, lack of a desire to eat. Pregnancy can be carefully revealed by these signs, just as it can be seen, some women said,
in "a woman's face." Self-knowledge, too, can be gentle and gradual,
always suggesting the risk of loss. Pushpadevi and her sister-in-law
said one cannot know for sure that one is pregnant after one missed
period, which may only signify "delayed period" or a bodily "block-
age." After two missed periods one is more certain but only knows
"for sure" if missed periods are accompanied by other signs—nausea,
weakness, lack of appetite or increased desires. Because of a fear that
babies will "fall" (be miscarried), many women, in partially disclosing
their pregnancies to others, may only tentatively embrace pregnancy
themselves. The extensive and consumption-oriented preparations
that characterize pregnancy in other locales (and in the fantasy
world of affluence in Hindi films such as *Hum Aapke Hain Koun*)—
setting up a nursery, amassing clothes, "baby showers," consideration
of names—are absent from this landscape. A few old cloths might
be collected, tiny t-shirts sewn from old sleeves, but otherwise, little
or no preparation happens—names are not picked, future life is not
discussed.

After a few missed periods, authorizing knowledge might be
sought—often secretly—from older women who can know by feeling
the belly. In wealthier families a trip to the doctor might be requested.

When, in what I imagined to be my third month of pregnancy, Shalini's Dadi felt my stomach while I lay on a *charpai* in a dark room
in Pushpadevi's house and Jawan's Wife kept watch at the door, she
said, barely audibly, looking up at Pushpadevi, who was sitting on
the floor behind me, "Yes, something is there. But I knew already
from her face. It is like this. The head is here." She tapped my stomach on the right side. "But it will move many times." When the elder
Chamarin felt my stomach she too had a quiet response. "Yes, *bitiya*.
It will happen. Eat good things. Take your iron pills. Move a lot."
And Chachi, as she prodded my belly, explained, "You can feel something soft move just below the navel. When you press your fingers
it slides away. That is how you know."

At a certain point, there are words to express these things. Euphemisms for pregnancy are many and colorful. Most common is to
say "her condition is not good," or "she does not feel well." But also,
"my feet are heavy," or "my legs are heavy." Speaking of others (often the pregnant one stays silent and a sister-in-law or female friend
speaks for her), *inko kuch hua hai*, "something has happened to her,"
and *inko kuch hai*, "she has something," "something is up." And also,
kuch lad gaya hai, "something has been loaded on," and *kuch garbar
hai*, "there is some confusion," or "something is wrong." *Kuch chakkar hai* or *kuch chakkar me phas gayi* convey similar sentiment; the
term *chakkar* is difficult to translate, referring to a discus, something
spinning or circular, a spiral, and implies confusion, being caught,
obsessed, trapped (*phas gaya* also means "trapped" or "ensnared"). In
the same vein, "She has become ruined," "my husband has ruined
me" also indicate pregnancy. The weight and meanings of seemingly
negative descriptions are multivalent, not necessarily indicating that
pregnancy is experienced this way, yet also pointing to the ways
pregnancy can be felt—its effects on the body, its ability to transform a life, its hold on the future and the self. At the same time, euphemisms point away, distracting attention from that which is good.

Such ways of seeing, Eck notes, are not things of shadowy otherness (1985). Rather, they are part of a form of visuality neither
"dark" nor "light," where seeing constitutes communication and truth
embedded in the *experience* of seeing. As Eck points out, this "seeing
is believing" is not the same "seeing is believing" as that which underlies medical knowledge, in which seeing provides access to a universal, objectifiable truth. Instead, it is intensely *personal*, communion
privileged over the knowledge produced. Yet "the shadow" can speak
to the particular convergence of gazes and lights: "And her eye has
become accustomed to obvious 'truths' that actually hide what she

is seeking. It is the very shadow of her gaze that must be explored,"
says Irigaray (1985: 193). For pregnant women in Sitapur, it is in
such a space that the pregnant subject takes form. Through management of both shadows and "obvious 'truths'," hiddenness constitutes knowledge. One must visually conceal the physical signs of
pregnancy, not only the early symptoms, but the eventual swelling
of the belly and rounding out of the body. I was, even before any
part of me enlarged, admonished to wear my *dupatta* (scarf) properly, hanging fully over my torso. Jawan's Wife, Pushpadevi's neighbor, said to me in a whisper, "You don't wear it right. I know you
don't like the *dupatta*, but now it is very important. No one must
see." Pushpadevi pointed out pregnant women on their way back
from the fields: "You cannot see. But I know. Look how well she
hides it!" As pregnancy advances, those who can bow out of field labor and retreat into homes—to rest, and effect a concealment no
longer possible behind the folds of a sari or scarf.

During my pregnancy I took bits of food with me on visits to
homes, unable to tolerate long stretches of time without something
to appease nausea. I often, with silly solemnity, I'm sure, held an orange peel to my nose to stave off retches. Choti Bhabhi told me one
morning, in the confidence of the kitchen, that I shouldn't eat my
fruit "outside the house" or "in front of people." I should take it into
my room, behind a closed door. When I misunderstood, thinking
she was giving another admonishment that I should not eat among
or share intimacies of knowledge with *"niche log,"* she corrected me.
"That's not what I meant. If you can be seen eating these good
things, then *nazar lagega* [the "evil eye" will adhere]. Others can't
get such nice things." Trying to protect me and them, prevent me
from making ostentatious show of my ability to buy oranges, and to
thereby stave off harm, she, in effect, sought to prevent my displays
of ignorance—what they might reveal about wealth and poverty,
the risks revelations can incur.

In these cases, concealment and delicate revelation of pregnancy
can be less about modesty and privacy and more—or as much—
about the dangers of too much visibility. Good and auspicious things
are attractive to threatening gazes, to the power of the *nazar*, often
translated as "evil eye." The dark side of *darsan, nazar* embodies the
notion that powerful emanations emerge from the eye. Sight, like
sunlight, can be a substance (Woodburne 1981: 56), instituting a de-
structive communion. Associated with women, its malevolent powers lie in the force of *shakti* (power associated with the feminine).
With respect to the call to consider the feminine subject within the

male gaze ("Woman has no gaze" [Irigaray 1995: 224]), concealment of faces, bodies, and names in rural Sitapur is not a sign that women have no gaze, but precisely that they *do*.

At the same time, *nazar* implies a cosmic balance between good and bad, happiness and sadness, such that exuberant joy inevitably attracts its opposite. One must protect oneself from too much beauty and goodness, mar it to prevent bad things from swooping in on the good, deaths from occurring to beautiful babies, illness to young brides, misfortune and loss to the rich. Precaution includes smearing lampblack on the foreheads of cleaned, combed and smartly attired children, tattooing crosses or marks onto faces, necks and arms, hanging an old shoe near something auspicious, and wearing black cords such as the one that Bari Bhabhi tied around my wrist. Protection comes by not complimenting beauty or health, but by saying nothing or, at times, making negative comments. Babies and children, especially vulnerable, are subject to the protection of certain objects—bits of iron, *kusa* grass, *tulsi* leaves. Some pregnant women carry or wear an amulet containing a combination of herbs and onto which a prayer has been incanted, a pendant into which is sewn a written verse of the Koran (worn by both Hindus and Muslims), or a piece of iron.

Disclosures are fraught because they involve threads (cast, stitched, tied, woven, severed) of desire. Desire is a binding force, at once fruitful and dangerous—an external, palpable thing which, not unlike *darsan* and *nazar*, moves between people, while also being an internal force with soteriological impact—that which stands between you and *moksha* (liberation), that whose metered engagement drives passage through the stages of life. The covetous nature of *nazar* (Maloney 1976; Pocock 1981; Woodburne 1981) means that the crippled, diseased, infertile, and deformed are especially dangerous, as are the spirits of those who have died with unmet desires (suicides, women in childbirth). *Nazar* may involve performances of authority, at the same time contributing to egalitarianism by putting "restraint on conspicuous consumption" (Maloney 1976: 134). While it may point to the difference between haves and have-nots, it does so on a fundamental premise of equality and, in some cases, may be less a threat between those of obvious difference in status and more so between those who *should be* equals (Pocock 1981: 208). Desires are dangerous forces that can be unconsciously put into effect, as the mother lovingly gazes at her own child, or an admirer looks, with stirrings of longing, but no malicious intent, upon a child. But such effects can also carry an "implication of a moral defect" (208). That is, as I slowly became aware, in pregnancy, concealment itself is equally as important as *demonstrating* concealment. Hiddenness may be on par with demonstrated lack of pride, lack of outward awareness that what one has is good, lack of the possibility that having means others have not (208).[3] The desires of others may be less tangible, however, than one's own longings. Pregnant women experience heightened desires of their own, and cravings should, women say, be met. She should "eat what her heart desires" and indulge in longings more generally as, as Ayurvedic texts assert, her desires are not entirely her own and denying them may harm the fetus, whose desires may be holdovers from a previous incarnation expressed through her.

While pregnant women embody the happiness that comes with, as one woman told me, "a house full of children," at the same time, their bodies are more permeable to forces transmitted by sight. Things gazed upon can affect the fetus, images of beauty and ugliness transforming its appearance. Inauspiciousness likewise seeps through. The impact of an eclipse, for instance, keeps pregnant women indoors; those who gaze upon gazes that seem "traditional" imagine, as one young woman in Lucknow articulated, "There is a scientific reason for this, but for those people it is just blind belief. The powerful rays of the eclipse can enter a woman's body and make the baby blind." Gazes, gazes everywhere.

Shame, like risk, is a figment of desire. At the same time, it is a necessity of adult consciousness. As both a punishing outcome of bad behavior and sign of proper behavior, *sharam* impinges beyond the self (Das 1995; Mandelbaum 1988). Shame can be modesty or metaphor for consciousness, a curtain of self-regulating affect. Amma, talking about Rohit, who was running around naked, said: "Children's emotions are different, in their hearts, from an adult's feelings. [Children] don't hide behind a curtain from anyone, not an adult, not a child. ... when they become teenagers then they acquire some *sharam*. But he is not conscious yet. There is no *purdah*."

When consciousness is not revelation or liberation but a kind of veil, a form of at once perceiving and not perceiving, being seen and not being seen, shame and desire complicate talk about subject-constitution that pits seeing as a rationalizing technology of power on the one hand, and a sign of fully realized consciousness on the other (maybe Foucault was a bit Hindu in questioning the purity of the gaze). Desire and shame (as elements of exposure) speak of a self ultimately occluded, while at the everyday level they come directly from the heart of subjects often considered effaced in/by regimes of seeing. In pregnancy, in Sitapur and elsewhere, such epistemologies are especially keen in the way they involve a middle ground between knowledge and ignorance, visible and invisible, when one can, contrary to the old joke, be "a little bit pregnant." In Sitapur, desire inhabits this middle ground as well; vision is one of its media, rather than or as well as a technique of institutional power, of governance and rationalizing law.

Freedom of and from sight

Thinking about how seeing is part of subjectivity requires a brief, and hopefully not too painful, trip back to the library. Because ways of seeing are understood by feminist writers, historians of science, and postcolonial historians to be ways of knowing, and visuality to say something about epistemology, approaches to colonial and post-colonial subjectivity have encompassed politics of disclosure extending beyond the visual. The subject (national, gendered) is considered for how she is constituted in sites less obvious to "Western eyes."[4] In a slightly different vein are those who, critiquing Western modes of representation, have pursued "alternate" or "marginal" realms of enunciation. This involves considering how silences, foreclosure, and concealment are sites of self-definition, in contrast with visions of emancipation in which subjectivity is predicated on full disclosure, visibility, and voice. The metaphorical focus of this conversation is on language and "voice," however, in the larger self-representations at stake, visuality and visibility are, perhaps, implicit.

Forms of agency involved in visibility are part of national identities, as postcolonial theorists question modes of subjectivity upon which European versions of nationhood, emancipation, and the colonial venture are predicated. In India, postcolonial historiographies are often revisionist of nationalist histories representing Indian history as a trajectory toward European models of nationhood and the kinds of singular, self-determining subjects the transition was felt to entail (such as Bhabha 1994; Chakrabarty 1992; Chatterjee 1993; Prakash 1999). In these accounts, distinctly non-Western national subjects are seen as crafted through gender categories, often against colonial regimes aiming to institute Western subjectivity precisely at the point at which they denied it. Anticolonial nationalism, Partha Chatterjee says, divided the world into parallel domains—the spiritual and material, the public and private (1993). It was in the private, spiritual realm that non-Western nationalism took shape, beyond the public spaces where colonial hegemonies held sway and visibility was high. Rather than being premised on a "conception of universal humanity," this vision of the nation was predicated on particularity and difference; it depended on certain ideas about women, their role in the family, and their absence from the public sphere— visions of interiority as the space of consolidation of identity and political consciousness (Chatterjee 1993).

Colonized women's autobiographies demonstrate this relationship between political identity and gender, as women's visions of self were constrained by both nationalist politics and Western colonial ideologies, even as they disrupted ideologies which sought to contain them (Chakrabarty 1992; Chatterjee 1993). Such elusive subjects might be, for historians, found in lacunae, places where self-representation diverges from the "confessional mode" of the European through a series of "self-constructed veils" (Chakrabarty 1992: 273). Alternately, autobiographical silences can amount to denials of subjectivity, to voices that are absent in the place where they should be most revealingly located (Chatterjee 1993). Where nineteenth-century Indian men constructed a nationalist self by establishing *themselves* as other to colonial power, women's autobiographies described only the alterity—the events, the framework into which a self would presumably fit, absent authorial expression (Chatterjee 1993: 193). Whether in autobiography or ethnography, the problem of reckoning subject positions beyond the terms of oppressors comes down to the critique that "other" subjectivities are largely absorbed and appropriated by larger narratives, reduced to pieces of an argument, their fullness effaced (shades of Irigaray). Such is evident in colonial and nationalist appropriation of victims of *sati*—ritual immolation (Mani 1985), post-Partition repatriation of female victims of abduction (Das 1995), contemporary efforts to curb "Eve teasing"—public harassment (Rajan 1999), ethnographic representation (Visveswaran 1994), and subaltern historiography (Spivak 1988b). Such examples beg the question of why so many sources of power—men, the colonial regime, the postcolonial state—have been concerned with women's visibility (less so their visuality), either with restricting it (by concealment), or with unfettering it. The answer may well be that this is so because sites of power ultimately assert a narrative that validates its own status—through national and family honor (Das 1995), ideals of free will (Mani 1987) and social restraint (Rajan 1999)—rather than acting out of concern for actual people.

In the broadest such critique, Gayatri Spivak asks how scholarly representation makes women the "ground" for certain discourses. In her essay "Can the Subaltern Speak?" Spivak suggests that in colonial and nationalist discourses a sought-after "collectivity" is continually "foreclosed" by the way gender is put in the service of subject-creation and national narratives—as, we might add, in narratives of intervention (1988a: 283). Such discourses render subjects incapable of self-conscious speech, making the "subaltern female" the most silent of subject categories, "even more deeply in shadow" (Spivak 1988a: 287). Spivak critiques historians on the same basis—for over-determining subjects as "peasants" or "insurgents," making categories stand for an "irretrievable consciousness," and "represent[ing] ... [them]selves through them" (1988a: 287). In the notion of a "sub-altern voice," Spivak says, the subaltern does not exist outside of a framework that disallows it from speaking. This critique has become methodology, even master narrative: it is far better to "read silences" than "give voice," to perceive utterances outside of the domain of what is audible, legible, or expected.

Anthropologists have leveled a similar critique at ethnography, particularly approaches claiming to "give voice" to the oppressed. Following from critiques of anthropological complicities with colonial and postcolonial modes of power (Clifford 1988), the impasse of feminist ethnography is seen as based on deep and troubling desires for disclosure (Visveswaran 1994). Partial disclosure may be interlocutors' prerogative, even necessity, "interrupting a Western (sometimes feminist) project of subject retrieval" and calling attention to unequal relations of power present in the production of knowledge (1994: 50). Resonating with Irigaray's gaze in/from the shadows, such critiques do not stray far from the notion that certain discourses (hegemonic ones) are established on the ground or effacement of others (non-Western, female). We are returned, as always, to the figment or fragment of the "original," that which stands to be "transformed" (or uplifted) and to the threat that the seemingly "blind" and "concealed" poses to the very stuff of certainty. For Irigaray the matter is a clarion call for recognizing "other" feminine ways of knowing and constituting the self, ways that *defy* assimilation.

Such approaches so often hinge on the silences of archive and interview, when, ethnographically at least, there might well remain voices to hear and gazes to follow. In this regard, one might ask whether "reading silences" might not *also* amount to "giving voice"—filling in gaps by putting lacunae into the service of certain discourses—scholarly or feminist. Perhaps these approaches might valorize "original," silent, evasive, crafty, and resistant subjectivities—other heroic subjects. In Irigaray's philosophical models as in chal-

lenges to ethnography and historiography, the "other" is beckoned
and evoked, but seldom "seen" (or represented beyond its capacity
to evade)—and this is precisely the point. It might seem that, contrary to enunciations otherwise, there is indeed no "other" subjectivity, only representations thereof. This may be the logical end to
Spivak's argument. All of this is a prelude to saying that such dilemma of subjectivity is, ironically perhaps, tensely and tenuously
embodied in the clinic, in which not only displays of emancipation
and morality but actual *care* are at stake, and revelation is part of the
contract on which wellness is based.

Seeing, knowing, and schismogenesis

*On several occasions I sit in on doctors' clinic hours at the monthly NAFPA
health camp. The doctor, Ruchi, is an unmarried woman in her mid twen-
ties who grew up in Madhya Pradesh and works at a private hospital in
Lucknow. Several times a month she is the visiting doctor for NAFPA. We
share a car to Sitapur on several occasions, and chat, in English, about conditions of reproductive health in Uttar Pradesh, about rural women, and
about the larger project of rural uplift. We talk about our families, our pref-
erences in Hindi films and music, our taste in restaurants in Lucknow. She
is, in different ways, a foreigner in these parts too. "Uttar Pradesh makes
you so burnt out," she tells me. "It's a constant struggle. In the south women
are eager to improve their lives. In Uttar Pradesh people are just lazy." But
still, I observe that she speaks gently to the women she serves.*

*On the third Thursday of February, I walk over to the school in a nearby
qasbah where I am told the health camp will be coming this month. Preeti
is there too. We are both a little bit lost. We wait in a school office, and I am
interviewed by some teachers until it becomes clear that nothing is happening, no one is gathering. I wander toward the bazaar where I run into Manjari with some women I don't know and some I recognize from Preeti's
group of CBDs. Manjari says she thinks the camp will be in a different place
this month. We walk to a mohalla just beyond the edge of town. There is an
old government building there. Manjari says it is a health center, but it is
not used these days. "Maybe the clinic will be in this room," she says, "I
thought I was supposed to get it ready for them."*

*The door is locked. We ask around, but no one has a key. A glance
through the window shows some hay and piles of old scraps of something or
other. "Well, we can't use this. It's filthy. Maybe it has become a cow shed?"
Manjari jokes. With a small crowd of eight or ten women, we wait by a wall.
Manjari sends a child for one of the CBDs who lives here. It looks like we*

will be using her house. We wait. A few more women come, and we wait some more. There is much talk about "the van." When it will arrive, mostly. While we wait, the CBD's husband brings us sweets from a recent wedding in the household. Most of the women refuse, but Manjari and I take them. One of the CBDs, a woman the others say is "not right," a bit crazy, talks about her health problems and her son's wedding. We wait some more.

Finally, the van arrives, jolting slowly into the yard beyond the government building. Manjari talks with Mr. Sharma while I greet Ruchi. It is established that Ruchi will see patients inside the house. While her instruments are brought out of the van and unwrapped from their white sheets by one of the CBDs, Ruchi is given sweets. She says to me, in English, "It's gross, but you really can't refuse, can you?" She smiles and says thank you.

The room for the clinic contains a bare wooden bed, a small table and two chairs, one for me, one for her. There is no electricity today. One of the CBDs is called in to hold a flashlight and Ruchi opens, slightly, the shutter on the window to let in a streak of sunlight. Outside, women are giving their names to Mr. Sharma and Gopal, who write them on scraps of paper. They call the names, and women enter the room in turn. Some come in with their CBDs— the ones who tell them about the camp, who supply their contraceptives and refer them for sterilizations. The patients seem nervous. Ruchi encourages them with "Jeldi karo, jeldi karo," hurry up, hurry up, though she is not unfriendly.

The first woman, her head covered, sits on the edge of the bed. Ruchi says to me, "She is here for me to check on her pregnancy." She tells the woman to lie down and pull down her sari, and then she feels her stomach. Even I can see a large bulge. Ruchi asks, "When did your periods stop?"

She does not answer immediately. Ruchi asks again. And one more time. The woman replies in a light voice with a hint of what sounds like nervous laughter, "Maybe three, two months ago."

Ruchi feels her stomach again. "You are at least six months pregnant. Maybe seven. Sit up." She gives the woman a tetanus shot.

"How many children do you have?"

The woman answers, again in a flutter so soft I cannot hear. Ruchi admonishes, "Get a [sterilization] operation. That is enough children. After this baby you can get an operation." The woman is adjusting her sari; she doesn't seem to be listening, though she smiles lightly.

The next woman comes in and Ruchi asks what her problem is. The woman mumbles incomprehensibly and Ruchi asks her to repeat herself. "My monthly has not come."

Ruchi asks how long it has been. She answers, "Four."

Ruchi tells her to lie down. She turns to me and says, "She wants me to tell her if she is pregnant. She has not had a period for four months and she doesn't know if she is pregnant." She rolls her eyes. I am not sure what I say—perhaps a "hmmph," perhaps a sad "oh my." I am aware again that I can hardly be considered not complicit here—I am part of Ruchi's presence, with her metal speculum and needles; she is part of mine, in the dark, on a chair, with a notebook. I sit straight, lean in, hold an instrument or two. Ruchi feels the woman's stomach, tells her she is four months pregnant. "Get a tetanus shot," she says, "And an operation after this baby comes. How many children do you have?"

"Char bhaiya." Four sons.

"You have four children?"

"Char bhaiya, do bitiya." Four sons, two daughters.

Ruchi turns to me. In English, "She has six children already and she doesn't know if she is pregnant. They are so stupid."

She tells the woman that after the baby is born it should get a tetanus shot. The woman says, "My other babies never had a shot, and they are fine."

"It is still good to get the shot."

The woman, looking down, mumbles that she will not.

Ruchi writes something on a little piece of paper. "Take the medicine I have written here." I ask what it is, and she tells me it is for iron and folic acid pills.

"Do I get them free from the government?"

"No, but they are very cheap and the benefit is great."

The woman takes the paper, folds it up, puts it in her blouse. When she leaves, Ruchi says, "They won't take any of the medicine, they won't get tikka *(vaccinations). Look at the way she says her other children were fine without* tikka. *These people expect everything to come for free. But it doesn't work like that. You have to give something."*

The next woman says her problem is "pain." When Ruchi asks where, she says, "In my stomach and in my whole body."

Ruchi asks if the pain is constant and the woman says it is. "Is there pain when you pee?"

"No."

Ruchi asks if she has "safed pani" (vaginal discharge or leukorrhea).

"Sometimes, but not all the time." Ruchi feels her stomach and asks how many children she has.

She says she has one son, but a few seconds later adds, "There are two children." When Ruchi asked if she wants any more, she says yes.

"Two is enough. In my family there are two, brother and sister, and in her family," Ruchi points to me, "they are two, sister-sister. And we are all

*happy." The woman says she wants at least one more child. Ruchi gives her
a piece of paper, saying, "Take these pills."*

*She turns to me and says, "She won't take them. She won't even buy
them."*

*I notice that Ruchi doesn't give diagnoses or explanations, except to say
"there is a baby," or "you are four months pregnant." She resolves queries
with a prescription or admonition to "get a shot." When I ask what she
thinks a particular patient's problem is, she tells me in English. She tells me
what she writes on the little pieces of paper, but does not tell the patients,
many of whom cannot read.*

"How to master these devilries, these moving phantasms of the
unconscious, when a long history has taught you to seek out and desire only clarity, the clear perception of (fixed) ideas?" (Irigaray 1985:
136). "Is there a baby in my/your stomach?" These questions seem
posed against one another in the clinic. The latter is posed by doctors to women, and to doctors and medical authorities by women—
subtly in the offering of the body, the symptom, the period that has
not arrived—in a way that leads doctors to suggest women are ignorant for asking on the one hand, and making them ask, on the
other. It opens up a ground for insertion of *sui-goli* and *operation*—
needles/pills and sterilizations—as a point of communication, signs
of state authority on the one hand and local ignorance and resistance on the other. In the "betrayal" (Visveswaran 1994) of "averted
gazes" lies the "illegitimate utterance" (Bhabha 1994) that may show
that voices of resistance are difficult to separate from the constraints
by which they are held. Or, in such a field of power, as Homi Bhabha
suggests, "indeterminacy" of speech may "constitute its importance
as social discourse" running counter to forms of power in which de-
terminacy, clarity, and volume are markers of significance (1995:
332). But how to reckon the overlapping and multiple sites in which
this occurs in a space in which techniques of intervention, or *kaccha*
and tentative "bio-availability" (Cohen 2005), are not bound by
clinic walls. For women, gazes run deep into the ways law interjects
the domestic world; as Ranajit Guha has shown in the case of an illicit abortion in nineteenth-century Bengal, "comprehensive … surveillance" of female bodies takes place within the home even as it is
denied in the "ruse of law" (Guha 1985: 161), making "subterfuge
and secrecy" necessary strategies (155).

The "clinical" scenes I have just described might be read as moments of a paradoxical overlap of surveillance and inattention, concomitant with evasion of the constant monitoring of reproductive

life and the moral burden of sterilization. They might also be read as points of incommensurability—the failure of communication at the point at which local modes of disclosure encounter medical ones, or mandates to conceal confront demands to reveal. These scenes might be imagined as sites of translation, where the medical gaze confronts and interprets the local enunciation, or in which both size up and categorize one another. But as moments of "contact" they evoke less translation than meshing, less divergence than convergence, in which shifts occur beyond the point of encounter and ways of broaching the subject involve different valences of power depending on where and to whom enunciations are made. In a range of readings, they suggest a troubling commensurability, something like what Gregory Bateson referred to as "complementary schismogenesis" (Bateson 1958, 1972). Schismogenesis, he says, is "a process of differentiation in the norms of individual behavior resulting from cumulative interaction between individuals" (1958: 175). It produces a dynamic and distorting equilibrium in which two ways of being affirm the other while promoting mutual exaggeration (1958: 188). "Selves" and "others," in this sense, blossom through conversation rather than mere production of discourse, found precisely *in* points of communication, not their absence, in convergence rather than obfuscation or overwriting. Thus, in pregnancies gradual and vulnerable, in which revelation is threatening and accomplished indirectly and having someone feel a belly to come into knowledge themselves is safer than saying, however gently, "I am pregnant," perhaps the best way to get someone to feel one's belly is to hedge the matter, be vague, complain of symptoms, pose an illness, refuse pills; or perhaps it is indeed ailments that bring women to the clinic whereas their pregnancy, in the gaze of Ruchi, takes over the encounter and the "presentation." Either way, hedging produces probings that hint at moral failure. The giggles and scoldings of the clinical encounter, perhaps dampened versions of the moans of pain and threatened slaps of maternity wards, can be spaces of emergent affect, neither entirely about essential ways of being coming into conflict, nor failures to "see" or "hear," nor "responses" to points of discord.

Pratima and I are walking through Devia on her rounds. We enter a household where some women are knitting in the courtyard. A woman lying on a rope bed asks in a soft voice, looking down at her hands, if Pratima has brought more birth control pills. "But don't give me pills like you did before—those were very hot. I don't want any hot medicines."

Pratima says, "So take them in the evening. If you take them and go to bed, what's the problem?"

The woman tells us, "No, they are so hot my period is not coming," but in such a low voice I am not sure I have heard correctly. Pratima asks what she said. The other women smile and stifle laughter.

"Three months," she says, holding up her fingers.

Pratima asks, "So is there a baby in your stomach?" and the woman says she does not know. Pratima tells her to lie back and feels her stomach. "You haven't had your period for three months?" The woman shakes her head. Pratima says, "There is a baby in your stomach. You shouldn't have any more of this," waving her hand at the packet of birth control pills. "Get two tikka [shots] soon." The women laugh. It is as though the joke is on us.

At the next house, before entering, Pratima tells me a baby was born here ten days earlier. "They are Muslims," she says. We knock on the door, which, oddly, is locked from the outside. Pratima mumbles to herself, "They have locked her in?" as a voice calls us in. Inside is a young-looking woman on a bed in the corner. In front of her lies a tiny baby wrapped in blankets.

Pratima and I sit on a charpai *across the* angan. *Pratima asks who the baby's father is. She stares at her hands. Pratima asks when the baby was born and she says, "Ten days ago."*

Pratima asks if she or the baby had gotten shots and the woman says no. Pratima advises that the woman should get shots for herself and the baby, and asks again who the father is. The woman says nothing. An older woman I take to be her mother-in-law comes in. Pratima asks her who the baby's father is. The older woman tells her, and she jots this in her ledger. As we walk away, Pratima marvels, "She won't even tell the father's name." I ask why.

"They are all afraid."

"Afraid of what?"

"Afraid of the government."

Enunciations are multivocal; and the clinic may hardly be the brightly lit space of all-seeing gaze. We cannot assume that evasive enunciations are *the same* in the home and in the clinic, that they—and the ontologies underlying them—move unchanged from site to site, or that women mean the same thing when they at once invite and defer recognition of pregnancy by kin, neighbors, and doctors. Indeed, doctor visits of all kinds are matters of visibility. In Sitapur, one does not "go to the doctor" or "go to see the doctor," but rather, "*shows* the doctor," making encounters with medical authority explicitly moments of revelation. Where, perhaps, "not knowing" can also be an act of revelation, of "showing the doctor," or encounters with institutions less about "confirming" pregnancy or finally, really "knowing," than efforts to seek recognition from authorizing—and health-giving—forces, entering the ledgers and numerics of intervention can also come with fears of different kinds of visibility. For those most marginalized, or stigmatized in a range of ways—Dalits, poor Muslims, lower castes—fears that the state aims to reduce their numbers by way of their reproductive bodies make clinic visits and visits by institutional figures moments of concentrated desperation and risk. The risk of visibility is as multifold as that of concealment. Drawing attention to fertility runs against the grain of multiple urges toward protection, against the grain of desire. At the same time, it is part of a pull *toward* institutions as sites of recognition and promise, another locus of desire.

From the perspective of authorizing agents—doctors, NGO workers—complex reluctances can only be signs of ignorance as they do not measure up to a particular vision of "knowledge." As an epistemological challenge, "Is there a baby in your stomach?" demands more of the patient than confirmation of pregnancy. Efforts to probe and illuminate provoke resistance; badgering about numbers of kids or about sterilization prompts reticence, validating fears of authority while enunciating the enumerating power of the state. This, clearly, is schismogenesis. As Pushpadevi put it, women's concealment is about recognizing and acknowledging authority—yet authority, in this case, demands both appropriate display and revelation. For many, seeking recognition and care on their own terms prompts those offering care to "see" them as *not* adequately calling attention to themselves, ignorant of their bodies, and morally corrupt for failing to say, or even know, what they want. Alongside ignorance is the " noncompliance" that, as Ruchi put it, denotes lazy disinterest. For those who define themselves as bearers of not only health but the empowered consciousness of health seeking, it is impossible to see "failures" to speak about the body as anything other than lack. Even for those sensitive to affects such as "modesty," "shame," and fear, such things—as elements of concealment—become obstructed gaze, "blind belief." Yet, like betrayals, evasions can be, from the perspective of their speakers, not only appropriate, but legitimate and necessary (Visveswaran 1994)—necessary for self-protection in spaces where reproduction is heavily monitored by the state, where pregnancies, infant deaths, condom usage, and sterilizations are recorded in big notebooks by women who come knocking at one's door, just as menstrual cycles are watched by affinal kin. Only misrecognizable in the clinical encounter—and at the same time constituted by their misrecognition—"illegitimate utterances" bespeak not so much lack of sight or knowledge, but the tangibility of seeing as *darsan* and *nazar*, the knowing critique of the gazed upon, the simultaneous dodging from and longing for institutional attention.

Just as voice and visibility can be made to stand for agency, they also stand for a framework in which experience marks the incommensurability of discourses. Kalpana Ram argues that situating "voices" within discourses oriented around Western feminist models renders those "voices" silent, inaccessible to interlocutors in such a frame (1998a). But, the threshold of visibility converges with subjectivity in the clinical encounters of the "health camp" less in the incommensurability of discourses or inaccessibility of utterances than in the socialities and embodiments that result from layered visions of vision. Women's voices are not necessarily "silenced" in the space of "encounter"; rather, both their silences and the things they say out loud can only be "heard" in a certain way, only invested with certain meanings. This may, in effect, amount to silencing, but my sense—and the benefit of doubt—is that something does get through. As schismogenesis suggests, conversation rather than obfuscation is the key issue. In being invested with certain moral codes, certain senses of freedom, citizenship, and right, the very utterances—translated into "silences" in the medical encounter—that were the "problem" in the first place become all the more necessary.

"How can we help them if they are so lazy and don't want to be helped?" Ruchi asked me in the car. "The problem in U.P." she said, "is demand. These women don't want to take care of their health. They don't want contraception and they don't want to come to the doctor, they don't want any of it. There has to be demand. Was there once this problem in America? Do all races go through this stage where women have to be taught to demand high standards of health?"

Putting aside the term "races," I replied that to the best of my knowledge, the women's health movement in North America got moving in a different way—through the encouragement of activists and through women's own demands.[5] "I don't think there was the kind of phase you are talking about. But the context here is different, don't you think?"

"No, it's not that different. It's probably an evolutionary thing. India hasn't evolved socially to the level you are talking about. Not U.P. anyway, not with SCs and STs [scheduled castes and scheduled tribes]. It's different in the south. There, women actually *want* these things. They come to doctors, they tell us things, they ask for birth control."

Women in Uttar Pradesh—especially those in low social ranks, "scheduled castes," "scheduled tribes"—fail to live up to certain ideals of empowerment, thwarting the efforts of those who know better. The women of Uttar Pradesh represent, simultaneously, extreme forms of female oppression and extreme forms of "ignorance." In such a vision, in which desire is central but, as Ram suggests, only accessible within a certain narrative, health-oriented, empowerment-conscious branches of feminist activity in India are situated on a vision of the rural reproductive body and the moral passivity of rural women. Such a vision, put in action and encased in clinical performances of state power, doesn't just *encounter* and misread the "local"; it *prompts and produces* it. Rather than ameliorating the clear fact that many women in rural Uttar Pradesh have less "choice" in their reproductive lives, and that health services here are a pale shadow of the way they appear in the south, the shape and coding of these efforts make a mockery of such inequities. Perhaps they are less "empowered" socially and politically than southern women; perhaps, whether "because of SCs and STs" or not, they are less present within the state, medical, and bureaucratic structures that do exist; but these structures are themselves arguably less visible and less predictable in Uttar Pradesh and other northern states than in what is considered to be the more modern, affluent, and developed south. These institutional, universalizing, self-consciously "modern," perhaps modernist concepts of empowerment are, like "blind belief" in *nazar,* very much matters of vision. As sites of schismogenesis, they play out as though scripted by Irigaray, such that medical authority seeks a mirror of its own socialities and values, and, when befuddled, erases syntaxes of desire by assigning (then filling) the "silence" with symbolics that render women mute, ignorant, "lazy," "stupid." But while for Irigaray and others silence is a tactic of "revolt" against male discourse, quiet enunciation, the near silence of concealment-as-exposure is already a strategy, part of already-present negotiations of gazes, forms already in circulation.

Medical *darsan,* medical *nazar*

Do we learn anything from the poorly lit clinic-in-a-household about the ways subjectivity may take a particular shape, or be inflected by power in a particular way, in pregnancy? There are clear analogies between the subjectivities entailed in reproductive ontologies in north

India and those of Western models of science and medicine, in which
a subject/object divide is gendered. R. S. Khare describes the concept of *mata*, mother, as being predicated on an explanatory framework in which women are "fields" (*kshetra*) to the male "seed" (*bija*),
and part of an "expanding analogic chain" of contrasts between action and inaction: "the sphere of effort (*karma, purushakara*)" and
that of "fate or destiny (*daiva*)" (1992: 157). Islamic models of gender
are not so different (cf. Delaney 1992). The chain extends to knowledge, and to the crux of the production/reproduction continuum;
"*bija* is the knower of the field (*kshetrajna*) while (*kshetra*) is the
field, the physical body itself." (Khare 1992: 158). The seed/knower
is to the field/known the "unchanging, superior cultural principle,"
even as the "logical and practical prominence" of the field grants
"sentimental priority (homage of the heart) to the conception of the
mother." Leaning curiously towards Irigaray, in this unfolding principle, male syntax is implanted on/in the female, as "Within the system, *mata* [mother] … symbolizes that entire cultural idea of the
process of transformation by which the seed decodes itself" (158).

Perception impinges, by way of extended analogies (seed:field ::
knower:known :: seer:seen :: man:woman), on gender categories
within feminist ("Western" and "Indian") concepts of gaze. However,
in Sitapur anyway, though seeing extends to knowing, it cannot be
easily assimilated to such analogies. When seeing and reproduction
intersect, they demonstrate that gazes—and by extension, knowing—cannot (always) be reduced to a subject-object divide in which
knower and known occupy the same gendered niches they occupy
in Western scientific frames or Hindu orthodoxy. Gazes are not always matters of male objectification of the female, and control of
women's visibility not always a matter of male honor. Indeed, they
are not always matters of knowledge.

As many scholars and critics have shown, regimes of the visual
and the visible constitute kinds of sociality. The kinds of seeing that
orient pregnancy in Sitapur represent socialities that pose challenges
to notions of individual rights, empowerment, and voiced "desire,"
while not being based on something entirely *other than* individual
identities. Rather than (or as well as) speaking to the need to recognize silence, they demand that we question the ways "silence" is
valued, observed and dismissed or valorized, by posing ontological
and moral and causal principles both *beyond* and *constituted by* the
hegemonic discourse in question (and here there are many). Such
ontological and moral principles are embodied in modes of percep-

tion and the active potentials of desire. Both perception and desire converge in sight in a way that upends the "passive"/"active" binaries by which so much social engagement is understood.

Pushpadevi, when I complain about feeling nauseous all the time, says, "Oh, Didi-ji. This is only the beginning. You think these are problems!"

I laugh. "Okay. Maybe it's the beginning of twenty years of problems. Until the baby grows up."

She stops laughing. "Why do you say you will only have twenty years of problems? You will always have problems. Now. For your whole life. Children bring work and trouble. They ruin your body. Look at me. Look at my face. And if your baby is good, 'normal,' then maybe it is okay. If your baby is not 'normal' then you really have troubles your whole life."

I write in my notes that day that Pushpadevi is looking different, even, perhaps, pregnant, but there have been no disclosures as far as I can tell, though she summons me to look at her face for signs of dilapidation. She prides herself, she says, on being open with me, telling me things others would never talk about, asking the things she is dying to know but others are too embarrassed to ask. But even though we talk daily about pregnancies, babies, bodies, and sex, there seem to be none of the usual signs—no careful revelation, no active concealment.

Except the mention one day that she "needs to see the Mishrein. I have some problems. The work is not finished."

What work? I think I notice her waist thickening, am annoyed at my own forms of surveillance. I write in my notes that she is "looking even crazier these days." Pushpadevi always seems a bit on the verge. Some people keep a careful distance because of it. Now her hair is messier, her eyes spill with sudden tears, her voice rises and falls. Her language careens from sudden harshness to gentle tones, and she lashes out at her children with her hand and the sharp whip of her voice. They run from her, sometimes laughing and ducking her blows, sometimes looking scared, sometimes yelling back.

"Local" ways of seeing, while they bespeak nonabsolute knowledge of the body and pregnancy, do not represent a shadowy, dark, mystical otherness which, as Diana Eck (1986) points out, is often taken to epitomize India and Hinduism, just as the clinic is not always glaringly bright and doctors give little information, only illegible prescriptions and admonitions to get a shot, get an operation. Likewise, one can regulate visibility, use gaze, revelation, and intimate knowledge as a key to the soul, and concealment to prevent bad things from happening. But one cannot, in so doing, ensure that goodness stays and badness stays away. One can barter with gazes, institutional and otherwise, but the rest may be "up to God," though exactly what God's power involves is not so straightforward. In Push-padevi's comments about her misplaced life it becomes clear that pregnancy and fertility are not always all about deferred and pro-tected happiness. Life gapes back.

Chapter 5

DYING
IN THE BIG, BIG HANDS OF GOD

The finished

*W*e are in the enclosed kitchen and it is dark outside. The pot of vegetables has finished cooking and rests idly on the clay stove. Warm coals
glow underneath, and long sticks of wood jut out, immodest and knobby like
legs made useless by polio. The cozy box of a room is tucked against the mud
wall separating our house from the Pasi neighborhood, casted from untouchable, upar (high) from niche (low). The weather is beginning to turn,
and we are no longer here to keep out of the cold. Soon the kitchen will be
moved into the open courtyard. Rohit shuffles in and out wearing my shoes
and saying, "Look at me, I am Bua-ji, I have a cold." He mocks my sniffles
and we all laugh. We wait for the men to come and take their meals. Choti
Bhabhi leaves and Bari Bhabhi folds herself over to put her head on her
knees. She closes her eyes. When Choti Bhabhi comes back we talk about a
family over the wall. Their newborn baby girl died this morning. I ask about
sadness and sorrow, and how people share it. Choti Bhabhi says a few
things, but mostly she listens. This is Bari Bhabhi's domain.

Earlier that day I go to the house where the baby had been born a few
days ago. I sit with the mother after she tells me, when I notice the empty in-
dentation in the hay, "The baby is finished." It had not drunk properly of
the water it was offered, she said. I am surprised. This had been the third
day of its life; nothing seemed dire when I visited the day before. I remember she mentioned the baby was weak; I recall saying she might consider
breast-feeding it, but the suggestion was waved off. "The baby won't be fed
milk until the water falls and the Chamarin finishes her work, and anyway,

the milk hasn't come in yet." I sit in the house waving away flies as women come in to recount exactly what might have happened. The baby girl was weak even in the womb, one says. "We massaged the placenta and warmed the baby thoroughly, but it was still weak." It was her fourth child, her third daughter. As we sit, she talks about her other children with a more animated voice and between talking stares blankly at the floor and cries a bit as she holds her older daughter in her lap. Another girl lies in the space in the hay the baby has recently occupied. She tells me that the girl is tired, that she never sleeps on this side of the room, usually on the other.

*The girl's foot has an oozing wound. An amulet—an iron washer—has been hung on an anklet made of twined goat's hair, and hangs into the open sore. We talk about the sore, about whether the amulet is irritating it or not, and I suggest it be washed and the girl given a tetanus injection. The foot does not look well at all. A young woman comes in and sits for a while, recounting the story of the baby's death, and sharing stories of other women who had lost babies. She asks why I don't have my camera. That takes me aback, and I think of Pratima's photos—is she mocking me or expressing a desire for something to be captured? Maybe both. When, after some time, I leave, Choti Bhabhi asks how the baby was. "She died," I say, using the phrase everyone uses to say such things—*qatam ho gayi—*it is finished.*

"Oh ho, what happened?"

"They said it didn't drink." I feel part of the circulation of stories.

"Those people never feed their babies right away," Choti Bhabhi says.

"But it must have been early." Bari Bhabhi walks over.

"No," I say, "They said it was on time. But they said it was weak from the beginning."

"Those people will never show a baby to the doctor. They never take their children to show the doctor," Choti Bhabhi says.

"Come off it," Bari Bhabhi exclaims, "Everything is in the big, big hands of God."

In Lalpur, the wall separating the courtyard of my upper-caste hosts from the backyard of a Dalit neighborhood took on great, if predictable, significance for me. In "our" *angan* I was in a space of self-consciously bourgeois longings mixed with firm assertions of an us-versus-them vision of the world. On dark nights like this one, I sat in the kitchen (in winter) or the open air (the rest of the year), talking and playing with babies, picking stones out of uncooked dal and failing miserably to roll nicely shaped rotis, listening to the ways this household was a protected space in which rationality thrived, and the dirty, funny, depravity of "lower people" was held at bay. On trips out of the village with Choti Bhabhi or Bari Bhabhi I heard about things that might only be said from one person to another, rather than from one to many—about longings extended outward like strings of spider web. Choti Bhabhi wanted to live in the city, she said, where life was cleaner and more composed, where Rohit could go to a good school, where one does not always live as though in the laps of others. In the kitchen, as on the road, I heard about the "heres" and "theres" of rural existence. We leaned against the wall, a proverbial world away.

To get to Pushpadevi's house, I could go one of two ways. Out the front gate, up the path along the high wall of the Srivastav compound, around the corner, turn right down a small path just beyond a cowshed, pass in front of a household into which I would surely be drawn, often against my interest, where, according to the Bhabhis, the "good" Pasi neighbor, Kulu's Mother, lived. I didn't like her loud teasing and punches in the arm, and didn't like this route. The other, more direct way went via the back. It involved trash and rotting smells and a hop over a gutter oozing with a cloudy soup of cast-off liquids. I would go out the back door into the behind-house area of the latrine, trash heap, and a barrier of cactus-like spiny plants. I would cross the gutter, go by the trash area of Preeti's and Kulu's Mother's household, past Jawan's Wife's grass hut a mere fifteen feet or so from the wall. From there it was just a hop over a gully to Pushpadevi's veranda.

When Jawan's Wife's impermanent, illegal hut caught fire and burned to the ground, taking with it much of Kulu's Mother's household and the rooftops of Preeti's house (Pushpadevi's house was made of brick, her roof tile), people in my household removed everything from their rooms and doused the walls with water. Because of the capriciousness of the breeze, their home was untouched, save for a scar of black on the wall. After this, the difference between the two sites was visibly marked. Before it had been a contrast of imagination, but now it was visible. "Our" space was intact, "theirs" a desert of the baked shells of mud homes, patches of black scarring the grey earth, a dearth of green. In the midst of her weary grief, Kulu's Mother, with her youngest daughter, molded a heart into her patched mud wall and painted it pink and white. Jawan's Wife and kids lived in the open for a while, then rebuilt the grass hut.

On Pushpadevi's veranda, I chatted and watched her kids play with batches of puppies in the time before the little dogs died or ran away. We watched people coming and going from the fields and passers-by on the back road into the village, and Pushpadevi interviewed me about life in America, about my marriage, and about marriages in general. Where the Bhabhis were enclosed in the courtyard safety of *purdah*, Pushpadevi's was a veranda with a view. Jawan's Wife joined us most of the time, as did Pushpadevi's *devrani*, who did not speak as much as Pushpadevi, carrying an air of upright morality in contrast with Pushpadevi's wild enunciations, over-full speech, absent husband, and out-of-control life.

In both spaces, talk sometimes came around to death. Bari Bhabhi and Pushpadevi both revealed and repeated their losses, as, even from their heavily casted realms, both spoke of divine intervention in life, a woman's lack of control, and each, in her own way, expressed outrage and sorrow. To say they shared loss when they shared little else would be a romantic falsehood—for the morality of blame, and insinuation of failed ethics shaded Bhabhi's language about Pasis and other "others," and flashes of injustice sparked Pushpadevi's talk. But to say that experiences of deaths of babies further deepened the entrenched differences of caste and class, of life above and below, would also mislead. Pushpadevi had too many children, Bari Bhabhi too few; the lives of both were profoundly marred by the deaths of children. Empathy, too, crossed barriers.

As for most women in Sitapur, for Pushpadevi and Bari Bhabhi babies who died were said to be "finished." That is, to say a baby has died they said *"Baccha qatam ho gaya"*—the baby is finished. Other, (to me) gentler-sounding phrases—*mrtyu ho gaya* (the death happened), *mar gaya* (died), *expire hua* (expired), *guzar gaya* (passed away)—were seldom used except as a means of translation out of the idiom of *dehat* and into urban, middle-class talk. For both Bari Bhabhi and Pushpadevi, as they said at varying times, "Everything is in the hands of God."

Infant death is always near to the experience of reproduction in Sitapur, so near that for many outside *dehat* it is its first order; numbers and mortality statistics are a distinct weave, a recognizable pattern of the fabric of reproduction in this part of India and the world. Numbers are often brought out for consideration, to introduce a topic with a punch of quantity that mere "anecdote" is not able to supply: in 1998, the infant mortality rate for Uttar Pradesh (defined as death under one year of age) was 86.7 (deaths per 1000 births), ranking Uttar Pradesh second highest in infant mortality in India (the highest rates were found in the northeast province of Meghalaya at 89.0; the lowest in southern Kerala at 16.3); the overall rate for India is 67.6 (Government of India [GOI] 2001). Across India, rates are significantly higher in rural (73.3) than urban areas (47.0) (GOI 2001). In South Asia, India's infant mortality rate ranks lower than that of Pakistan (74), Bangladesh (79), and Nepal (83) (though Uttar Pradesh itself exceeds the averages of these countries), and significantly higher than Sri Lanka (18). In North America, Europe, and Japan the numbers are in the single digits.

This is one way of naming death. Michel de Certeau says that "death is not named. But it is written in the discourse of life, without its being possible to assign it a particular place" (1984: 197). In saying death is not named, de Certeau refers to the speech of the dying person in the context of biomedical narratives of progress, in which death is an unspeakable affront to the conditions of reality. Within such contexts, he says, "death is an elsewhere" and can only be "given over to" religious discourses already emptied of substance and a claim to the real. Like the uncanny moment, death too moves back and forth across the threshold of visibility and consciousness, returning, de Certeau says, as a "wound on reason" (192). Such is true in speaking death. But in "writing" it, that is, as I understand it, in transforming it into discourse, it is revealed that death is always present as a condition, "written in the discourse of a life" (197). Its unbearable constancy can be made over, he says, to express "the marvelous and ephemeral excess of surviving" (198)—the fact that life can be capricious amid the certainty of dying. In the framework of his thoughts on modernity lies a notion that death can constitute "the index of all alterity," and at the same time the core of discourse (de Certeau 1984: 192; cf. Stewart 1996).

In considering languages of grief in relation to languages of certainty, there is a tension in the ways death can be thought of in connection to modern knowledge. On the one hand, we can consider death as that which underlies the possibility of knowledge, as that end point to the fostering or disallowing of life that stands for the modern configuration of power/knowledge (as Foucault had it [1978]). On the other, we can imagine death as de Certeau does: as that which cannot be spoken in languages of modernity. Put differently, this is the distinction between death as the ultimate condition of biopower, the "absconding presence in the institution" (Chatterjee et al. 1998: 189), and death as the final *affront to* the certitudes of knowledge-power, that which speaks the limits of human effort (de Certeau 1984). Yet, when death is spoken in spaces of poverty and intervention, where it is made to speak about the overwhelming quality of everyday life and where it is that around which claims *to* knowledge and norms are built, perhaps it dwells in both realms. Death can be both affront to and outcome of certainties about normality.

Ways of naming death, of allowing for its return into language, bespeak a political subjectivity constituted as a factor of loss. More to the point, it refers to subjectivity as a factor of not just any death, but infant and child death. Nancy Scheper-Hughes (1992), in her devastating account of infant death in Brazil, suggests that infant mortality produces certain subjectivities, and she pursues the contours of that experience, the forms of affect involved, and, perhaps most importantly, the material, embodied, and structural conditions that produce them (hunger, poverty, labor structures, racism). But in the favelas of *Death Without Weeping*, the gaze of the state is, as Scheper-Hughes says, turned resolutely away, and the state's capacity to ignore and discard part of the picture of dying (1992). In Sitapur, the situation is somewhat different—for one thing, it involves not quite the level of poverty and abjection described by Scheper-Hughes and others writing on marginality and social exclusion in Brazil (e.g., Biehl 2005). More importantly, however, infant death in Sitapur happens under the gaze of the state, a gaze at once committed to enumeration and also picky and distorted. The very nature of intervention, the ebb and flow of temporary schemes alongside the unreliable—but not absent—quality of state institutions and infrastructures, gives infant death and women's responses to it an ability to stake claims on the paradoxes of intervention, as well as on the broad structures of poverty. As such, the recuperation and rehearsing of memories of death, like the experiences they reference, are part of multiple subjectivities, the reverberations and disjunctures of simultaneous worlds in which the demands of the state ("have fewer children," "two is enough," "small is happy") are at odds with the conditions of lives.

Where infant death is a key part of the way institutions represent their own activities in rural Uttar Pradesh by assigning the region the dubious distinction of being a flagship for infant mortality rates in Asia, at the level of persons and experiences infant death is also part of socialities in and of authority. Like reproduction more generally, it is a way men and women relate themselves to institutional structures. In this regard, stories of infant death are part of an ongoing conversation about power. They are constant references to the vagaries of higher forces, whether of fate, God, the state, medicine, hospitals, injections, pills, ghosts, jealousy, or gazes. Fate replaces karma here. Indeed, karma is notably absent from these stories, though even where it is unspoken, it might retain a place within other causalities, even those that leave it all "up to God."

Death is not the only "elsewhere" (de Certeau 1984), and at times it is not really an elsewhere at all. In stories about lost children, women refer to God, medicine, the state, fate, and "nothing at all"—all sites in which an outlying power is reckoned in the conjunction of grief, outrage, and longing—at the same time that they speak of their own actions. One quality of the web of alterities is an immobilizing pairing of its unapproachability and power. But there is also something more mundane here. Following recent trends in ethnographic syntax, I might be tempted to refer to this element as "haunting," but something about the feel of stories of infant death is at once more overpowering and more graspable and pedestrian than the translucent shimmerings of ghosts and other uncanny things. I am struck in rereading, rehearing these stories, by a sense of constant drawing near to and backing away from this alterity, from the way movements of *people* (not, or not only, haunting others) shape experiences of suffering.

At a group singing for a birthday, a woman is passed the drum. She hands it back and says, "No, since the death of my son I do not sing." Women nod. The drum is passed to another singer. What, then, are the ways that death can—and cannot—be named in the spaces just at the edge of institutional certainty, the ways that stories open up an unsteady normality?

"This also happened to me..."

One weekend afternoon, Pratima Srivastav comes by the house with a female cousin. They are offered chairs in the angan, and Bari Bhabhi comes out to touch their feet (Choti Bhabhi is visiting her maike).

Pratima and her sister discuss with Amma how they are related, and what relatives lie in the degrees of separation between them—who is the wife of whom, how many children each has, whether the children are boys or girls. The maps involve many I have never heard of. When Amma says that Bari Bhabhi has one son, they stop kin mapping. "Only one? Why?"

"There were two others, but they died," Amma says. Bari Bhabhi stands nearby.

"Oh ho," Pratima says and looks up at Bhabhi.

"Yes," Bhabhi says, "One at three months, the other immediately, meaning at that exact time [of its birth]."

Amma repeats this information. "One right away and the other at three months."

Pratima and her sister ask at the same time, their voices overlapping, "Did you give the babies the t.t. tikka [tetanus vaccine]?"

"Yes, we gave everything," Bhabhi says.

"Did you give the tikka *shots then, at that time?"*

"Yes, we gave everything."

"And before, meaning when you were pregnant? Did you get the tikka *then?"*

"Yes, everything. Both times. We gave all the tikka. *But sometimes it just happens like this. That something is not right."*

"Yes, yes. Sahi bat. It's true."

Bari Bhabhi goes into the kitchen to bring the tea. Amma says in a low voice, "And that baby was so healthy. It was this big and in good health...."

Later, while Bari Bhabhi is moving around in the angan, rinsing dishes at the hand pump, sweeping up ginger cuttings, Amma whispers to Pratima and her sister about one of the ill-fated deliveries. "There was some kind of confusion. The water broke, but then the baby did not come right away. It didn't come for a long time."

Pratima's sister whispers, "If all that water is there and the cord gets twisted the baby has to take in that dirty water, so it dies." She looks at me and nods her head.

"What can it breathe? It has to take in all that dirty water," Amma repeats, "Its eyes weren't even open." Then she raises her voice to a speaking level and glances at Bhabhi, "Sometimes this is what fate gives us."

At Bari Bhabhi's maike, during the preparations for one of her brother's prewedding ceremonies, she tells me that the naoun will be coming by later to help with the preparations—organizing and dividing the gifts, doing women's hair, applying red paint to feet and mehndi to hands. "While she does this," Bari Bhabhi tells me, "She will tell you all her life's sadness." Telling grief is part of the work of marriage, reproduction, and anticipated sexuality. Like postpartum workers do when massaging a jaccha, they will tell you their life story. "How many babies have died, how difficult their lives have been. They do this to get your sympathy and a better payment," Bari Bhabhi laughs, though at the same time, I sense, it is in the nature and timing of their work to evoke the complex affects of reproductive life.

On the evening of the day the neighbor's baby died, Bhabhi tells me about grief. Telling it is supposed to help, though sometimes it can, she says, make it worse.

"If you don't talk about it you might start thinking about other things and gradually forget, but here people don't think that. They think that if something bad has happened, someone has died, a baby or a man, then they must go to that house and sit with the people and talk to them about things that have happened to them, how this pain also happened to me and to tell the story."

I ask if this means that people feel that by talking about it the pain decreases.

"Yes," she says, "If someone dies and people don't go to the house to sit and talk, they will be offended. People think that if tears come a lot then the pain will be drawn out, if you feel more sadness you will feel better, but also you will feel that other people feel sadness and have experienced sadness. When my second baby died I just wanted to be alone. To be in my room and not sit with anyone, but so many people came and what happened? They said, 'Where is the bride? We heard that her son died.' And they came into the room; all day people came—from this village, from Devia ... people heard Bapu-ji's grandson died, and they came that night ... he died that night, I couldn't sleep at all. Not a single second of sleep came. Not a moment passed when I was not thinking about the baby and feeling pain. I could not sleep for all the pain I felt. I did not feel like living. In the morning people began to come and did not stop until evening and I wanted to be left alone."

Pratima takes me to the home of two sisters-in-law known for their skill at delivering babies. In the middle of the conversation a neighbor woman and her daughter come by. Like Pratima, the neighbor works for NAFPA. They divide the clients in the village. Her daughter is wearing a maxi *and is wrapped in a shawl. Her head stays bowed to the ground. Her mother cuts in to tell us a story; it is confusing and its temporalities are circular and difficult for me to follow, but unlike other death stories, this one is interjected into a* pakka *"interview" already in progress. Unlike others, it is "caught" on my tape recorder.*

"Her baby was born one month ago. There was so much pain, so much pain and still the baby did not come. So the baby was not born here in the village. We went to Munniabad. The baby was born there. The pain was so great that I thought my daughter wouldn't survive. The baby was stuck. It was not coming out. We tried laying hands, many people put on their hands, doctors and nurses, but there was so much pain that she could not go on any further. She would have to be cut."

Another woman cuts in and adds, "It was stuck, and nothing could be done."

The mother continues. "It was stuck, we could not say if it would be alive or dead so finally there was an operation. After so many days of pain. Fifteen, but the really bad pain and trouble was three days. So much difficulty that we said, 'Let's take care of her,' and we took her to Munniabad to that hospital. We went in a [hired] Maruti [van]. There was pain up to 5:00, but the doctor was not there. But then she eventually came and there was an operation. The baby was born with the operation. The baby was very tired and weak.

Someone else adds, "But the baby was very good," which I take to mean it was large, plump, healthy.

"Yes," the woman says, "But the baby was tired and weak, and they [the doctors] didn't know that the baby was weak, so I told them and said, 'Can't you do something?' There was nothing, they did nothing. They said to us that sometimes a baby is born like this. What else? [Afterwards] she [the daughter] said she did not want to live without the child, she could not endure. The sadness was too great. She said, 'I had a good baby.' There was so much sadness, she could not go on any further. She said this to me, 'My life is trickling out.'"

In Sitapur I heard very few birth stories. Women often told me that they just could not remember, or asked, "What's the point?" But stories about infant death were common, detailed, and specific. While it might be tempting to write that to have babies in Sitapur is to risk unspeakable sorrow, what is paramount to this grief is its spokenness, its presence as open and exchanged talk. Rather than feeling private or protected, such memories have a public, traded, and ever-present quality. Tales of death—of one's own children, of other people's children, of children's children—circulate through households and villages, arising at predictable times and inserting themselves at others. They are varied, though they also follow patterns, even genres. In some tellings, they assert a brand of morality, one based in difference. In others, they are less about diacritics than complex causalities, even soteriologies, of infant death, in which morality is defied rather than defined.

As part of social "transactions" (following Das 1997), stories about past losses speak of a conversation with death, and, more broadly, of what it means to think of "healing as a kind of relationship with death" (1997: 78). Likewise, they mark intersubjectivity, most vividly in the cotelling of stories, the taking over of someone else's story for a moment. Pushpadevi interrupted her sister-in-law's telling of her own daughter's death to finish out the story, and her own story about her son's death was begun (briefly—it was difficult to stem the tide of Pushpadevi's talk) by her sister-in-law. Mothers told daughters' stories, mothers-in-law told the stories of daughters-in-law, daughters recounted mothers' losses and those of mothers-in-law. Sometimes stories cropped up in places I might have expected to hear them ("Tell me about your children's births…"), other times they interjected in discomforting ways. Some were told as a means of introduction, their layers meshed into the bisections of self- and other-presentation, the layers of subjectivity that arise when two people meet. Others were not so much introductions as interruptions.

At the risk of sounding glib, I draw on de Certeau in considering ways of telling infant death, like the physical walls and gutters between houses, to be frontiers, dividing and marking points of difference and convergence in which things like morality and causality are reckoned. For de Certeau, stories "found spaces" between people and moral topographies in which boundaries are marked out and crossed. Frontiers, he says, are not a "nowhere," but spaces between, with a "mediating role," a "sort of a void," a "middle place," a "narrative symbol of exchanges and encounters"—with all the differentiating and coming together such meetings may entail (de Certeau 1984: 127). As frontiers, stories about infant death are sites of uncertainty, or of tentatively postulated certainty. At the same time, they are points of reckoning with the ambivalence of memory—as at once an unreachable beyond-space and intimate presence.

Educating desire

A few days after the promotional navtanki *(play) put on by NAFPA in the village just to the north, I am walking on the road between the villages and pass two men. We get to talking. One recognizes me from the show. "I remember you. The* navtanki *about children and babies. You went with Tulsiram."*

"That's right."

"Now I remember. They were right. It is good to have only two children," he says, half to me and half to the other man.

A third man stops and gets off his bike to join our conversation. "Two or three is good. Three is good too." There is a pause. Then his voice rises, "But look, they say 'have two children, have two children,' but I had two children and they both died."

The other men look at him, "Really? Two and both died?"

"What happened?" I ask, and another man asks the same thing. "Were they sick?"

"No, no illness, nothing. Sometimes it is like this. The first one was born and then three days later he died. Then the younger one was born and he lived a few hours but died the very same day."

"Oh ho," says one of the men. "Were they born here in this village?"

"Yes."

"So sad," we all agree.

The first man says, "Did you do anything?" but I am uncertain what he means.

The man on the bike snaps back, "Like what? This is all given by the one above. It is out of our control, isn't it?"

Visions of morality are at stake in the way the presence of loss, the telling of greif mark a presence in society and to the state. For many, there is a ring of fatalism to statements about everything being in the domain of some "other" force—be it God (women refer to the more general, less personified Bhagwan in these cases, never to storied avatars such as Ram, Krishna, or Shiva, or to the goddess Devi/Maia, to whom they sing and pray on other occasions) or fate. The relief heard in such phrasings is part of urban narratives about rural women, just as it is often assumed in public health circles that the sheer commonness of infant death is brought about by a numbness of response to it, a circular lack of affect and lack of urge to "do something" brought on by a basic misperception of "normality."

In the 1980s medical anthropologists writing about infant mortality described modernity as a condition in which "the dialectic between fertility and mortality has lost its edge" (Scheper-Hughes 1987: 1). Noting that childhood mortality was not considered a social problem in Europe prior to the twentieth century, Scheper-Hughes paralleled early-modern mortality patterns in Europe, as described by Arthur Imhof (1985), in which deaths were concentrated in infancy, with what she called "old" patterns of reproduction, in which higher numbers of births and briefer intervals between them went along with uncertainty about child survival. Accompanying uncertainty, Scheper-Hughes wrote, was a protective pattern of parental disinvestment, "allow[ing] ... a certain emotional distance that is psychologically protective" (1987: 11). But in this essay, and in her later work, Scheper-Hughes makes clear that this "old" pattern is hardly premodern, but is embedded in economic and political structures and is familiar in locales of intense poverty characteristic of industrialized societies. However, modern or not, the framework of "investment" and "strategy" models of childbearing and, by extension, parental affect may also foreclose certain understandings of how not only conditions of global capital but histories of intervention and their attendant structures of meaning *themselves* render lack of affect a pathology characteristic of subaltern women. The loop of missing emotion that is "fatalism" can leave little room for attention to languages of grief and the ways they may in fact speak directly *to* (rather than being muted by) complexities of living and caregiving amid state and transnational structures. What sounds like fatalism may be protective, but it may also bear political and critical weight, affect and critique instead of their absence.

Where infant mortality is a modern phenomenon, the pedagogical and subject-transforming nature of reproductive health intervention makes "awareness" central to framing the healthy citizen. In the early documents of the World Bank's *Safe Motherhood Initiative* (SMI) (Hertz and Meacham 1987), quantitative statements about the malaise of women in developing countries introduce a text situating both the need for and means of intervention, one firmly situated in the economic and political flows of the 1980s. Numbers are mustered to show basic lack of consciousness and affect. Worse than what statistics demonstrate, the text states that women and men in Asia "don't notice" such "high rates" of mortality and morbidity because they are ignorant of global standards; they don't, in other words, know their numbers. The "risks" of pregnancy and childbirth "go almost unnoticed" because "women have always died in childbirth" and because risks are "overshadowed" by other "disadvantages" (1987: 1). Third World women, the text tells us, "don't understand" that early childbearing and repeated childbearing affect health adversely; they don't understand, in effect, that ill health is bad (4). An outcome of "adherence to tradition" (4) such ignorance produces suffering without the ability to take its full measure.

Before we come to this exposition, however, a path has been cleared for intervention, one based on teaching desire. The preface to the 1987 SMI document describes "self-help programs" by which women are instructed to "want help" (Hertz and Meacham 1987: vii); evidence of successful outcome lies in observations that women who "understand health and the causes of ill-health" will demonstrate their understanding by "demanding" services (4). Such assertions, based on a kind of market logic, are confirmation that maternal mortality can be prevented through use of "known technology"; solutions need only be desired to come into being (1). This logic of educated desire is the reverse of development logics in which ignorance is a form of lack—notably of Cartesian rationality (Apffel-Marglin 1996). In terms the framing of rural women's affective and perceptive abilities, an imagined lack of sensitivity to "true" suffering grounds intervention; ignorance is a positive state, a matter of the choices women make.

The SMI asks, "Some women within reach of modern health care do not seek it. Why not?" The answer is that, as well as persistent ignorance and "disempower[ment]," whether or not women make the right decisions "hinge[s] on their *perceptions* of quality of care, accessibility and costs" (Hertz and Meacham 1987: 5, emphasis added). Indeed, "demand may be weak until quality improves." But the SMI

does not dwell on this point; the next sentence returns to the need
to "educat[e]" women to understand "the benefits of modern health
care" (5), regardless of the quality of existing care. Such emphasis on
demanders (rather than suppliers) of care, and on the psychological
source of desire, embeds intervention in a neoliberal logic in which
health is a private good and responsibility largely that of individuals,
largely matters of consciousness. With goals to make women "consumers" of health care, the SMI notes that "an informed consumer
can use whatever resources are available more effectively," whereas
an ignorant one will be adrift in a sea of unfamiliar, copious commodities (Hertz and Meacham 1987: 18).

It might seem reasonable to locate this moment of policy firmly in
the decade of its production, or at the cusp of an even more broadly
liberalizing decade. But the logic of privatization that continued
through the 1990s, coupled with the overt shift toward "target-free
approaches" and efforts to rid programs of the stain of the Emergency
by adopting languages of "choice" and human rights make the individualizing and affect-oriented logic of demand persistent. Likewise,
the circulation of texts separate from contexts, the filtering out of
sound bites and snippets of logic at a remove from the development
ideologies that might (in academic circles, perhaps) otherwise enfold them, means that the idea of "fatalism" in the face of infant
death, like harrowing images of placentas left attached and dirty
dais with dirty hands, provides emotional and moral urgency to interventions. "They think everything is brought about by God" is a
common enough observation in local development circles, requiring no further explanation. As one doctor involved in dai-trainings
told me, "They consider it normal to lose a baby or two. They are
always surprised to hear that I gave birth to only two children, and
to this day still have two children. They must be taught that [infant
death] does not need to be normal." The "peasant fatalism" Scheper-
Hughes refers to as a fundamental misunderstanding by "secular
anthropologists" (and others) of local ways of coping (1992: 363) not
only establishes relative subject-positions and socialities, it also establishes the way care will, in the end, be provided.

Whether things repeated are compulsive or meaningful, in practice as in policy such comments speak to the security of numbers, of
enumeration. Ways of framing feminine emotion in relation to the
purdah of ignorance have long described the veil lifted by knowledge of universal modes of accounting. To return to Katherine Mayo's
Mother India (1927), which gives so much to marvel at, ignorance involves lack of perspective within conditions of poverty at once nat-

ural and traditional. Responses to child death, for Mayo, involve both insufficient perception and inadequate speech, within a predatory vision of the natural world that is counterpoint to the rational world of enumeration: "If a baby dies, the mother's wail trails down the darkness of a night or two. But if the village be near a river, the little body may just be tossed into the stream, without waste of a rag for a shroud. Kites and the turtles finish its brief history. And it is more than probable that no one in the village will think it worth while to report either the birth or the death. Statistics as to babies must therefore be taken as at best approximate" (Mayo 1927: 110).

In a particular mode of modernity, utterances imagine the "world-as-picture," as a promise of "the immediacy of the really real" in contrast to abstraction (Mitchell 2000a: xiv). Such maps may also open up spaces in which meanings subordinated to the larger whole return as symptoms of social disarray. At the NAFPA *navtanki*, a play written with the intention of providing health messages in a "traditional" performance idiom, a long skit involved the silly sufferings of a man described as "Kaddu Ram" (something like "Pumpkin Joe"). Ignorant, bound by the strings of his desires, this marionette-ish figure produced endless numbers of children, and along with them, sufferings associated with lack of food, lack of tidiness and cleanliness, and general malaise in life. In an uncanny similarity, for Mayo the core of Indian women's suffering rested in the unchecked sexuality of "their" men. Mayo described Indian men's inability to control sexual urges as giving rise to broader suffering through sins such as child-marriage and overpopulation. Within this framework, as in the histrionics of Pumpkin Joe, laziness and lack of affect situate both excessive birth and attitudes toward death. Offered as an alternative is the "happiness" of the small, nuclear family.

There is a transformation here. Through individualizing causalities and converging crises of over-sexuality and lack of enumeration, a picture of modernity's crises leaves grief out of the experience of loss. Such suffering is negated in the production of new signs essential to the myth of development: the fatalistic rural woman, the oversexed Indian man, the senseless peasant. As nonspecific tropes of hygiene and disengagement locate whole groups on a national-(ized) and biologized map of threat and value, split-off specificities make the language of population, hygiene, and compliance create out of infant death a discourse on limited humanity, at the core of which is a misrecognition of death. Rural people, it seems, must be taught not only how to see but how to feel.

Sometimes the production of the abject feels accidental and inevitable. Manjari takes me to a meeting with her CBDs after which we will march through the community promoting family planning. She has been given a large banner and a list of rhyming couplets to chant to remind people that family planning is important, that they can get "copper-T's" implanted to prevent pregnancy, that "goli" (pill, not bullet) will promote happiness. With a group of about ten women—NAFPA workers and some just along for the ride—we wind through the neighborhoods. After not too long, our small but raucous group is trailed by a bigger crowd of children, listening to our chants about condoms and IUDs, and looking, it is hard not to observe, as Manjari and I do to each other, extremely poor, barely clothed, unkempt. In their appearance as in their number they lend a kind of ridiculous proof to our messages. In all these signs, shouted out, glued and painted on walls, blasted through scratchy loudspeakers, we hear about the devastation that comes with too many children. That children should be an investment, little nuggets of "capital," as Bari Bhabhi put it, products of "quality not quantity." But the man on the road after the navtanki *had a different idea. A visiting auntie tells me that children bring pleasure and joy, "It doesn't feel good to live in a house without children." Dev's Wife and sister-in-law remind me that, "Homes should be full." In our couplets and posters and signs, this burdensome sense of love works through a different relationship to the world, to time.*

Children and loss

To walk through the fields, one must balance along mer, *the stretches of raised, grassy ground separating one field from the next. And to walk on the* mer *is to tread on burial places of children. "Children have not reached the age of* shayani *(knowledge)," Pushpadevi tells me. Their rawness in terms of the way sexuality, reproductive capacity, and worldliness converge means, as she said, "They are not cremated, but we bury them under the edges of fields," in the lines of demarcation between plots and crops, at the edges of fertility and production. I wonder sometimes as I walk out to see Tulsiram's family working in the sugar cane or planting peanuts in the dry dust, what is under my feet? I imagine, but perhaps I am wrong, that it is not only for mothers and fathers, but for all who inhabit this space, that child death is part of a basic topography.*

When Shalini's sister is born, her family—and those who discuss them— are often reminded of their loss. Several years ago her older brother fell into the well outside their house. "It was a hot night," her mother tells me. We are talking about her baby's recent birth, but there is not much to say about it and talk turns to this. "We were sleeping in the angan, and some men and boys were sleeping outside near the well. He was sleeping on the ledge. It was a wide ledge, wide enough for a child to sleep on. He slept curled around like this. I don't know why he slept like that, up on the wall. He was this high [about seven or eight]. He must have fallen in in the night, while sleeping. In the morning the men woke up and didn't know where he was. They looked all around. Finally someone looked in the well and saw him."

"They are poor from lack of capital," *Bari Bhabhi tells me, speaking later about Shalini's family,* "And you can consider that boy the family's capital." *Three, now four daughters, three small fields shared among feuding brothers, a jobless father, a lost only son—the situation is related to me many times. Many women in the neighborhoods near Shalini's home tell me they like to give her a bit of work, even if they don't always need it.*

One morning, I ask Shalini where the boy is buried. She points and says he lies at the edge of the family's field. "There are three people there," *she says,* "An aunt and a grandfather." *But it is their burned remains that are there.* "On holidays we bring them food."

"They are here," *she shows me a few weeks later when we go for a walk in the fields, pointing to an undistinguished mound of grass-covered earth.* "I bring the food on Holi. On other holidays. Deepawali. When we make good food."

"Is there a puja here?"

"There's food, there's water, there's a puja. Everything."

Choti Bhabhi's younger son, Dilip, falls ill shortly after his first birthday. On a cold night he begins throwing up and spewing diarrhea. His parents comfort and coax him to drink rehydration fluid all night, and a kaccha doctor is summoned early in the morning to give an injection of antibiotics. That afternoon he begins to improve, but he is listless and pale for days.

A few nights later Rohit is playing on my bed as I type notes. I stop my work to play with him. We roll a lemon back and forth, and throw an imaginary ball. Rohit takes one of my pillows, puts it next to him, pats it and leans over close, as though listening. "My boy is crying. Comfort him," *he says, tapping the pillow with his hand and making a* "ba ba ba ba" *sound the way his uncle does to turn Dilip's cries into laughter. He hands me the other pillow.* "B-bua, B-bua-ji," *he says, Auntie, Auntie, with his usual stutter,* "Your baby is crying. Comfort it." *I pat and make cooing sounds to the* "baby," *and we go back to rolling the lemon. Between catches, Rohit comforts his* "baby." *First, he repeats,* "My baby is sick," *and then, with growing intensity and specificity,* "My baby is vomiting," "My baby is shitting," *each time his voice grows louder and shakier.*

The lemon is no longer interesting, and the "baby" requires full attention. "My baby is vomiting, my boy is vomiting. Give him an injection, give an injection." He gives the baby an injection, then grabs my arm to make me give one too. As the "needle" goes in, he grimaces. "Give me an injection too, Bua, Give one to me." I pretend to give him one as well.

The game goes on. New ailments, new remedies. "My baby is crying, comfort him. Your baby is crying too—comfort it." "Give my baby pills, give your baby pills, give me pills." "Isko bubu pilao, isko bubu pilao," he turns to an imaginary mother, beseeching her to breast-feed the baby. It becomes a desperate rite, and Rohit gets more and more distraught: "My baby is shitting, my baby is vomiting, my baby has a fever, give him pills, give him an injection, breast-feed him." I try to distract him with the ball, but he plays for only seconds before his crumpled face turns back to his pillow. I begin to repeat, "Rohit, your baby will get better," and he repeats, "He will get better," but he doesn't believe me and slips back into the worried effort.

"Look Rohit," I say, "your baby is sleeping, your baby is better." I am not convincing.

At this point Choti Bhabhi puts her head in the doorway. "Are you bothering Bua-ji? She is working. Come into the house and get some food." Rohit follows her. His terrible anxiety dissipates.

You cannot hear without crying

Some tellings unfold slowly over time, then suddenly come tumbling out. The night of the day the Pasi baby girl died, we sit in the darkness waiting, waiting, waiting until Jawahar, Sunderlal, and Raju take their meals, until the women will eat. Bari Bhabhi tells her story. A coherent, in-time narrative, different from the talk of introductions or self-situating ("I had three sons; two died"), it resonates with the dangerousness of details. Choti Bhabhi listens in silence. She has not heard this before, or not in this way.

When the second one died ... it was terrible ... I cannot even tell the story without feeling so much pain. You cannot hear without crying. I was all alone that time. The baby was born in February. We were living in Munniabad, me and Arjun, and Arjun's Papa [Sunderlal], and the baby lived for three months, and then it got diarrhea. I had the baby ... was in the village for one month, then it got sick and I went back to Munniabad. He was very sick and for two days we gave this doctor's medicine and that doctor's medicine, and that doctor's medicine, and nothing worked. He became very, very skinny and weak and we were told to go to Bishwa because there is a doctor there, a good doctor, he is a baby doctor. He's Punjabi. Bishwa is close, right? It's not too far, so we went by train. There's a morning train and we two people went by train [she and the baby] and I took the baby to the doctor and he gave some medicine. So that night I slept.

Look, for three days I had not slept at all. I had been awake all night taking care of, looking at the baby, worrying would it get better or not. I hadn't slept at all, and that night, I don't know from where, but finally I could sleep. I felt, we have shown the baby to the doctor. He is a big doctor, and now everything will be okay. That night I fell asleep with my hand like this on the baby, and in the night I woke up and my hand had come off the baby. Was separate. I was very worried and right away woke up and put my hand on the baby and I felt it and I thought, oh the baby is so cold. But I didn't think it had died, because I don't have any experience with this, I didn't know.

It was hot weather, weather for the fan. After Holi. The baby was born in February, and February, March, April. We were staying with some Mami (aunt) who lives in Bishwa and it was hot so the fans were on. I pulled a blanket over him. The fans were on him and so he got cold. And then went to the other room to get some medicine. I tried to give him the medicine but I could not open its mouth. I still didn't know he was dead. His eyes were closed. I went to the front room and called Mami and said, "Mami, come, look, there's something wrong with the baby. I can't get it to eat the medicine," and Mami came and felt him and went into the front room. She didn't say anything to me, but she knew the baby was dead. I was in that room and I heard her outside saying to the other people, "Dulhan is in there. Her baby has died, but she doesn't know it. She says the baby is cold, but he is dead. She doesn't know."

[I interject—"My god, you heard her saying that?"] Yes, that's how I knew. So everyone woke up and what could we do? It was the middle of the night, so we all sat up and first thing in the morning I got the train back to Munniabad. I had to get back somehow, right? And Mami took me to the train and everyone said, "Hold the baby close, keep it hidden and don't cry. If you cry people will know that something has happened to the baby and will kick you off the train, and then if you get on a bus it will be the same. People will be even closer and will know and won't let you stay and how will you get back? So hold the baby, hide it, don't let anyone know."

So I sat on the train and a little closer there was a woman with a baby, but I had to sit far away because I knew if I sat close to her I would begin to cry. And I was sitting there and I don't know how, but I held the baby and I stayed quiet. The baby was completely hard. There were these other women, Muslim women, in burkhas, and they saw my face and recognized something was wrong and said, "The baby is not well?" and I said, "No, he is not well." And then I got off the train and got a rickshaw, to go to our house, and I passed the milkman who comes to our house and he saw and he said, "The baby has died?" and I said yes, and he went to get Arjun's father and he must have said, "The teacher's son has died," because when I got to the house there was a big crowd. Mamis, Mamas, Chachis, Chachas, everyone, asking what had happened. And sitting there.

They all said, "Should the burial happen here or in the village?" and they were discussing this and I... I hadn't been able to eat a thing and of course hadn't slept, and hadn't even been able to cry because of the travel and the people and I said, "Look, how can I reach Lalpur? I could barely get here with the baby, and so how can I go on another journey to the village?" If we had a phone we might have called and told someone to come pick us up, but what phone was there? So the baby was buried there in Munniabad and then Bapu-ji came from Lalpur and got a car and Arjun's Papa and all the relatives went to Lalpur by bicycle and I sat in the car with Bapu-ji. And when we arrived here there was even more of a crowd than in Munniabad. Everyone had heard that Bapu-ji's grandson had died, and they came from everywhere, the house was full of people. And when I arrived I don't know what happened to me, but it was like all my breath left my body at once, like I couldn't breathe from below, the breath was gone from the inside. I just collapsed and couldn't breathe. And then there were all those people. Men came and they won't come inside the house, but they will stay outside, and the women were inside. So all day people came and sat and talked and at night I lay down but I couldn't sleep. They gave me liquor and medicine, medicine to make me sleep, but still I could not.

Like the breath was gone from the inside

Let us locate a quality of movement. Grief, like lives, can be mediated by the constraints and imperatives of daily life. Death can come in motion as much as stillness, a distinction about which, the Bhagavad Gita reminds us, even the wise can be confused (Bhagavad Gita IV: 16). In the seeming human vulnerability of "the hands of God" may lie commentary on the instability of the action/inaction binary. Such statements, their intersubjective demands for an agreement ("Yes, it's true," a nodded head) and their meaning-consuming gulp seldom stand alone, coming instead at the end of often complicated stories of desperate action and institutional failure.

Writing on women's grief in India focuses on the tension between internal and external suffering, what is told, and what is withheld. In her powerful accounts of women's grief in the wake of the violence of Partition, Veena Das describes the interiority of women's suffering, using womb-like metaphors and recognizing the construction of pain as "a transaction between body and language," in which "grief is articulated through the body" (1997: 68). Enunciations, Das says, after the subject-shattering violence of rape, speak of "healing as a kind of relationship with death" (78), a sustained rather than absolved relationship to deaths physical and social. At the same time, expressions of grief are "the work of the collectivity," vitally gendered, embodied in the female as "the one that will carry this pain within forever" (80). In constituting a subject through grief, laments—and the presence of those who have suffered—are a continued commentary on a political reality, situated at the heart of the existence of the Indian nation. For Das, both laments and the containment of grief have reconstituting power, relocating suffering into the flow of life. In lamentation, the "inner state" is made visible and "is finally given a home in language," making the world livable again, "transforming its strangeness [as] revealed by death" (68). Yet this wholeness, this mitigated strangeness signifies the ever-unfinished project of healing.

Infant mortality is a different kind of crisis than the brutalities of rape, signifying a different rent in the flow of life and locating the grief elsewhere in relation to body, kin, and nation. Likewise, the ability to speak or not speak violence constitutes a qualitatively different dilemma than that posed by speech—or constraints put upon it—about infant death. For one thing, the latter aims less at nationalized politics than at a transnational, even when nationalized, structure of intervention, law, and biotechnique. However, in its description of the shape of grief and its ability to be sustained as commentary on the political condition, Das's account gives us material for understanding grief as a relationship to power—and, indeed, a necessity to juxtapose it to the very languages meant to intervene in the site of loss. In particular, we can emphasize, as Das does, "work" that runs, perhaps eloquently, against the grain of healing.

As moments of suspended resolution, stories of infant death occupy a political and moral space that speaks to things akin to the structural violence described by Scheper-Hughes (1992), but under the wobbly presence of state and transnational attention. Infant death's symbolic place in the apparatus of intervention in India, the structures of governance and hierarchy in which death becomes meaningful as a "Third World" problem, and, most importantly, the diffuse causalities of infant mortality mean that, in repeated stories of loss, while certain things are being made—or kept—visible, other things are "swallowed whole," rendered part of social life in a symptomatic way. In such a context, perhaps, rather than transforming the strangeness of death into something more comfortable, women's stories of loss obscure the certainties in which medical practice is supposed to exist, speaking to long-standing rationalities meant to account for the suffering of the poor, the "internal others" who threaten the well-being of the nation.

Freud's concept of melancholia might enter here, in the way that it makes it possible to imagine what suspended—or sustained—grief might sound like in the flows of speech. In a "devouring" (Freud 1963: 171), which is counter to the integration characteristic of mourning, the grief of melancholia remains an "open wound" (174), and the loss of an object is identified with the self (168, 170). As the lost object is taken in, swallowed whole, the self remains entangled in longing and it turns upon itself. It is at this moment of consumption that fatalistic-sounding statements may dwell. What was spoken—causality—is devoured, replaced by a singular agency. Narratives of infant death involve a language of the entangled subject, ending with a gulp of causation that consumes the locatedness of death. But rather than abrogating causality they up its ante. A broader contingency emerges from what the narrative swallows whole, through the grief consumed and the consuming grief.

Put in simpler terms, while some sites, stories, and ways of telling take the listener into the "margins," off the radar of institutions, in other stories the state and its agencies, the stuff of medical authority, are part of a rough weave of life and death. Institutions provide a fantasy of stability amid radical uncertainty, but wither when approached. Accounts often describe such failures, the pinball movement of people from one institution to another, failure in the midst of approaches and withdrawals, appeals and rejections. Where authorities represent infant death in rural India as a matter of failure to desire institutional engagement, rural women remind each other—and reminded me—that death can take place precisely *at* the point of engagement with institutions—hospitals, doctors, *kaccha* and otherwise, and ANMs. They confound the idea that one either does or does not engage biomedical models and institutions, describing at once the unstable presence of institutions. They suggest, angrily, that something larger is at work, and institutions are not God.

These frontiers are places where causality is dealt with. While it is clear to me that stories of infant death, in their circulation and in being tucked away or saved for later presentation, do not all "do" the same thing, one way they differ from lamentation is in *not* (or not only) transforming the strange into something more comfortable. A theme of mourning ritual, Das says, is "to absolve the living of responsibility for the death that has occurred" (1997: 81). However, in the case of infants and children, death's connections with modern institutions and conditions enter into discourse as already morally loaded. There is no one way to hear, "Everything is in the

hands of God" or "Sometimes it is like this." Its use by the man on
the road rebuked and made flimsy state claims that happiness comes
with fewer children, while its use by Bari Bhabhi in response to Choti
Bhabhi's comment, "those people never take their babies to the doctor" was surely meant to absolve blame. Were we to consider such
statements separately from the narratives from and into which they
erupt, then we might sense the same freedom from responsibility
referred to in the languages of colonial and postcolonial intervention. But thinking about ways memories are exchanged and retold
requires constant reevaluaation of what it means to act and to grieve
in a specific context.

Such stories' orientations to the past unsettle the terms of life and
death into which the "fatalism of the poor" is often cast, persistently
begging the question of reality – what experience, what form of affect, what mode of remembering is, or conveys, what is going on?
The rehearsed memory pushes offered-up futures into a relationship
with the past, with the very sites of instability within those offered-
up promises. Without the consuming moment of the narrative—in
which specific causes are absorbed into larger Causation, in which
objects of loss, including that which is the moment of explanation,
are absorbed into the subject—futures, or visions thereof, might become forgetful.

Certeau writes, "In this combination between subjects without
action and operations without author, between the anguish of individuals and the administration of practices, the dying man raises
once again the question of the subject at the extreme frontier of inaction, at the very point where it is the most impertinent and the
least bearable" (1984: 191). But the death of the child may push that
frontier yet further. Birth's potentiality of action and the child's ability to embody the future mean that in loss—at this edge—when the
distinction between inactive subject and authorless practice breaks
down, perhaps one cannot speak except in a crush of time, cause,
and effect. With a slight tweak, a modest tuning out, it is easy to hear
ignorance and laziness. But retune, and it is not so uncanny that the
only thing to say is "sometimes it happens like this" or "everything
is in the hands of God."

Talking statues

*On one of my last weekend mornings in Lalpur a traveling sadhu (holy
man) comes through the village. He stops first at the house next door, sits out-*

side their door and speaks with a few men. I go into the kitchen in search of some company from the Bhabhis. Bari Bhabhi tells me about the sadhu. "He will come here next," she says.

"What will he do?" I ask, "Tell stories?" There have been others like this, deep-voiced men reciting tales that end with a moral punch line sung in rhyming couplet.

"No," she says, "This one will read your palm. To tell the future."

This is the time of the wheat harvest. The air is thick with the dust of its cutting and people are moving in and out of the village—family members coming from cities to receive their allotment of the harvest, village men leaving for days at a time to make deliveries to relatives in Munniabad and Lucknow. "Sadhus also come out at this time of year," Bhabhi laughs. "The wheat has been cut and they come for their dan (gift)." She doesn't recognize this one, but says it doesn't matter. He will wander the countryside, staying in people's homes. "Families will give him a bed and something to eat, and he will sit in the house and read palms for whoever comes by. People give him a bit of money, too."

Bhabhi says this one has probably come here because he heard this family would give a substantial donation. He is from Ayodhya, but she does not know which temple. Being from this spiritually and politically important city will no doubt appeal to Sunderlal, I think. Over the last several months he has become more and more vocal about his rightward leanings, his belief that India is on the brink of a "world war" with Pakistan, and his support of the construction of the Ram temple in Ayodhya. His brothers disagree with him, and no one pays him too much mind.

"Will you have your palm read?" I ask.

"No," she says. "I won't show my hand to anyone. I don't want to know my future. I don't want to know if something bad will happen."

We go to the outer yard. Bari Bhabhi and Chachi, who has been hanging around, squat in the doorway, within earshot. Bari Bhabhi pulls her ghungut low over her face. I go under the veranda and sit at the edge of the men. It is not easy to understand. The sadhu is partly deaf and speaks with a strange frog voice punctuated almost to the point of stutter as he clicks his mala beads. He is tall and skinny, wearing a faded orange lungi and undershirt. The yellow stripes of Shiva are crusted on his forehead, and he carries a canvas bag from which he pulls a small, shapeless murti (statue). Sitting on an upright chair, he holds Sunderlal's hand and peers closely at its lines. Intermittently he holds the statue to his ear, nods his head, and makes soft conversational grunts as he listens to what it has to say.

"Three boys. You have one now and two who died before." The men nod. He listens to his murti and clicks his beads. "They died. Yes, hmm... they died." His speaks in bursts of a few words at a time, as though by effort, and

occasionally his blunted pronunciation is clarified by men sitting nearby.
"Two boys who died. Do you know why?"

"Illness," Sunderlal says.

"They died because a spell was put upon them. A spell. Something very
bad. One son now. You must look after him closely so the same does not happen to him."

I am called over. I sit where Sunderlal sat, and one of the men says,
"Didi, record this so you can tell your husband what is said."

"Husband?" *the sadhu says to Sunderlal.*

"Yes," *the men nod.*

"Children?" *he asked.*

"It will happen," *Tulsiram says, in his subtle avuncular way.*

*The sadhu turns my hand over and looks at it closely, his eyeball inches
from my fingers.* "A son. A boy. There will be more. Three. But first will be
a boy." *He listens to the* murti. "You will get a job. You will have an important job."

"What kind of work?" *I ask, but am not understood. Tulsiram translates.*

"Something with the government."

"She is from America," *someone says.*

"The American government will give you a job, and you will return
here." *A son, a government job, all signs of stability, happiness, and a
morally upright life.*

"And her husband?" *someone asks.*

"He is good. He is a good husband. You will have a happy life. You will
work hard. Life will be hard. But you will be happy." *I take a five-rupee note
from my bag and give it to him.*

Sunderlal says, "Now you will read her hand." *Bari Bhabhi is summoned
from the doorway. She sits on the ground in front of the sadhu. He begins
with children.*

"You had two sons. Finished. Grabbed." *He speaks facing Sunderlal and
does not look at Bhabhi, who keeps her head and much of her face covered. Sunderlal nods. He leans forward with a look of intense concern and
concentration.*

"One son. He is big now. You will have a bahu *[daughter-in-law]. The
son will get a government job. The* bahu *will be from the city. She will be a
good* bahu. *Do you keep* vrats *[fasts]?"*

"No," *Bhabhi says in a strong, clear, almost careless voice from under the*
ghungut.

"Vrat rakho! *(Keep your fasts!)" Sunderlal reprimands loudly, using the
same voice I hear when he threatens to hit Bhabhi if his tea is not made
quickly enough (the same voice to which she rolls her eyes and often snaps
back).*

"Keep vrat *on Thursdays. A full* vrat." *This means foregoing food and liquid, including water, while continuing to fulfill the day's household responsibilities—no small effort.*

"One son. Look after him and keep vrat. *What has brought harm to your other sons may also harm him. Do* puja, *keep* vrat." *After this, Sunderlal tells her to go back inside the house. Bhabhi touches the sadhu's feet and goes inside. She returns with a plate of recently milled flour, raw dal, and unground rock salt. The sadhu dumps it into his bag.*

Not long after, Sunderlal invites the sadhu into the angan *to discuss further means to protect Arjun from the deaths that befell the siblings he barely knew. The sadhu sits on a wooden bed and calls for a small brass cup of water and a dish of black salt to be balanced on top of it. He tells Sunderlal to put his hand over them as he clicks his beads and speaks once more to his* murti. *Bhabhi stands behind with a look of bland concern on her now-exposed face, while Sunderlal looks more intensely worried and effortful than I have ever seen him, even in the heat of his tirades about Pakistan. Bhabhi calls Arjun over.*

"To fully protect this boy, fully, totally, you must give a sum of money to the temple."

"Which temple are you from?" Sunderlal asks, and as the sadhu explains Sunderlal registers slight recognition.

There is some discussion of the amount to be given. Eleven hundred rupees (thirty-five dollars, a substantial sum for such a donation) is suggested by the sadhu. Sunderlal agrees.

The sadhu takes from his wallet photographs of two children, his own. "They died when they were young," he says.

Bhabhi shakes her head, "How sad."

"Yes, it is very sad when a child dies," he replies.

Sunderlal is told to put his hand over the lota *and* kitori.

"Say, 'I will pray to Shiva.'"

"I will pray to Shiva."

"Say, 'I will pray to Shiva.'"

"I will pray to Shiva."

Sunderlal sends Arjun to fetch his wallet, and then pulls five 100-rupee notes from it.

"Where shall we get the rest from?" he says softly. His gaze flits to me but does not land. The sadhu, however, looks up, into my eyes. Bhabhi does not look at me at all. I find myself for the briefest of seconds torn between anger and obligation—the former of which had begun to take shape when the sadhu read Sunderlal's palm, at what to me seemed to be manipulation of profound sadness, a sadness at once collective and intensely personal—conveyed through the tweaking of ever-latent fears and the circulation of images.

Belief, disbelief, and the suspension of both are impossible to parse in this performance and its reception. I look away, overcome by the way the at-all-costs fear of losing a child finds a modicum of relief when attached to institutional promises of protection, of well-being if only a connection is maintained. It is not anything like irrationality that enrages me, but the thinness of the veneer on which the sadhu is operating.

"It will come," Sunderlal says to the sadhu of the money, "We will send it to you." He writes the address.

"You will say after I leave, 'We won't give the rest of the money.' Or you will forget."

"No, no, we won't forget. We will send it when we get it. I will send it in a registered letter. I run the post office in this village, so I'll send it myself."

The sadhu pauses. "No, no. Don't send it. I will come back in a few months to look after you, to see to your safety. I will pay special attention to you." He looks at Arjun, "And to his safety. You can give me the money then."

He leaves after a few more pleasantries. Feeling I can stand it no longer, I leave too, out the back door.

Health institutions, like *sarkar*, are sites of alterity, massive but evasive, enticing with promises of healing, enfranchisement, encompassment, attention. Stories about them describe, in almost Lacanian terms, the structure of desire constituted as lack by evading the object and referring constantly back to points of absence, to the illegitimate, incongruous spaces a dead baby places one in. But such "lack" is not quite, or not only, absence, but can involve the *failure* of certainties when present—the familiarity (not the paradox) of presence and absence. Like Rohit's frazzled fantasies, stories of infant death become "written in the discourse of life" at the margins of institutions, making death part of other narratives—some about the morality of involvement with medical institutions, some about gods and higher orders of causality, some about things that cannot be known.

As with doctors, it might not matter so much whether a healer— of bodies, society, or fate—is real or fake (though, to be sure, there would be plenty of Lalpur residents who, when told this story, would suggest that any sadhu demanding so much is surely "fake"). Where quasi-institutional medical practitioners engage the magic of bureaucratic and medical institutions through rehearsed, naturalized practices and the imaginaries of their clients, the sadhu engages an equally potent experience of death. We can bring the following to Sitapur and its crumbling hospitals, sporadic health camps, foreign-funded state "schemes," come-and-go NGOs, *kaccha* doctors, and prognosticating holy men: a sense of what Taussig calls the "literalizing"

power of the state—and, I add, its institutions of intervention—
"staging intermittent exposure to the abject" (1997: 128). This is the
power of the claim staked on the *surface* of the real, of transactions
with the explicit aim of eliciting desire that create the broad expanse
of what it means to try to make things better. If claims about fatalism repress the grief present in women's stories, then, in the figures
of haphazard infanticide and willful laziness, the sting of a grotesque
"performed hiddenness [is] achieved by a disingenuous insistence
on taking things at face-value and materializing them" (128). The
promise of cure effaces the ability to provide it; outcome of engagement doesn't matter nearly so much as the surface of the engagement
itself. This is the magic of institutions. In more basic terms, babies
die in hospitals, and after meeting with "big" doctors, just as they die
after sadhus have been engaged, *vrats* kept, prayers recited, and sums
paid, or "just like that," "for no reason," just because "it is like this
sometimes." Or, to paraphrase Amma, "What's the big deal with hospitals? Babies die there too."

Phenomenological anthropology approaches the efficacy of healing ritual by suggesting that religious causalities do not operate
solely on the basis of "belief," but rather through a matrix of cultural
rationality and experience, and as such are not reducible to biomedical explanatory frameworks (the placebo effect, for example) (see
Csordas 1994a, 1994b, 1997; Desjarlais 1992; Jackson 1989). In India,
because God can be interlocutor as well as distant omnipotence, to
say "Everything is in the hands of God" situates causality in a balance
between engagement and overwhelming causation of which human
action is only part. In interactions and transactions between person
and deity—as between people and doctors—life and fertility can be
brought into effect (Goslinga-Roy 2002). In a sense, such a perspective "realities up" (to borrow a trick from Marilyn Strathern [1992])
religious or nonbiomedical systems by not pausing on "belief" versus "rationality." One could say that in Sitapur deities and cosmological forces should be considered, if not absolutely "real," then no
less real than medical institutions. Indeed, "the real" may be inde-
terminate here.

But if there is "reality up," there is also the reverse. We can think
about the ersatz, cynicism, and suspicion, and their marked absence
as part of the way "magic," "prayer," and "medicine" take shape; we
can use both the veneers of biomedical and religious rationality
alongside impasses of causality to "reality down" certain claims. We
can imagine that women lodge their "rational" and "magical" longings, powerful memories, and utter devastations upon doctors, hos-

pitals, sadhus, *car-sau-bisi* (con men), quasi-doctors, each other, and
visiting anthropologists with equal force. Just as those people (doctors, sadhus, anthropologists, etc.), at once ersatz and legitimate,
cast their lot with the longings and emotions of rural women, with
both legitimate concern and ulterior motive, to heal and to take advantage, further blurring the distinction between what is "real" and
what mere "imitation."

A longish quote from Taussig sums this up:

> What is not a trick? What for instance is the opposite of a trick? Is a
> technique the opposite of a trick? Is reality the opposite of a trick?
> And why do these pairings effectively eliminate the ethical issue in
> trickery, that it's somehow dishonest and amounts to a dishonest
> technique, a phony reality, reality in disguise, and so forth? The very
> notion of the trick, we might say, seems to sabotage binary logic, let
> alone reality, and does so most pointedly by making a clever mess of
> good and evil in relation to ontology and technology. Might it be that
> reality itself is one big trick, and the professional responsible for re-
> lating to this, such as the shaman [or, this author wants to add, the
> doctor or ANM or sadhu or quack or trained dai] entertains such cos-
> mic trickery while extracting a small profit in the form of healing
> power and sorcery? (Taussig 1998: 251)

It makes sense to think of sites and spaces that are the self-de-
clared alterity to magic and "fatalism" (biomedicine, for one) as not
only equally mimetic but no better able to avoid deception than
conjurers and quacks. We must not, Taussig says, "let reality off the
hook" (1998: 251), and should instead, as some people in Sitapur
seem to do, question claims made to it. Where the conditions of institutions make them evasive in a physical kind of way, and where
the promises of privatization are part of the very temporariness of
care getting, suffering is both an outcome and condition of the
range of tricks that is healing, intervention, and redemption. As
women who have lost babies after seeking health care—"doing the
right thing"—know, and as those who have lost babies after refusing the long arm of the state—also "doing the right thing"—can also
tell us, "reality will always out-trick human trickery modeled on reality so as to deceive it, but the seduction provided by the attempt
is awesome" (Taussig 1998: 250). The claims of talking statues are
part of why devastating and common stories, stories which fling accountability in many directions, stories that suggest the abyss over
which the poor seem to hover, are so often bracketed by the "hands
of God."

In whose hands

In India, at least, languages of journey show that anthropologists, develop-
ment workers, health workers, colonial officials, and missionaries share(d)
a basic way of spatializing—and narrating—the world. With a sense of out-
ward motion, of leaving home, we say we put behind us the securities of the
city for the "the field"—the productive space. And, thinking with city-self
about village-self, passages into the rural can also mimic, in hollowed-out,
kinless fashion, a return. The journey home. Ways of talking about the ru-
ral as "the interior" suggest something within the self. Putting them together
with the "backwardness" so often evoked, even solidified into law in terms
like "backward castes," we get the "real," the wild me, the place of origins that
disturbs notions of inside and outside, home and jungle. Language shapes so
much about what feels "real," I suppose, and it can also be so wrong.

In the reverse of what Ashis Nandy calls the "ambiguous journey to the
city" (2001a), the van that carries me and my stuff to Lalpur "at the begin-
ning" (which is really more like the middle), is diverted off the road by an
end-of-season storm. A fallen tree blocks our path. We go onto a perpendi-
cular side track. At the edge of a village, we stop in the narrow space between
road and field to let a lorry pass. While we wait, I watch out the window as
rain washes mud off a small bit of grayness sticking out of the ground. I fi-
nally recognize the shape. A rib cage, a small pelvis. I think of police stories,
of crime, of "something is wrong." I point it out to the driver. He says, "Yes,
it must be a child." Wrongness recalibrates into the familiar, homesickness
into home, home into field, life into decay.

For de Certeau, writing accomplishes something that speech cannot. If we can take his sense of "writing" less, well, literally, and
consider the repetitive production of after-the-fact narratives to be
ways of naming death, then we are left with a powerful response to
refusals to name death de Certeau claims are part of biomedical rationalities and narratives of progress. As frontiers between persons,
death stories are also frontiers that demarcate the unstable ground
on the edges of institutions. As frontiers, these stories do more than
speak to the differences and sameness between persons, cultural
zones, and moral domains. Kleinman, Das, and Lock say: "because
of the manner in which knowledge and institutions are organized
in the contemporary worlds as pragmatically oriented programs of
welfare, health, social development, social justice, security, and so on,
the phenomenon of suffering as an experiential domain of everyday
social life has been splintered into measurable attributes. These attributes are then managed by bureaucratic institutions and expert

cultures that reify the fragmentation while casting a veil of mis-recognition over the domain as a whole." (1997: xxv)

If the "veil of misrecognition" is cast by fragmenting complex so-cial worlds into separate domains of action—medical and religious, rational and irrational, legitimate and fake—then the everdayness of loss, and the inherent critique it poses, can, like the near-silences of the pregnant women of Chapter 4, only be misrecognized as nor-malizing the "truly" pathological. But by making everyday suffering out of extraordinary grief, these stories and their speakers are doing just the opposite. Rather than normalizing loss, it is as though they are saying, "*Look* at what is normal."

Speaking death in places where it cannot be spoken, stories are not only elements of a discourse—part of the *chakkar*—but also a kind of work upon the way institutionalized certainties depend upon disappearance. Scheper-Hughes argues that infant death (not just sto-ries about it) produces subjectivities embedded in dire conditions—the raw experiences of poverty, hunger, exhaustion, and love (1992). In Sitapur, the constancy of memory involves the meaning of action and inaction and the fragmentation of worlds, maps, and promises. Worlds might not be separated at the points one might expect—cer-tainly not at the points intervening discourses of social science and biomedicine expect. Where stories fragment some worlds, they su-ture others; there are, they reveal, few firm distinctions between re-ligious and biomedical causality. "The hands of God" encompass biomedical rationality just as Dumont might have predicted, by de-valuing and relativizing it, rendering it part of a larger story about certainty, just another tired production of the real, rather than ren-dering it mute and/or incommensurable.

Where children grow up in the shadow of lost siblings, and mothers routinely count among their own those who no longer ex-ist, "God's hands" are countermythological. Such stories may trump the promises of "intervention" by evoking less the distance between birth/death and the center of power and rationality (or other insti-tutions which hold the promise of life) than the condition of their nearness. Resonant with rural lives and words in other parts of the world (cf Stewart 1996), and perhaps with overdetermining dis-courses about "ruralness," stories of infant death in *dehat* pose re-membering as the work of the local. They offer, in the face of healing narratives that have no time for movement and no place for failure, a *motion through*, within, and around enmeshed elements, a pulsing of exposure and devouring, a map of the world in desperate human movements.

Where similar tellings in other rurals might be ways of bringing everyday life into "the space of big meanings" (Stewart 1996: 168), the stories I have described are evasive about "big meanings," bringing to bear the many smaller things that create such stories in the first place. Too *much* causality makes for a particular soteriology of death, one that looks like "fate," but is just a bit different. Concepts of fate, Stewart says, "address the order in disorder, and the weight of immanent meaningfulness surrounds the narrative recounting of events" (167). Das, too, suggests that evoking God—or fate—gives reason and order to suffering. But in the cases described here, listeners are not impressed by an offered sense of order or larger meanings; they are hit with the pain of the jumbled and everyday.

As Stewart says, signs can provide the relief, not of coherence, but of "the structure of desire itself—the sense of an absent presence that leaves behind its traces." In the way traces can offer "clarity" on the structure of desire, it becomes possible to "read the 'really real' out of the contingent, the accidental, and the senseless." (Stewart 1996: 169). The way authorities make promises in *dehat* may pose "presences" more tangible than the term "traces" suggest, resonant in both the shape and structure of care as in the permanence of one or many losses. In this way, perhaps what Lacan said about the importance of the object for the child can be transposed into a political statement (that is, that the importance of the object is not its objectness, or meaning, or the thing itself, but its way of evoking presence and absence, the shape of desire). That is, speaking infant death demonstrates that the structure of desire not only forms the subject and its relationship to object(s), but constitutes a way of being in relation to specific alterities—law, institutions, authority, the stuff of "modern" reproduction and modern medicine particular to *dehat*. These alterities are the things that claim to offer care and life, to offer the future. In Sitapur, if there is relief in these stories—in "sharing the load"—perhaps this is also where anger comes from, for desire so mapped is—not by definition, but as structured by the state, global "policy," urban stakeholders, and their promises—desire diverted, contracts deferred. It is the nature of such longing, it seems, to be located upon sites always slipping out of grasp. The "really real" is, in these cases, not just "read … out of" the contingent and the senseless, it *is* the contingent and the senseless, both.

This, again, is where the soteriologies of infant death come in. To say it one more time, "the dying man raises … the question of the subject at the extreme frontier of inaction, at the very point where it is the most impertinent and the least bearable" (de Certeau 1984:

191). So too the dying child, in the space of memory and the embodiment of retelling, in the zones in which action and inaction wear one another's cloaks, pierces teller and listener with both culpability and impotence, and then sends its arrows out to a world of contingencies, to settle in the hands of God, where all contingencies are equated.

Chapter 6

IDEALS
CIPHERS OF TRADITION

Radha lives in Ramgadh village. She is a dai (traditional midwife). She has actively assisted in births of all children in Ramgadh. Radhabai learnt this from her mother-in-law. Women respect Radhabai and she also cares for them. Men also respect her and seek her advice. She is warm and friendly towards all children. They play in her aangan (compound) throughout the day. Radha is warm and supportive when she assists in childbirth. She gives a massage and hot fomentation. She also gives herbal decoctions for safe and easy childbirth. She asks women to squat during delivery so that the baby comes out faster. When Salma was having pains, she provided a lot of support and encouragement. Her loving touch and soothing words were like balm to her pains. Sometimes Radha prays to the goddess of childbirth and performs certain rituals for ensuring a safe childbirth. She speaks positive things related to childbirth, which has a good effect on the mind of women.... She also advised Champa on how to take care of her baby and some home cures for baby's illnesses. She knows that she cannot handle certain complications. She sends such women to the PHC and discusses with ANM for care during pregnancy. When the people came to know about the reservation for women in panchayat, they cajoled Radhabai to contest elections. On popular demand, Radha contested elections and was elected the sarpanch. The village people have arranged a function to honour her. Radhabai has already trained two women.

Women's Health—Towards Empowerment:
District Level Training Module, 2000

You study what, dais? I think they should all be killed.

Obstetrician working in Delhi

In the "outsides" to life in *dehat,* in whose hands is blame for loss placed? In whose hands are promises for the future felt to lie? What happens when blame is written into such promises, such imagined futures? Let us pull back from Lalpur and move now into the stream of languages of intervention. If fatalism is the way we are used to hearing grief, then knowledge and its lack are how we are used to hearing reverberations of caregiving in rural settings. If intervention talk—and the structures that make it so important—are as much internally (re)produced "outsides" as things that enter from "other" spaces, then what interiors and exteriors inform such talk *in* those spaces? Returning now to the "dai," or the idea of what a "dai" might be, we see that a particular kind of figure, indeed, a particular sensation is concurrent with institutional efforts to grapple with death. In the embattled "dai," loss is negotiated by producing a target of intervention; and "knowledge" is the idiom of these productions. According to Arthur Kleinman, the "local world" and the "moral world" are domains in which it becomes apparent what is "really at stake" for people (1999). Even as institutions and the *pakka* sites of intervention impose moral frameworks on the local moral worlds of Sitapur, they contain their own visions of morality, conversations about and perceptions of what is at stake—for themselves and, more overtly, for their "targets" and "recipients." But even as "knowledge" is so often a driving category of subjectivity and intervention, "knowledge" as such may not be what is, in the end, "at stake," either in rural births or the places and policies in which so much seems to depend upon it.

Few things boggle the mind when entering into official, health-oriented settings in north India more than the range of discourses—often meant to counteract one another—on "the dai" and her role in health care delivery. This debate, while on the one hand seeming to involve new discourses, efforts, and ideas, is part of long-standing uncertainties about meanings of "tradition." Taking as starting point an argument central to critiques of development, that social categories are constituted (and power relations deployed) on the ground of "change," dissent over whether dais are "good" or "bad" involves something more than difference of opinion. Health interventions on the basis of education, or more specifically "training," emerge *through* this dichotomy, not in spite of it, as the persistence of a logic involv-

ing more than "contests of knowledge." Conversations about epistemology, valuable though they are, which are predicated on distinctions between local and interventionist (biomedical, usually) ways
of knowing, may, as they refract into the policy settings they critique,
set terms of engagement *as* matters of difference. In these refrac-
tions, this space in which (perhaps critical) academic voices merge
with (let's call them proactive) interventionist voices, conversations
about women who do birth work in rural communities extends only
as far as questions of value. In the process, conversations about loss
and culpability involve the shaping of subjects.

Elements of discourse circulate in sites of intervention rather
than operating as monolithic structures of meaning. They are perhaps more conversation than narrative—mutable, internally inconsistent, internally contested. But in spite of a dialogic quality, they
remain—in effect more than essence—representative of condensed
logics, though not necessarily representing "a self-generating, for-
malist system," and not easily reckoned as either orientalist and objectifying or not (Tharu 1989: 128). The ambiguities in these dia-
logues are crucial. They are interesting for more than the mere fact
of *being* ambiguities. They are strategic and productive rather than
marking points of rupture or contestation. Even as they are "battle-
grounds of meaning," such ambiguities efface contrasts and nullify
power and can be as effective as they are indicative. In response to
the way most institutional conversations about dais in India are oriented around value, I am *less* concerned with such matters as the
worth (of knowledge) or the existence or lack of sensitivity to dais
than I am with the socialities that emerge out of the visions of time,
space, and society in which such debates are situated. Among these
is the sense (as much as observation) that something called "the
dai" embodies conflicts over something called "tradition." With a
mea culpa for *chakrivit tark,* I observed in the socialities of intervention the ways policy scripts social life by establishing gaps and am-
bivalences as much as by solidifying identities, setting in motion
relationships imagined as "encounters," either potentially antagonistic or potentially fruitful. Policy stories and the worldviews of implementers construe health care in developing countries precisely *as*
an encounter. But the everydayness of interactions within institutional frameworks and the structure of idioms placing blame for a
range of ills in the black box category "dai" destabilize the very notions of encounter on which they rely. Scripts are variously adopted
and ignored.

The troublesome dai

By now, contrasts between policy visions and the "local picture" in Uttar Pradesh should be clear. This discussion goes, I hope, beyond reiterating that local realities confound policy universals (though this is true) to consider the conceptual gaps into which "targets" and "agents" can fall. In reproductive health policy in India, at the time of my research, three aspects of local talk and sociality were inter-weaving with the terms of global policy: (1) a vagueness around the term "dai," (2) vilification of birth workers, and (3) efforts to recuperate "dais' knowledge" and validate "tradition." Part of the conceptual gap surrounding the identity of "the dai" involves her debated status in these terms. Historical shifts in efforts to deal with dais reflect these themes as well as long-standing debates establishing that "tradition" can—and should—be characterized by its "value."

Though currently dai training is represented as a "new" or "innovative" component of reproductive health campaigns and family planning programs, the training of dais has taken place in central Uttar Pradesh (as well as in other regions of India) since the 1860s. The long history of dai trainings, their limited success in reaching stated goals, and the equally long history of considering such interventions "innovative" demonstrate that "training" has been problematic for over a century yet remains part of the fabric of institutional intervention. In the late nineteenth century, before the acronym "TBA" took hold, colonial policies and imaginations of gender, caste, and reproduction construed the dai as the "Indian midwife" and a concern for public health and social policy. "Training" of "traditional" figures became part of colonial medicine and the basis of many rural women's relationships with the state. Across the territories, "training" established a ground for modernization on the basis of enhancement of "skills," setting a precedent for policies that continue to this day.

While dai trainings did not begin until 1866, focus on female medicine and the education of female medical practitioners became important components of colonial medicine after the watershed point of 1857, when colonial policies and ideologies were affected by revolt and questions about the role of colonial forces in relation to local populations (Fitzgerald 2001; Forbes 1994; Harrison 1994). By the end of the nineteenth century, the provision of medical care to Indian women became a means of entry into the secluded space of the *zenana*, the women's realm considered by historians a guarded site beyond the reach of (colonial) hegemonic forces (Arnold 1993; Chakravarti 1997; Chatterjee 1993). Such efforts were informed by

aims to promote hygiene as a means of "civilizing India," and operated alongside other medical efforts such as vaccination campaigns
and "lock hospitals" (the latter targeting prostitutes and aimed at
addressing venereal disease in army camps) (Arnold 1993). Across
India, colonial and nationalist authorities considered the professionalization of obstetrics an "antidote" to the conditions birthing women
faced (Van Hollen 1998: 49), making education central to the extension of the medical establishment. Dai training figured in this form
of intervention, as dais, like indigenous practitioners of Ayurveda
and Unani trained in Western medicine and pharmacology, came to
occupy a mediary zone through which European medical culture
could be communicated to the hinterlands (Harrison 2001). At the
same time, elite Indian women were being trained as doctors and
nurses as British women began to enter the medical profession (often practicing in India when doors were closed to them in Britain
[Fitzgerald 2001; Lal 1994; Qadeer 1998b]).

The emergence of dai trainings in India coincided with debates in
Britain on the regulation of midwifery practice and the emergence
of the field of obstetrics as a medical specialization (Donnison 1988).
As midwifery became regulated and professionalized in the West, in
India a schism was created in birth practice. By the late nineteenth
century, elite women were trained as professional midwives, nurses,
and doctors in medical colleges, while "traditional practitioners"—
dais—became targets of different kinds of training, in part because
of their lack of literacy and low social status, thus falling into a vague
and shifting set of strategies for bringing medical care to working
class and nonelite women. It was these trainings that were fraught
with difficulty and, arguably, met with little long-term success (Forbes
1994).

In India, the Countess of Dufferin Fund, or the National Association for Supplying Female Medical Aid to India, involved dai training as part of a large-scale effort to improve women's health more
generally. Begun in 1885 at the bequest of Queen Victoria, it involved
a broad effort to educate and employ women as medical practitioners and generally improve the medical care of women. Other initia-
tives followed, some, such as the Victoria Memorial Scholarship Fund,
having a more direct aim at training dais (Qadeer 1998; Van Hollen
2002), and included a range of programs begun by colonial authorities, British missionary groups, and Indian women's organizations.

The history of obstetrics and midwifery training in India has been
described extensively elsewhere (cf. Ahluwallia 2000; Arnold 1993;
Forbes 1994; Harrison 1994; Jeffery et. al. 1989 Lal 1994; Qadeer

1998; Van Hollen 2002). For the purposes of this discussion, it is important to point out that while colonial and elite Indian discourses continued to depict dais as dirty, dangerous, and backward (Forbes 1994), dai training remained central to efforts to improve the lot of women, stall population growth, reduce maternal and infant mortality, and extend medical care into the private domain. Training paralleled developing relationships between indigenous and Western medical systems, and between the professionalization of medicine in India and Europe. But dai training differed from these efforts in that dais represented women of lower caste and class groups. Unlike practitioners channeled into medical certification, Western and indigenous, strategies for approaching them were markedly less standardized.

Although colonial health programs appear to have considered "the dai" a unified category—the "traditional midwife"—ethnographic observations undermining the category erupt into many accounts. As signs of defiled categories, divisions between baby delivering and cord cutting were used to demonstrate India's deficiencies with regard to hygiene and basic human sensitivity. Early 20th century accounts engage, at times with puzzlement over the distinction between "midwife" and "sweeper," the presence of different and divided birth-tasks. Colonial ethnographer G. W. Briggs described the "midwifery" performed by Chamars and its divisions as analogous to the divisions between caste and sub-caste. Among subcastes of Chamars, he noted, could be found a group designated "*Nālchhinā* (one who cuts the navel cord)" (1920: 56). Connected to the low status of the "untouchable" caste group whose practices he documented, was the fact that "The practice of midwifery is looked upon as most degrading. The women who follow this sort of profession employ methods of the crudest sort. Sanitary conditions are almost entirely neglected and no attempt is made to prevent infection.... The whole technique of the practice of midwifery is directed by custom and superstition (54)."

More scathing, as always, was Katherine Mayo, writing of the group called "dais" (without reference to one particular caste group,) "Therefore, in total, you have the half-blind, the aged, the crippled, the palsied and the diseased, drawn from the dirtiest poor, as sole ministrants to the women of India in the most delicate, the most dangerous, and the most important hour of their existence" (1927: 92). Preceding Mayo's account were decades of writing in which the dai was vilified. As Forbes notes, it was in the second half of the nineteenth century that the dai was transformed from "the appropriate person to assist in childbirth" to a "wizened hag" in British colonial and elite Indian discourses, and among Indian women's organizations, the colonial medical establishment, and reformers concerned with the conditions of the poor (Forbes 1994: 153–54). For all-India women's groups, abolishing the dai became a "stated goal" by the 1930s (167), as increasing demand that dais be trained and licensed were voiced but not necessarily pursued (168). Amid these social programs and aims, the scandal of birth work in India consolidated in the scandal of the dai. That the dai was constituted as a "social problem" for colonial and Indian authorities in the late nineteenth and early twentieth centuries is true, though understates, perhaps, the level of scandal associated with divisions of labor behind the category "dai"—scandals posed to maternity and, indeed, humanity on the bases of the presence of persons rendered "unspeakable," tasks rent asunder. Referred to in Chapter 2, Mayo's words warrant repetition here, in the way that her emotionally charged language associated a division of labor with Hindu orthodoxy, locating the scandal at a conceptual distance from "the West:" "In Benares, sacred among cities ... the unspeakable *dhai* brings with her a still more unspeakable servant to wreak her quality upon the mother and the child in birth" (Mayo 1927: 96).

As shifts in values attributed to Western medicine blamed the dai for high rates of infant and maternal mortality (Forbes 1994: 172), languages of social observation found in the dai—and, indeed, in the difficulty of containing "her" to a single entity—the essence of danger and pollution. As the figure—"the dai"—witchily overflows its claim to a single person, the social location and specific praxes of birth work become "unspeakable," person becomes "quality." As part of a trajectory toward institutionalized birth as moral principle, programmatics involving "the discrediting of the traditional systems and practices of Dais" and associations of "*purdah*" with ill health (Qadeer 1998: 271) drew from such social imaginaries a visceral urgency. Through the Dufferin Fund, maternity hospitals served upper-class clientele (1998) even as primary caregivers for lower-class women were vilified (Forbes 1994), giving a symbolic moral structure to the triage of care that left those on the lower ends of the spectrum ambiguously victims and to blame.

But the women known as "dais" also spoke back. According to Forbes, the Dufferin Fund's initial intention to train dais to act as professional midwives fell flat—women wanted to be paid to attend trainings, trainings interfered with their work, they did not recognize the superiority of what they were being taught, and courses were taught in English. To these complaints, Forbes observes, administrators of the Fund began to envision (she quotes) "a class of nurses or midwives who ... would in time supplant dhais" (Forbes 1994: 168). Indeed, as medical centers for the urban working classes were being imagined and constructed, the dai became for urban elites "an embarrassment," "the symbol of superstition and dogged resistance to change" (171). What this says about power, Forbes says, is that "Hegemony operated, not to change the system of health care, but to describe the dai as a social pathology.... Proponents of Western science, face to face with the dai, had created an ideology, not a system of medicine" (172). This ideology contained not only the vilification of a group of people or form of practitioners, but a particular architecture: the ability to, in a moment of speech, transform discourse on persons into discourse about "qualities," to change social location into moral attribute, indeed, the social world of people into an abstract world of effective and affective essences.

Where some languages, plans, programs and goals in relation to women's health have changed over time, such architecture proves more difficult to dismantle. It remains intact in postcolonial efforts to train dais as well as in interventions related to reproductive health care and "family planning" (see Chapter 7). It has been argued, following Lata Mani's approach to colonial efforts to end the practice of *sati*, that dais became the "ground" for colonial and nationalist ideologies and performances, rather than being subjects in whose welfare the state had a genuine interest (Qadeer 1998; Van Hollen 1998). But as "ground," their status as entities requires further consideration and may, indeed, be contained in the very consolidation of social complexities and actors into a singular "they." While postcolonial efforts struggle to determine whether trainings should create a new breed of practitioner or absorb dais into the medical system as "upgraded" but "traditional" practitioners, the "dangerous" and "dirty" quality of dais persists in everyday talk, as does the architecture of this form of the abject. Urges to eradicate their practices, even to "get rid of them," are present in everyday talk, even as these ideas clash with global public health interests in incorporating "TBAs" into the structures and referral hierarchies of primary health care in the developing world. It is as objects of affective attention, as points of slippage between person and quality, that "dais'" long-standing role as trainees lends additional irony to their position as both objects of blame and agents of change. This convergence of blame and agency points to a broader structural imaginary of the subject of intervention. Likewise, in colonial India, the idea of "the dai" at once challenged notions of "the traditional midwife" (though these challenges were relatively marginal, at least in colonial texts) and took shape as a point of contrast, a colonial trope according to which health "policy" emerged. The Indian "dai," constructed by and through colonial intervention, confounded standards of intervention and ensured the need for future interventions, making dai training a permanent fixture of state programs aimed at rural populations and creating not just a category for development, but a particular sort—odious yet embraced.

Where "professionalization" through colonial or postcolonial training programs may have the potential to provide legitimacy and legal recognition to those whose work takes place outside of formal market and professional structures, trained dais remain in ambiguous spaces on the margins of the professions. The linking of "training" with professional validity and hierarchized institutional structures may have *prevented* low-caste women from entering certain kinds of institutional legitimacy while creating a niche in state structures largely on the grounds of caste and "untouchable" or subaltern status. Since Independence, dai trainings have aimed to incorporate an aesthetic of professionalization into projects oriented around knowledge transmission. Signs of professionalization operate as free-floating signifiers, unhinged from the institutional support that would allow for professionalization. They include training kits, identity cards (intended to facilitate referral at hospitals), encouragement to charge "fixed rates," signs proclaiming one to be a "trained dai," and vague linkages to NGOs and hospitals by means of naming and interpellation, but only rarely through payment or long-standing involvement.

While post-Independence trainings have not differed significantly from their colonial predecessors in structure (and, in all likelihood, in much content), the structure of maternal and child health (MCH) services has undergone a number of critical shifts since 1947. In the first post-Independence decades, maternal and child health, and thus, interest in dais, was an important concern, marked by the Bhore Commission's report and recommendations for training of women health practitioners, and subsumed into interests to establish a health care infrastructure more generally. This resulted in the establishment of medical practitioners such as ANMs and LHVs (lady health visitors) as permanent features of rural life and government health structures. But the fact that goals (to train doctors, ANMs, midwives, and dais) were consistently unmet marked the state as permanently behind schedule (Qadeer 1998) and made ANMs and LHVs signs of the state's failures to meet its own ideals. Responsibilities for dai training were absorbed into larger concerns about developing state infrastructures, educating professional practitioners, and improving technological facilities—that is, with modernization. Indeed, dai training was not part of the first Five Year Plan. In the 1960s, though dai trainings were mentioned in Five Year Plans, the consolidation of primary health centers and enhancement of specialization took precedence over training auxiliary workers and maintenance of subcenters (outposts of PHCs) (Qadeer 1998). In 1967 MCH services were integrated with the GOI's family planning program.

Concurrent with these shifts, the onus for dai training has moved through government departments and the standard length of (ideal) trainings shrunk from six months (in the 1960s) to six days (presently in most Uttar Pradesh schemes). In the 1970s a reinvigorated interest in the use of TBAs more globally meant renewed attention to dai training in India. After the disastrous family planning efforts of the Emergency, the 1980s were a time in which emphasis was on reducing infant mortality, linking sectors in health planning, establishing comprehensive primary health care, and reducing poverty. But in the 1990s liberalization meant that, on the one hand, the state relinquished interest in basic health services, while on the other hand, the intense focus—of the state, NGOs, and international funders—returned to population. The 1990s also showed an invigorated emphasis on reproductive rights and matters of choice (as well as a "target-free" approach in response to the nightmares of "targeting") (Qadeer 1998). Likewise, dai training was placed largely in the hands of nongovernment organizations and voluntary groups, though the state now keeps a foot in the door through integrated family planning/ MCH programs that channel GOI and international funds, personnel, and "modules" through the state while utilizing NGOs and private organizations for implementation. In many ways, by funding and participating in short-term training operations and primary care measures meant to fill gaps in infrastructure (like heath camps) the state has become, for rural women, just another NGO rather than a source of long-term, dependable services.

Concurrently, feminist activism has made matters of reproductive rights elements of dai training and family planning measures, in both impetus for and content of trainings. "Reproductive rights" can be thought of largely as referring to a person's stance as childbearer within larger constraining hegemonies that restrict choice; yet the discourse of reproductive rights' appearance in development health policy associated with dais is so overwhelmingly individualized that the firmest hegemony appears to be the one inside women's heads. Its use in policy and everyday life means that, in this context, "reproductive rights" can be thought of as the ability to successfully assert free will and choice (which, it is assumed, will mean the choice to limit reproduction) in one's childbearing, parallel with availability of means to do so. In India, as well as in other parts of the world, at policy and everyday levels of feminist activism, "choice" is a key idea and symbol of emancipation. As an individualizing aspect of "reproductive rights," it is potentially at odds with emphases on factors such as poor infrastructure, shoddy and demeaning health care, and structural forms of inequality and violence, marking a central tension in the politics of "access." In many ways, though "reproductive rights" discourses locate "choice" centrally, recent MCH policy recommendations have given the lie to public health and development programs that make morbidity and mortality entirely matters of private, individual, and moral concern (as do those I describe below). Though dais remain vilified in many spaces as antithetical to enlightenment, individual expression, and "choice," the language employed in TBA-related policy can be heard to emphasize that rural women lack access to institutionalized health care, that state infrastructure is insufficient, and that poverty is not only linked with ill health, but that these things are themselves part of complex national and global flows of capital. In other words, it is not so easy to demonize. There is no unified or easily characterized "apparatus"—or ideology—at work.

At the same time, efforts to promote cultural sensitivity and the "value" of "indigenous knowledge" have made their way into training policies, producing a new vision of "the dai" that, while it presents a happier picture and more generous language, also may simply shift the stereotypes. In a recent training manual, we find the story of Radhabai (meant to be shared with trainees to validate dais and present a positive picture to those who might aspire to such a role). Radhabai is a fictitious rural woman who demonstrates an ideal blend of traditional and modern qualities, and who, in return, is so highly regarded by her community that not only is she respected with their health needs, but also is elected *sarpanch* (head of the local government). This well-meaning tale, offered to counter the frequent debasing of dais in a range of discourses, is part of a training module to be used at the district level. The manual includes trainings for a range of gender-related issues: "Me and My Society: Promoting Understanding on Gender, Self Esteem and Empowerment," "Access to Government Services Focusing on Health Care," and "Traditional Health and Healing Practices," along with the more standard sections on care before, during, and after pregnancy.

Demonstrating a commitment to cultural sensitivity, the module presents an idealized view of health care delivery in rural areas, a vision of a fully functioning (if confusing) matrix of state and NGO institutions. It contains a section I found, personally, extremely useful: a module explaining the complex chain of command and institutions where health care is concerned, a flowchart of agencies and government officials demonstrating the ideal "map" of care—so complicated as to require its own "module." It is uncertain whether this module's clarifications are meant to describe how things are or how they should be. But clearly, both the map of agencies and figures and the gentle portrait of the local dai are out of kilter with situations in Sitapur (where dais are neither patently valued nor stigmatized, though none could realistically imagine being elected to public office). While dais' "traditional knowledge and practices" are considered things of value, there is no mention of what would most likely be Radhabai's low caste status, or of the question of postpartum care (does Radhabai cut cords, or is postpartum work done by others?). Clearly, such a possibility could not be "the norm." Politics, bureaucracy, and hierarchy work in favor of the "valued traditional practitioner" here, producing a soft-focused rendering. There is no sense of struggle.

NGO workers, scholars, filmmakers, and independent activists are now the primary champions of dais, and just as it is not uncommon to hear cowboyish statements to the effect that the only good dai is an absent one (one of my students tells me her father, a doctor from India, thinks "they should get rid of the dais" and "hopes they all just die off"), it is also not uncommon to hear NGO workers listing the importance of dais to programs and public health as a whole. Not all go so far as to emphasize the value of dais' "knowledge systems," some stopping at the point of their utility to institutional structures. But there remains a growing community of activists, advocates, artists, and policy makers who assert the importance of "preserving" dais' knowledge, while recognizing their disempowered place in caste hierarchies and institutional structures. There is some evidence— through the presence of things like the Radhabai story in training modules, as well as through the circulation of talk, pamphlets, published articles, and people through the South Delhi drawing rooms, dining rooms, conferences, offices, private club poolsides, and cocktail parties in which policies are discussed—that "new" renderings of dais may impact the shape of dai training. Yet, as much policy has become "funder driven" over the last decade, through the turning over of implementation to NGOs, the shape of policy slips further out of grasp, becoming at once more diffuse and at the same time more subject to flows of capital and corporate/transnational interests. Even where they may affect training modules, the extent to which views impact the socialities of intervention on the ground is up for debate. But the shape of debate—the good or bad of the "traditional"—and the unstable space between person and quality remain intact.

Development discourse and tradition: The imagination of the TBA

Shifting gears, I turn to ethoses of training found within a handful of global(izing) texts. Traces of these documents can be observed in ideas about TBAs in circulation in India over the last several decades, during which time dai training has demonstrated that, in spite of shifts in valuation, it is here to stay. Disjunctures between the above history and textual genealogy are as telling as connections. Yet, as "dais" have had ambiguous relationships to institutional structures and dai trainings are shifting, even failing, it is necessary to ask how broader ideas about the "TBA" impute meaning onto the category of "dai," the assumed local variant of this universal entity. In the argument that "reality is colonized by development discourse" (Escobar 1995: 5) lies an approach to intervention in which development as a set of cultural representations involves global relations of power that allow "development" to be put between inverted commas (Ferguson 1994). Immediately confronting the curious person interested in languages of improvement and intervention is the observation that, in its internal critiques, shifts, and ambiguities, so-called "development discourse" is as variegated a literature as any. It is not to any imagined whole or totalizing system of meaning, then, that I turn, so much as to flows and bursts of speech, reiterations, and harped upon themes that give shape to points of dissent and departure as much as, or more than, gluing themes into consistencies.

Thus, because "development discourse" on TBAs cannot possibly be addressed as a singular thing, I focus on four texts, spanning three decades and four of the larger institutions involved in "TBA training." First is *The Traditional Birth Attendant in Maternal & Child Health & Family Planning* (to emphasize the power and play of acronyms in this "world," let's refer to it here as TBAMCH), published in 1975. This document is a policy recommendation, outlining guidelines for maternal and child health programs in developing countries (Verderese and Turnbull 1975: 5). A compilation of results of an international survey, it was written in response to recommendations made at a World Health Organization-sponsored seminar on the role of the midwife in maternal and child health care, held in 1970. The goals of TBAMCH are to define and describe the TBA and to promote her inclusion in MCH and family planning projects. The second text, published in 1986 by the World Health Organization (WHO), is the introduction to a collection of articles entitled *The Potential of the Traditional Birth Attendant* (PTBA) (Maglacas and Simon 1986). PTBA presents analyses of TBA training programs in various developing countries, primarily in Africa and South Asia. The introduction culls these results into a set of recommendations at once descriptive and prescriptive. The third text is the SMI (Hertz and Meacham 1987) referred to in Chapter 5. It is an introductory description of the goals and philosophies of the Safe Motherhood Campaign, a World Bank initiative channeling resources and ideas to state and NGO schemes in India, as well as carrying out promotional activities of its own. Its posters, banners, and documents appear in a wide range of places in urban and rural India. The SMI's policies and recommendations have had a large impact in shaping specific programs, ideologies, and methodologies in reproductive health care in India, and I regard this text as emblematic of a larger web of ideas and languages that have had great impact on maternal and child health in the developing world. The fourth text is *Traditional Birth Attendants: A Joint WHO/UNFPA/ UNICEF Statement* (TBAJS), published by the WHO in 1992. It represents an effort to link and homogenize existing approaches to MCH and was intended to "constitute an example of the common purpose and complementarity of programmes supported by WHO, UNICEF, and UNFPA" (WHO 1992: 2). While each document might arguably represent a distinct "moment" in a genealogy of policy, read together the effect is hardly one of linear development; they reflect on and through each other, at times diverging, often expressing common frameworks—though seldom explicitly so.

Understanding "tradition" in these documents is essential to locating the TBA. As part of the creation of subjects of reform (Escobar 1995: 41), the idea of "tradition" is at once that which characterizes TBAs and that which the TBA helps to define. Indeed, in these texts, even as TBAs are identified as reformable subjects, the idea of the TBA says more about "tradition" and its imagined relationship to development than about women who do birth work. "Tradition" takes shape in several ways in these texts. It is imagined in terms of the things people in developing countries do and think. In defining TBAs, the documents juxtapose *modern* ways of being and doing against a set of praxes that are variously called *traditional practices, cultural habits,* and *local practices/ideas.*[1] Tradition is coterminous with *local, cultural,* and *indigenous,* all of which are primarily defined by being neither modern, scientific, nor universal. Lists of *traditional practices* denote the kinds of things development may encounter.

In the most recent document, the TBAJS (WHO 1992), the TBA, as compared with the *doctor, nurse-midwife, midwife,* or *health worker,* is defined through the distinction between *profession* and *practice*— doctors and midwives are *health professionals,* TBAs are *practitioners.* They *work,* but do not perform "labor" or a "job." More often, they play *roles,* have *practices* and *beliefs* that are also referred to as *activities* and *habits.* Being traditional precludes the possibility that she be a *professional,* while status as a *practitioner* is part of what it means to be traditional. As such, in the 1992 document, the TBA's gradual *phasing out* is a crucial part of attaining the goal of *professional maternal and child health for all* (1992: 17).

In earlier texts, while tradition is defined as being not modern, attitudes toward tradition are more ambiguous. Because the TBA embodies tradition, it is unclear what development is supposed to do with her. The introduction to TBAMCH (Verderese and Turnbull 1975) illustrates these crosscutting ambiguities, beginning with a reference to the flexibility of tradition: *As the network of the centrally organized system of healthcare has not yet reached everywhere, populations in remote rural communities and in many periurban shantytowns have learned to rely on one another for help in gratifying their respective health needs. They have built systems of folk medicine and traditional care to deal with the burden of their health problems. Included in these systems are several kinds of traditional practitioners* (1975: 2).

In this passage, tradition is both a timeless, premodern reality and a response to the effects of modern relations of power, or, more specifically, the unfinished business of modernization. The subsequent text calls for sensitivity to *local understandings.* This may indicate the authors' sensitivity to relations of power underlying *cultural beliefs* and *practices.* It also demonstrates an ambiguity based on the *un*ambiguous idea of the secondary, even incidental nature of *traditional* and *folk* categories. It sets the stage for what will later emerge as a response framework oriented around *consumption* and devoid of politics (cf. Ferguson 1994). In any case, the story soon changes. For, while traditional practices are said to represent systems of *common understanding,* they are also found in communities where births are attended by *untrained personnel* (Verderese and Turnbull 1975: 2). Reference to the dangers of *untrained personnel* follows calls for sensitivity to *traditional practices,* and is itself followed by a list of the ill effects of *lack of prenatal care* (1975: 2), leaving two things unclear:

Should interventions defend or eradicate *traditional practices?* And what is the difference between *traditional practitioners* and *untrained personnel?*

The next section of TBAMCH, "Possible Constraints in the Mobilization of TBAs," begins with TBAs' imperviousness to change—*refusal to alter cultural habits* (Verderese and Turnbull 1975:3). Misunderstandings can result from the fact that TBAs have different *cultural* concepts of health, one of which might be *no concept of health as a positive state of well-being* (4). Thus, while we should be sensitive to *traditional practices, community understandings,* and *cultural habits,* these things are also detrimental. *Sensitivity* is a precursor to eradication at worst, and transformation at best, making *cultural understanding* an instrumental rather than general principle. Equally importantly, rather than demonstrating reified boundaries, this logic obscures distinctions between the relative (changeable) and the essential (unchangeable).

Discussing development practices in Nepal, Stacey Pigg describes the antimodern as a key idea for development discourse. Labels such as "the village," Pigg argues, reduce sociocultural diversity to a generic category of backwardness (1992: 504), posing "the village" as the opposite to "development," and supplying "an authoritative social map for Nepalese national society" (492). The category of "TBA" orients a similarly reduced terrain of "progress," as she addresses in another paper (Pigg 1997). Ambiguity may be equally important to its functioning as a "target" category, in particular for the way the "traditional" (the "T") denotes both staticity and plasticity. Thus, as well as establishing boundaries between tradition and modernity, the idea of the TBA as a vehicle for development identifies tradition and modernity as not just separate, but different *kinds* of entities; tradition is nonuniversal and relative (on the one hand) and a sign of immobility and fixity (on the other), while the totalizing nature of modernity makes its changeability a nonissue.

In the earlier text (Verderese and Turnbull 1975), the shifting nature of tradition is part of the construction of progress. In later policy texts progress takes shape as a constellation of "choice" and "demand," posited against their opposite, "risk," reflecting larger moves in health policy. As part of a move toward imagining reproductive health in terms of "risk" and "choice," both population control policy and the Women in Development (WID) movement employ totalizing strains of feminism based in concepts of individuality and self-determination (Apffel-Marglin and Simon 1994; Morsy 1995). These ideologies locate tradition as pathology, symptom of female subordination, and hindrance to development (Apffel-Marglin and

Simon 1994: 32). Reflected in texts on TBAs, this logic of "choice" provides specific rules for how to be a modern woman, rules positing a baseline of ignorance and the redemption of demand.

Within this framework, ignorance characterizes TBAs as much as does tradition. As Chapter 5 illustrates, this is wrapped up in a quality of fatalism that is part of lack of awareness of universal standards. With such lack of perspective, the SMI document asserts, women are incapable of *noticing* not only *risk* but suffering. Such ignorance, constitutive of their ill-being, is an outcome of *adherence to tradition* (Hertz and Meacham 1987: 4), that is, to a kind of knowledge that is, by definition, no perspective. As TBAs are taught these markers, they are to become agents, *identify[ing]*and *refer[ing]* women *at-risk* to a preexisting health infrastructure. They will become the voice of the system, "promot[ing] better family health and nutrition" (viii).

The logic of ignorance, in which women must be taught to make *demands,* is not so easy; women must ask for the right things. *Evidence* that women do not yet fully *understand* comes in the form of women who *seek help* during childbirth from the wrong category of person—identified as a *TBA, family member,* or *friend* (Hertz and Meacham 1987: 4). Limited by *long-standing ignorance* and dangerous *attitudes ... many pregnant women have no choice but to turn to TBAs or others ill-equipped to handle obstetrical emergencies* (5). By referring to the "ill-equipped," a discourse about education is also one in which the ultimate answer is technology—of which "training" is but one. Education means a pairing of global awareness with internal drive in learning how to choose technologies. While the logic is difficult to refute, it also poses an individualized sense of change that is nothing if not a mode of desire and action. Who can argue that a well-equipped, well-staffed, clean, accessible clinic will perform any technique more safely than an ill-equipped practitioner? The imaginary suggests bright, clean, hospitals filled with shiny new equipment, doctors waiting eagerly for patients to come through the door. Except, laws of supply and demand so often bolstering the desire side of the equation (at least in these texts) mean that demand must exist in order to bring such facilities into being. Material concerns become individual responsibility, and choosing a "TBA" (choosing tradition) amounts to no choice at all. The idea of consumption embeds the language of choice in a neoliberal logic in which health is a private good. As the figure of the consumer becomes a sign of the modern, at once a foreign idea needing to be taught and the end result of a natural teleology, "awareness of global conditions" (and the

inequalities they point to) falls away. Consciousness is turned inward toward the self rather than outward at the world.

We might ask which is worse: lack of choice, or making the wrong
choices? The logic of the SMI says that as ignorance is defined as the
lack of ability to choose (a particular technology of the self) making
the wrong choice is the same as making no choice. Women as consumers are stuck in a loop of tradition until they make correct
choices, thereby demonstrating their modernity through expanded
"options." But simultaneous to this is the phasing out of traditional
practitioners, practices, attitudes, and beliefs (by atrophy, as women
do not choose them), such that modernity, inextricably linked with
expanded choice, can only happen when range of behavior is nar-
rowed. Gertrude Fraser describes this situation in early twentieth
century United States: "For most [American] women, it may have
become safer rather than riskier to have a child at home under the
care of the midwife. Physicians could easily be called and transpor-
tation found to take the woman to the nearest hospital. But the structuring of the discourse over the earlier decades had all but closed off
that possibility. Women chose 'progress' when it became defined as
the only, as well as the best, alternative" (1995: 260).

Published a year earlier than the SMI document, *The Potential of
the Traditional Birth Attendant* (PTBA) refers to TBAs as *resources* (Maglacas and Simons 1986: 7). In contrast with the SMI, in PTBA, TBAs
are considered *untapped*, ignored by development projects that
would be better served by incorporating them into their infrastructure. Disagreement over the value of TBAs is less important than
the consistency with which both texts place TBAs in a framework of
demand, efficiency, use, and consumption. When the TBA is a commodity, debates about her merit can relocate her work in the supply-
demand matrix. Glorified or vilified, she remains the lesser of mere
options.

In all texts, the subject-positions of TBAs are obscured. In TBAMCH
(Verderese and Turnbull 1975), the *needs* and *desires* of TBAs are to
be elicited, but not so far as to ask what TBAs may actually say; the
final authority to determine *needs* lies with health workers (1975:
39). Further, TBAs are expected to speak for the *needs* of the community, but not their own. Where health of TBAs is addressed (in
these four texts I found mention of it once), it is considered only insofar as it affects their ability to serve as health workers (e.g., bad
eyesight or communicable diseases) (1975: 40). The line between
producers and consumers of care distinguishes TBAs from those
they serve, treating each as different kinds of subjects.

Where the TBA represents tradition, women-as-consumers cross from tradition to modernity through *choice*. Where some critics charge that development pedagogy requires certain people adopt unfamiliar worldviews (and thus a call for "culturally appropriate interventions"), this suggests the opposite: so-called traditional peoples are in a category incommensurate with modernity. Within a call for cultural sensitivity, TBAs (as opposed to rural women) are not expected to recognize the universality of modern rationality because as *traditional practitioners* they are, by definition, *local*. Rather than foisting modernity upon them, these texts affirm the TBA's identity as traditional, while transforming their *roles*. Neither ignorant nor modern (in a framework that pits ignorance against modernity), the trainee is more like "tradition trained."

The SMI, in particular, establishes a logic characteristic of development discourse, "implicitly (and perhaps unconsciously) reasoning backward from the necessary conclusions—more 'development' projects are needed—to the premises required to generate those conclusions" (Ferguson 1994: 259). In the case of the SMI, the conclusions are the SMI itself, an international, and largely educational, project. Where the solution is education, a repository for pedagogy must be created, and complex—and global—problems situated at the level of the individual. As such, the TBA's ambiguity charts a never-quite-completed shift in policy. Broadly speaking, the more recent TBAJS argues in favor of gradual, passive fade-out of TBAs, while the earlier PTBA and TBAMCH recommend their inclusion, if not full incorporation, into a modern system. In the introduction to PTBA, the training of TBAs is presented as one of the *daunting problems of attemps [sic] to change long-established customs among the poor in developing countries* (Maglacas and Simons 1986: 6). Though a vehicle for incorporating TBAs into "modern" health care, training does not mean absorbing these *people* into a particular infrastructure. Rather, it entails a transformation that begins with ambiguity about the *untrained* TBA, rendered both obstacle and resource. Ambiguity is reshaped in the trained TBA, as tradition is redrawn.

Where the *untrained* TBA is a consistent, if vague, category across texts and time frames, as a subject of development the *trained* TBA is also debated. Her role remains ambiguous even where clearly laid out, as in TBAJS (WHO 1992). In this text, two main features distinguish the trained TBA from her untrained colleagues: her skills have been *upgraded* by way of a short passage *through the modern health care sector* (1992: 4), and her role in the community is expanded to include new tasks and responsibilities (6). However, in a later section, "The Limitations of TBA Programmes," TBAJS reminds us that *the trained TBA is not a substitute for the professional midwife because the limited depth of her training makes her less able than the professional midwife to make critical judgments* (14). TBA training is an *interim measure.* At the same time, the TBA has a place in modern medicine, articulated through the positing of a persistent lack: *For so long as women give birth without the assistance of a trained birth attendant, TBA training will provide the potential to decrease maternal and child mortality and morbidity, by dispelling ignorance, decreasing harmful ritual practices, and promoting safe practices and use of the modern health care system* (16). Whereas, *TBA training should not be viewed as a permanent solution to meeting the healthcare needs of mothers and children, and neither should TBAs be considered a substitute for the disappearing midwife* (24).

Here we meet someone new: the *disappearing midwife*. What is a TBA in the face of efforts to eradicate the "need" for her if not a disappearing midwife? Indeed, (in 1992) it was the hope of the WHO that the TBA would disappear as tradition atrophies and modernity progresses. *Full integration* [of TBAs into health care systems] *is probably impossible since the TBAs would assume more of a technical character, removed from their cultural context* (WHO 1992: 16). Thus, TBAs are always defined by the *T*—one cannot be a true *traditional* birth attendant and part of institutional medicine because such inclusion removes them, by definition, from the "T." Though they are *utilized,* they can not be integrated into infrastructures. Instead, they enter a relationship that renders their work redundant.

This is not to say that material needs may not outrank what the WHO defined at the time as *cultural* needs, or vice versa, but is meant to note the doubleness of tradition—at once an essential category representing modernity's other, and valued alongside other subordinate categories within the larger framework of modernity. Discursively designed to disappear, but also to remain linked to the system that will disappear them, trained TBAs become at once *interim category* and health care *option*. In this regard, the next and final passage from TBAJS is the most telling: *In any event, there will always be a need to keep what is best in TBA care: the sense of caring, the human approach, and the response to cultural and spiritual needs. For a long time to come, even when women have access to modern health care and the services of a professional midwife or physician, they will also seek the care of the traditional healers and birth attendants for advice and complementary care until the modern health care system can meet the needs of its clients* (17). Thus, need for TBAs does not diminish as need for tradition diminishes, but rather as tradition becomes a subset of modernity, a catalog of practices reduced to the most benign. *Tradition* (the *local, culture*) is transformed from existential state to part of a set of *needs* women have at the time of birth. As traditional practitioners become *complementary*, they stay the same while the structures orienting their work and world are transformed. The TBA is not transformed into a new subject; instead she is kept an ambiguous figure while the nature of tradition is transformed around her, is appropriated. As part of a catalog of secondary needs, "tradition" becomes ancillary to more fundamental needs for "professional" or "trained" care. When seen in terms of relative value, the social context of TBAs and their "traditional knowledge" is obscured, but more importantly, so too are the social contexts of poverty, ill-health, and poor birth outcomes. These are reconceived as they are absorbed into the obsession with "tradition" and the imaginary figure of the TBA. As historians of colonial medicine in India tell us, this is a familiar process, but with new language, technique, and, in the form of "cultural sensitivity," a cunning subtlety.

The Janus face of tradition represents two phases of the teleology imagined as "modernity." Tradition-outside-modernity is what some people are, while tradition-within-modernity is a quality a modern person can choose to augment her modern self. Through the category of the TBA, development discourses perform an operation on tradition, reducing it from essential characteristic of some to choice for all (as though no elements of "tradition" were "chosen" or mocked or scoffed at or desired or rejected before such a worldview came along). The untrained TBA represents the essentialized version; the trained TBA signifies culture-become-lifestyle choice. Embodying mollified, decontextualized "tradition," the trained TBA embodies a transition from a choiceless world to one supposedly full of options.

What I have noticed as a splitting of tradition, Akhil Gupta describes as the "twinning" of "tradition" with "the indigenous." While modernist development constituted tradition as a "residual category which contained everything that was devalued for not being modern," a concurrent movement to valorize the "indigenous" *against* a pathologized modernity renders the antimodern an ambiguous category (Gupta 1998: 179). Gupta says, "The modern project thus becomes one of constant displacement of 'the traditional' to ever more constricted domains" (180). Perhaps this is also the case with development discourse on TBAs. However, rather than being broken into two separate movements within a larger project, through the figuring of desire and the near-tyrannical (as Rapp [2000] and others point out) notion of "choice," development discourse condenses the two contra-

dictory attitudes into one argument, and reconciles them according
to a logic in which both the "good" ("indigenous") and the "bad" ("tradition") of the antimodern can be signs in a chronology of progress.

Ambiguity and power

*In Lucknow, I make an appointment to see Dr. Patel, who works for the
agency that trains trainers for NAFPA programs and other NGOs. It has
taken me ages to figure out exactly what her office does, and its own acronym
is vague and nonspecific. It seems to be a key middle agent in the flow of
"modules" (i.e., training structures) and trainings from transnational and
government sources to dai trainings. I cross paths with a number of her
trainers in my movements through rural Sitapur—at other NGO offices, in
health camps, the times I go to trainings invited by NGO directors or to meetings along with CBDs. I had spoken with Dr. Patel and another doctor, Dr.
Varma, in this office a year earlier, before I moved to Lalpur. This time I am
trying to get my hands on some training modules and to ask her more of the
same questions. She is very busy, and I am grateful to have managed to find
a time we can both meet, a time that—now that I am pregnant—will overlap with my better times of day.*

*"The TBA is a term of two meanings," Dr. Patel says, when I ask her how
she understands the term and the acronym. She brings to the foreground the
between-the-lines meanings of the policy statements I had read in New Jersey. "It means traditional birth attendant, and trained birth attendant. It
can involve the two meanings at the same time." From her enthusiasm, I get
the sense that this bivalence is one of the exciting things about the term,
making it encompassing rather than vague—a different reading of the ambiguity than mine.*

*She goes on, "TBAs are the best social workers in the country. ANMs
come from the outside, like other people from NGOs, but the TBAs have a
sense of responsibility to their communities and so they are more dedicated."*

*She goes on to say that "our" main role in this regard is to encourage
"village women that someone must be present at births. Otherwise, they see
it as just a normal thing. We must teach them that there must always be an
attendant at birth." She shifts to talk about the normality of infant death,
and I recall earlier conversations in which Dr. Varma had said, "They are
always surprised to hear that I gave birth to only two children, and to this
day still have two children. They must be taught that [infant mortality] does
not need to be normal."*

*In this earlier conversation, I recall, after some discussion of matters like
the timing of cord cutting and the roles and responsibilities of NAFPA work-*

ers, Dr. Patel says, "What we are teaching is informed choice. We have a cafeteria approach." Dr. Varma agrees, "The basic idea is education. About what they can get, what their rights are, and what is good for them. In all of this we are creating a demand. We must teach them what is normal, and what is not normal."

Dr. Patel cuts in, "We must teach them the impact of not doing something, like taking the iron tablets, and must teach them their risks and rights. Especially their reproductive rights."

"Overall," Dr. Patel goes on, "Dais have a hit-and-try method. There is no system. They just try something and if it works, if they hit it, then they keep it. Hit and try."

I ask whether women face family resistance when they become ANMs. Dr. Varma says, "No. It is government work and earns a reliable income."

"Do dais ever become ANMs?"

Dr. Varma laughs. "No. The minute she becomes an ANM she is no longer a dai."

Dr. Patel clarifies, "The main reason why dais do not become ANMs is because to be an ANM one must be literate and have an educational background."

The later conversation covers much of the same ground, and I worry that she is finding me boring and repetitive, but the conversation feels channeled into the same flow. She offers a slightly different description of the work of the "dai" this time—not "hit and try" but "push and pull," and a failure to know "real" from "false," the same dichotomy I have sensed that rural women struggle to ascertain, here contained in the body's trickery. "The dai's main work is push and pull. They can't recognize real versus false labor, so they don't know to wait until a baby is ready to come. We train them to be janm sahayika (birth attendants), the person who is attending the birth, not pushing and pulling.

"It is the same with the family planning. They know about family planning, but they don't know which one to choose, or how to get it. They have no selection criteria."

Later, pathologies of normality come up again. "Ninety-nine percent of rural women have either PID [pelvic inflammatory disease] or leukorrhea. They think that this is part of being a woman, that it is natural. So we teach them to know about their rights. They don't know about their own reproductive rights. So we teach them."

"How do you define reproductive rights?" I ask, but she does not hear my question. She says, "Dais can give messages to the community, they can be middlemen from us to the community."

In our first conversation, Dr. Patel had mentioned the "taboo" on cord cutting and the dirtiness of the placenta. "Eighty percent of births in this

*area are attended by family members. Dais are just sweepers. They also do
some* malish *(massage).... In trainings an aim is to get dais to attend more
deliveries. People don't want to accept the dai doing the delivery. If the dai
comes to my house she is not allowed to cross the threshold, so for a dai to
touch a woman and be in the house at any time other than after a birth is
undesirable." I have a bit more experience in Sitapur, our shared "field," by
our second conversation, even, I imagine (though I am wrong) a smidgen of
authority now, having lived in "the village," something that people in Lucknow often comment upon. So I explain the division of labor as I have observed it, and say that I don't always find it so useful to think in terms of
"dais," at least not in Sitapur.*

*"Yes!" Dr. Patel says, "That is why we focus on dais. This is why we can-
not make a dai in six days [the length of the training]."*

*So much for the clarity that comes with "understanding the local." I am
even more confused. When I leave, I wonder, is a dai something that exists
already or something that is made? Why do incisive scholarly critiques (the
"target" is a "product" of intervention!) make unproblematic common sense
to interveners?*

The presence of TBA/dai advocates in India and the confused sen-
sitivities of policy documents bear intriguing connections and dis-
junctions with socialities of development on the ground. It is not by
chance that I refer to "old" documents rather than more current
ones. Many of the themes threading through changes in policy in
the 1970s, 80s, and 90s remain in contemporary conversation, even
as things debated change (slightly). As is clear from the above texts,
"cultural sensitivity" is a subset, or instrumental component, of larger
reifying narratives. In spite of some of the differences between international policy and images of dais in contemporary talk, beyond
Delhi the tropes of global genealogies have loud echoes in everyday
interactions. A main point of contrast remains the question of whether
dais are valuable or a hindrance. Public awareness (by policy makers, implementers, and academics) that models of "choice" and "demand" are insufficient to account for the health of the poor does not
necessarily filter out to everyday happenings in MCH and family planning programs. These relations remain overwhelmingly characterized
by themes of choice, education, and demand, reflecting a series of
critical ambiguities. The tension between good or bad dais, good or
bad traditions, collides on the ground with ambiguities at the heart
of global policy. The structural and symbolic ambiguities of TBAs and
"tradition" restrict the ways women are brought into institutional
structures as, or to become, dais.

Development practitioners in Sitapur are hardly a uniform bunch. Though many subscribe to a set of ideals based in, if nothing else, the very idea of their universalizability, their presence in the field (field of implementation, as well as "the field" in terms of the career of a health worker) involves fluidity and, often, self-critique. As such, specific figures in Sitapur and Lucknow are hardly cogs in a larger apparatus, so much as, like the very folks who are their "targets," they are nodes in circulations of shared language. The content of such language involves imagining people (health professionals and trainees) in time and space, as parts of society and moments in teleological flows. Imaginaries of urban and rural situate such language as they situate its speakers; many urbanites have ties to rural communities in practice and imagination, ties that can involve aversion and distancing as well as nostalgic remembering, regular visits, evocations of the hardships of rural life, and sometimes romantic imaginings of its placid contrast with urban life—or its opposite—dirtiness, crowdedness, and noise. At the apex of such complexities are imaginaries of the rural as the site of the "other," while it is the specificity of that "other" status that is most important, not the fact of its otherness. Whatever it is to be rural is very often precisely the flip side of whatever it is to be urban and middle class. It is also its buttress. "Dais," as a unified category applied to a more complex set of practices and persons, enter this rendering as objects of so many affective claims.

On the ground, terms of participation described in global policy remain consistent regardless of practitioners' opinions about dais, even as there is little clarity about the meaning of the term itself. For me, the most satisfying answer to the question, "What is a dai?" came in a conversation with a Delhi-based public health specialist conducting evaluations of past dai trainings in Uttar Pradesh. She described two projects in which NGOs were confronted with distinctions between baby delivering and cord cutting, and with the disjunction between these "local realities" and their own models. In light of this, she said, almost as an aside, "Really, there is no such thing as a dai.... Calling someone a dai does not mean that that is all they are, or that it is a fixed category. It indexes an activity or set of activities." Likewise, in the director of Mahila Seva Sansthan's comment that "Dais here don't do deliveries" was a complex of language and practice that, as he said, posed an obstacle to their goal of increasing the attendance of "trained practitioners" at rural births, a challenge to the inherent structure of intervention. He said he had asked himself if training should take a different form—aimed at rural women more broadly, not just those imagined as "dais." But such an overhaul would require reenvisioning not only the NGO's purposes, but also enshrined elements of policy and ideas of funders. Though the term "dai" would be central to his organization's programs and philosophies, it was one he used with personal ambivalence.

If the term "dai" is distinguished from "traditional Indian midwife," and if its imagination as such can be linked to colonial efforts to understand, transform, and regulate birth work, then a circularity emerges: through development-oriented trainings that include "educating dais" to attend births *and* cut umbilical cords, it is not just a "trained TBA" (or modern practitioner) that is created, but an idealized dai. A true TBA is made through modern intervention; in a recognizable pattern, the performance of modernity creates tradition. Despite variation in the ways health workers talk about their jobs and their "targets," moments of consistency between policy aesthetics and everyday speech speak to the categorical differences between "traditional" and "professional," in which "traditional" status precludes (for some, at least) full participation in institutional structures. This is *not* the case for other "traditional practitioners"— Ayurvedic practitioners, for instance—for whom there are institutional structures of regulation into which they can enter *as* professionals. Other avenues for institutional work exist for "dais"—such as becoming menial workers in hospitals. But these preclude participation in birth work as part of professional status. At the same time, "village dais" are encouraged to professionalize *themselves:* set up clinics in their homes, demand fixed rates (to become, in effect, quasi-legitimate medical practitioners). All such efforts are described as giving them a modicum of self-respect, enhancing their social status and sense of self-worth by promoting professional behavior.

The second moment of consistency with TBA policy statements is confusion over whether or not by entering "the modern" the TBA-as-TBA is meant to disappear or remain part of what it is to be a "dai." This ambiguity, in which it is assumed that all in the position of "traditional" will eventually be reformed (or will evolve), is based on the maintenance of a fundamental breach between some modern folks and others. "As soon as she becomes an ANM she is not a dai"—difference is encoded into the status of the "traditional" and disappearance into the "modern" (and perhaps both difference and disappearance written into identities associated with Dalit women). The differences between the elite/modern/bourgeois and the subaltern are reaffirmed and grounded on the "limited humanity" of the latter (Escobar 1995: 53), the core of which, for birth workers, is a perceptive quality glossed in the notion of "knowledge." Such perception can only be taught: recognition of the abnormality of ill health, and poverty, of the difference between quality and quantity, between "hit and try" and science. Likewise, in order to expand the scope of their humanity, women must be taught their rights (whatever they are) and enter into the cafeteria of choice (as served up by the state). As part of learning they have rights and choices, they are taught which choices to make, which ones demonstrate knowledge of rights, and which show lack of awareness.

Notions of subject constitution that attach to education-oriented health interventions and the forms of surveillance and self-regulation they involve (Foucault 1977a) can suggest a near-universal process in which while some will be defined as the opposite of the idealized subject, subject transformation can, in theory, extend to all. It is easy to imagine this as a force of homogenization. Yet, while the subject-constitution of rural women involves overt training of perception and bodily management, the fullness of this subjective position is not open to all. Indeed, it depends on being closed off to particular categories on which it depends—the ambiguous objects of blame and agents of change.

It has been observed that development discourse often makes social evolutionist claims in India (Van Hollen 2002). However, in Uttar Pradesh, we encounter social evolution with a Victorian twist—some people can only ever evolve so far. Or, to "evolve" means to be incorporated into another framework yet remain "other." A birth practitioner becomes not just trained, but a "dai." As such, her subjective possibilities are delimited by the way she is a cipher of tradition, even where she acquires new epistemologies and praxes. Becoming all the more fixed, her place in the scheme of things according to institutional authorities is said to change (though to what extent it does is open to discussion). That this happens largely to Dalit women is not to be dismissed.

Dais and resistance

At a meeting in a village outside of Lucknow with a Mahila Seva Sansthan representative (Deepika, a young woman with a Master's degree in social work), seven village health workers, and three trained dais, we sit in a nicely painted brick home on a concrete floor under a (moving!) fan. The village health workers (young, married caste Hindu women) have been made responsible for disseminating information about family planning to local women. We all attended, a while back, a distribution of foreign government-

donated "rations" in a nearby village, during which women who came to family planning meetings and brought babies to be weighed could get free grains and oil. The purpose of this meeting is to discuss the next ration distribution, and to hand out the necessary equipment—a plastic funnel, a dipper, scales, and cloth slings.

Deepika goes through the agenda. Women talk about who will take which items, where they will meet, what time they should tell women to come. A few of the dais, sitting toward the back of the room, complain about being under- or unpaid by clients, about the distance they are required to travel to attend the distributions. Deepika listens to them with a slightly amused look. I don't quite understand what they are saying and she says that "they don't want to leave their bahus *home alone." One woman, sitting in the back of the room, leaning against the wall, complains more than others. She says they (the dais) should be paid for taking part in the rations distribution because of the distances they travel and because of the frustration of being frequently accused of stealing the food goods. The ration distributions are chaotic, she says. They are really frustrating and everything is crazy. They take a lot of work.*

The health workers look at each other and giggle; they look at me and roll their eyes. Deepika says to me, "She is a little bit crazy. She does this all the time." After the equipment is given out, as complicated scheduling and logistics are worked out, the old, "a little bit crazy" woman sits silently in the back of the room—with a plastic USAID funnel on her head. With no hint of a smile, no look around to see who might be watching, she wears the funnel for the rest of the (long) meeting. Later I ask Deepika what she thought of it. She says she didn't notice.

So, it seems that both certainties and ambiguities can be rebuked, especially by those who enter these homes-become-institutions as "trainees." In meetings and trainings and follow-up meetings moments of clarity can take the form of the ludicrous amid both chaos and good intentions. Such acts, on the part of "dais," fall into the register of the irrational and inexplicable, in which ideas about old age, gender, and caste filter through social marginalities. Or, for the visiting anthropologist, they fall within the register of parody and critique in which nothing is without a little bit of meaning.

Not long after this meeting I am introduced to Mr. Sharma through links in this world of interconnected agencies and overlapping institutional "agents". I visit a CBD training at the local office Mr. Sharma runs—Pratima Srivastav, who will later be so important in my life, is there being trained. One of the young trainers, Smriti is pregnant, but for now trying to conceal it. We share a room and she complains about the way some of her superiors don't let their trainees talk, and don't listen much to her either. The next day I participate in an exercise in which women stand in a circle and Smriti tells us to say in turn "big fish, small fish." While we say "big fish" we must hold our hands close together, and as we say "small fish" spread our arms wide apart. This, she explains with a contagious and smiling enthusiasm at odds, at least in mood, with the confused glances of trainees not used to such management-training fun, is to help us learn to think beyond what is predictable, to be creative and work outside our preconceptions.

Later, Mr. Sharma takes me to Lalpur and some other villages to meet with "dais." Many months later I want to return to Lalpur, thinking this might be a good place to settle for a while. I ask if he minds taking me back—I can't remember exactly how to get there, and would prefer to have some formal introduction to people. He knows that I want to live with, or at least near, some "dais," and that I have met some of the "trained dais" from Lalpur already.

Manjari meets us there—she lives here too, which makes it all the more ideal, Mr. Sharma says. We visit a few places, including the home where I will eventually live, where I meet Choti Bhabhi (though of course I don't call her this yet) and Amma. Choti Bhabhi asks me what my jati *is, and I have trouble explaining. Manjari says I am "Christian," which doesn't seem quite accurate, but is, finally, the right answer. Hit and try. Saying I have "no jati," is like saying I don't exist.*

After I meet Sunderlal who has set up his post office desk to meet with me, we go back to Mr. Sharma and his assistant who are waiting by the van. I say I would like to look around the dais' area to ask if there might be a room there I can rent. They both say this won't be possible. "It won't be good for you," Mr. Sharma says, "It will be very dirty. And they eat different kinds of food that won't be suitable for you. The post office-walla house is very close to their neighborhood—just along this path, so what is the problem?"

I ask if we can just wander over to see if something is available. Gopal mentions a pandit's house a bit closer to the Chamar mohalla. *"That might have something." We walk in that direction. We stop at what I later learn is Rakesh's Mother's well. Mr. Sharma and Manjari and Gopal stand around, and ask someone about renting a room, but it feels like a bit of a show. "There isn't anything, is there?" Mr. Sharma says. A man—whom I will later know as the schoolteacher Rohit imitates so well—gets off his bicycle to see who we are. Mr. Sharma explains. "I told her it would not be a good place for her over here." In the end, nothing is found. Mr. Sharma asks a child to run and get her grandmother. A few people gather around. When she comes out, Mr. Sharma says, in a loud voice, that I have come to learn about their work. "You must help her," he commands. "Take her to your cases; answer her questions." I am horrified by the tone and volume. I see in my mind a stack of carefully underlined and notated readings about the ethics of fieldwork and the politics of the production of ethnographic knowledge turning to white cremation ash. Mr. Sharma asks how her work is going and says she should be demanding money from her clients. "Make sure you are getting a fixed price. Have you been collecting fees?"*

The woman I will eventually know as Rakesh's Mother says she wants to get a tankhah *(wage) from the government. Mr. Sharma shakes his head and waves his hands up and down. He looks angry. "This is not a matter of wages! The responsibility to collect fees is yours. You can't expect money from the government all the time. Those days are over." She argues that she should get money for her services; she describes the amount her family had had to put toward her training—the transport to the St. Cecilia's center, the loss of her labor around the house. Mr. Sharma continues to insist she demand money directly from clients.*

He points to the schoolteacher. "I do my work for St. Cecilia's and they give me money. And this man does teaching for the school and they give him money. So you too, when you do your work for people you should ask for money. You should make sure they pay you." There are now at least seven people from her house or community standing behind her; some older men, her devrani. *It begins to feel like a* tamasha, *a spectacle. Mr. Sharma is waving his arms; Rakesh's Mother is tilting her head up at him, squinting her eyes as she tries to interrupt. Mr. Sharma says something about "those times have gone," and initially I interpret this incorrectly to mean something about "tradition," channeled as I have been into thinking all such encounters are shaped around the yes or no of this concept. But I am wrong. I say something about "are those times really gone?" And, to my great embarrassment, he corrects me with a different kind of past. "No, not that kind of thing! I am talking about the days when the government funded projects and TBAs could expect some kind of money to come from the government. Those days are gone, those days of always expecting something from the government. We have entered the time of privatization," he says, and he and the schoolteacher explain to me about India's shift toward privatization. "Just like in America where any man can have a post office, any man can have an airplane, any man can have a private airport."*

"Yes, I know about that."

Privatization makes a handy weapon. Mr. Sharma says, half to me and half to Rakesh's Mother, "These women can't keep expecting the government to do everything for them. They must learn to do things for themselves, to collect money for themselves, not to be dependent. There are some people who just repeat the same thing over and over again, Sitaram, Sitaram, Sitaram, Sitaram, demanding something from the government, these women are like that—they are just parrots."

The parrot, once again, speaks across the breach between parody and critique. While in official contexts parrots are meant to signify the value of communication across difference, in everyday speech the parrot takes on a different meaning. It is an insult. It represents the one who knows only by rote, the economic immorality of mindlessly reiterated demands *on* the state, the opposite of the creatively thinking, self-motivated entrepreneur of privatization. In a context in which, as Drèze and Sen state (2002), care becomes yet another commodity in a global economy, efforts to transform obstreperous subjects take many forms. In the roving, indeed multivocal sign of the mimetic parrot lie alterities organized in terms of right economic/ moral engagement and an ability to prove that one is *not mimetic* (the logic of big fish/small fish). These are the subjective dilemmas underlying the suspended clarities about the term "dai," located at the point at which person becomes quality.

In games of parrots and fish, as in ideas like "illiteracy" and "lack of education," the idea of *demand* falls into (or crawls out of) the slender gap between quantifiable realities and discrimination. It is made into a key aspect of citizenship, of both individuals' and groups' relationships to the state, and of the sense of belonging (or not) that comes out of engagement with state institutions (themselves lurching toward privatization in the hybrid monster of intervention—so many agencies, state and private, patched together and given life). Clearly, one must demonstrate the right kind of demand, one "privatized," directed at "clients" rather than institutions, one in which accountability points inward not outward. This theme, presented by Mr. Sharma as social truth and as the train of history, underscores rumors of noncompliance (see Chapter 7) and points to the moral value placed *on* "demand" by policy texts: do marginalized people demand too much of the state, or not enough?

Mr. Sharma's lecture demonstrates the bold, even hackneyed ways reproductive outcomes and bodily praxis—not to mention social disempowerment—are made over into individualized moralities. This discourse entails a techno-morality, and exemplifies the way the technological (and thus depoliticizing) focus of development (Ferguson 1994) enters into the production of socialities and subjectivities—by becoming "creative thinking" and "taking some responsibility," by being transformed into the requirement that persons participate in a range of "appropriate technologies." The more middle-class and bourgeois of rural women anticipate the requirements state-supported modes of enfranchisement place upon subjectivity. But the most marginalized of rural women carry a burden of blame even in their demands and, especially, in their mockery of techno-moralities—in which cooking funnels become hats and no one listens when you use the voice you are told you are supposed to have.

A touch of madness

I arrived in Lucknow with an outlook shaped largely by conversations *about* "dais"—in texts, in interviews and everyday talk among policy and public health types in Delhi—and thus expecting to find a reiterated obsession with "tradition." "Those times are gone"—Mr. Sharma's statement—on the surface involves a sense of space temporalized that had formed much of my own approach to what it means to value and validate "dais' knowledge," to value and validate the local. But even in the local and institutional spaces, the "local moral worlds" (Kleinman 1999) where talk has a veneer of interest in "tradition," even where the focus is on the endless argument about the "good" or "bad" of "dais," the sustaining of that critical ambiguity involves a moral stance that is about citizenship, about participation in society at once opened up/offered and foreclosed. "Knowledge" is not at all of interest at the point at which women actually do enter into engagement with the state as "dais," and neither, in fact, is "tradition." The rejected past has nothing to do with "practices" or "beliefs" in relation to bodily practice, but everything to do with a stance toward the state. Not surprisingly, discourse on TBAs is not about women who deliver babies, just as talk about (and to) trained dais says more about imaginations of citizenship than about women who participate in birth work. But at the same time, development talk and everyday practices act out not so much "hierarchy" but raw power in diacritical terms, difference according to certain rules, those bespeaking citizenship more than modernity. They do so by way of the shifting (and invented) imaginary of "the dai," and the way those imaginaries are performed on and with real people—almost invariably elderly and low caste.

To reiterate, one of the most important correlations between TBA and dai (as imagined categories) is not their stereotyped frozenness or their position in particular hierarchies, but their critical ambiguity and plastic otherness to those things the state claims to offer. Ambiguity is not always bad; the mixed identities of the postcolonial are at times elegized as spaces for disruptive and creative subversion of master discourses (Bhabha 1994). North Indian agriculturalists have been seen as "in-between figures," the "'not-quite-indigenous' and 'not-quite-modern' [who] disrupt the complacent march of progress implicit in discourses of growth and development" (Gupta 1998: 233). Likewise, in shifting "global ethnoscapes," difference can involve both domination and "imagination as a social practice" (Appadurai 1996: 14). Of course, the "ethnoscape," or, more awkwardly, "intervention-scape," does not stand to be engaged by everyone on the same creative terms—indeed, in the case of trainings, an undeniably global scape is not *intended* to be engaged by everyone creatively, though "creative" and "independent" action is part of its pedagogy. The trained "TBA" and trained "dai" are defined as something like hybrid categories, but the ambiguities that make them so are part of structures of meaning that constrain their participation in all that modernity is about. Perhaps because the TBA is a continually re-invented category (we might say the same of the dai-as-midwife), the critical potential of the in-between space the trained TBA occupies is repeatedly closed off, as in-betweenness is given a particular function in the progression of development.

Circulating ideas about dais situate much about reproduction in rural settings. Such conceptualizations are not merely aimed *at* rural women, but are part of programs that will come to be part of everyday life. At the same time, rural women's ideas about what it is to be *them* are in conversation with this set of suppositions. Some are more vocal, crazy, or angry about it than others. But what seems to happen with some consistency is not unfamiliar to the production of dissent in other parts of the world, in other modes of power, in other times and spaces. That is, perhaps especially for the old, low-caste women who are made into "trained TBAs," what might be seen as "creative" deployment of ambiguities or clever or ironic or argumentative assertion is cordoned off as irrational and immoral. Such women may evade tired, circling debates about whether they and their knowledge are "good" or "bad," "valuable" or "dangerous." In part this may be because their enunciations fall outside the logics of development, but not through any recognizable "traditionalness." But as old untouchable women accountable to state logics of intervention and citizenship, their tirades and sacrileges become mere insanity—not insanity in any grand or disruptive way, not a "different" rationality of "local culture," and certainly not creative thought. The dai before and the dai after training is always just "a little bit crazy."

Chapter 7

TALK
CASTING DESIRE

Pushpadevi

*P*ushpadevi asks me frequently about birth control. The topic comes up
again and again. She and Jawan's Wife ask, "So tell us about the single pill that can be taken to prevent pregnancy."

I say I know of no such thing, but there is a pill you take daily, and another one you take weekly. "No, those don't suit us," Pushpadevi says. "They're
too hot."

"What about operations?"

"Those don't suit us either. They suit some people and not others."

Though most people refer to her as Rambal's Wife, or Rambal's Bride in
local parlance, she is one of the few women who tell me her name. "Even
my children don't know it," she says before whispering it to me. In my notes
I can identify her as I can identify Pratima, Manjari, Meena, Deepika—
agents of change or unmarried women. She says she doesn't mind if I write
it down. In one of our earliest conversations, as we sit on the grass in the afternoon, when I say I want to hear people's birth stories, Pushpadevi says,
"Stories? What is there to tell? It is like this. There is a lot of pain."

Pushpadevi's devrani, whose name I never learn, tells me then about the
daughter who died. "She was this big," she says, holding up her hand. Three
years old, I imagine, though translating these presence-in-the-world, this-
big estimations into years seems beside the point. I write in my notes that she
looks suddenly "very sad" as she speaks.

"What happened?" I ask.

"Who knows? She just died. Sometimes it is like that." She waves her hand. "She was this big, and I don't know what happened. She was sick—"

Pushpadevi cuts in, "She was this tall. Her mundan had already happened. No one knows why she died. It was so sad. She was buried out in the fields because she had not become wise yet, you know, had not begun to menstruate."

Her sister-in-law nods, "And her son died too—"

Pushpadevi cuts in again. "I had seven, now I have six."

"In about his third year," she says, "when he was this high, he became ill. His face and back went stiff like this." She contorts her mouth into a grimace and arches her back into the telltale sign of tetanus. "He got completely hard. Poor thing, he was only this big. He got completely hard like this, and after only a few days he died. Around here people call it jamooga. It is a spirit, like a moth, you know? It grabs you and causes this illness. In cities they call it tetanus. You can call it jamooga, you can call it tetanus. Now they give an injection for it. But none of my children have had injections, not a single one."

There is a measure of pride in her voice.

She now has five girls and one son. The oldest looks about thirteen or fourteen, though none of the children know their ages, nor does Pushpadevi—"We people don't remember ages or celebrate birthdays like big people or people in cities do," she says. Her children run around us, yelling into my tape recorder, running away, flopping into the hay piled up around us. Pushpadevi points to her eldest daughter. "She helps," she says, "She is very strong."

Months later, and after many conversations about birth control, Jawan's Wife says, "Hey, I've heard that you are really a very big doctor. You say you aren't, but I have heard that you are. And you can tell people what kinds of medicine to take."

Pushpadevi nods. "It's true, Didi-ji, isn't it?"

"No, no, I am definitely not a doctor, and I don't know much about medicines. Maybe some little things for headache, but not real medicine."

"Well, this is what we have heard," Jawan's Wife says. "So tell me, I have three children already, and I don't want any more. What kind of pill should I take? Tell me what pill there is that I can take so I never have children again." Again the miracle cure, the one-shot fantasy pill.

"Well there is the birth control pill, but you take that every day," it comes like rote to me.

Pushpadevi cuts in, "No, didi-ji. One pill. You take it once only. And after that no more children. We know about those daily ones and we don't like them. They are very hot. They don't suit us."

Jawan's Wife says, "That daily pill suits some people and does not suit others."

"I've never heard of a pill like this. A one-time-only pill? I don't think that it exists."

"No, there is one. We just don't know how to get it. Don't you know?"

"Why don't you talk to Preeti. She does the work for the state and she can arrange an operation for you." The logic of NAFPA, of the "cafeteria" is over-powering—I can't manage to talk about one technique without mentioning others, or, more ominously, without things coming around to "operation."

They wave their hands to dismiss the idea, and Jawan's Wife says, again, "Operations suit some people and they don't suit others."

But Pushpadevi says, "I would have an operation, but how can I?"

"Why not?"

"My husband won't allow it, and then you need to rest for some time af-terwards, and you need to eat good things—milk, meat. And how can I rest, how can I get those good things, with all these kids? A pill, one pill, that would be good"

If I ever think that Pushpadevi's talk about medicines, pills, and needles not suiting her are meant to imply that they are bad, I stand corrected. When I tell her I am nervous about the pills I have been given for my nausea, the effect they might have on the fetus, she tells me not to worry, "No harm will come of it." She says with vigor that all of her children were born "without a single needle or pill," but when, in the middle of a conversation about "needles," I mention that injections to bring on labor pains might be dan-gerous, she insists they are "a good thing. There is no danger."

"But there is," I say, feeling that I am entering the pedagogical frame I find both distasteful and, like a vortex of money, education, and outsider sta-tus, inevitable, "The womb can burst."

But pedagogy can be refused as well. "No, no such thing can happen," she says. My lack of experience, in dehati terms, with birth and babies trumps certain signs of so-called authoritative knowledge. Such things might not "suit" her—or many dehati women, she says—but their intrinsic value is undeniable. How can I argue? I am chastened.

Blame, causality, culpability flit about in Pushpadevi's talk, never land-ing solidly in one place, but also not leaving any site untouched. Pushpadevi is angry about her life, it is clear, enraged at her husband, her poverty, her lack of education, herself, her kids, and me at times.

There is an air of self-destruction to her approach to life. About condoms, she says, "Here the man has to do everything. If he doesn't like it he won't use it. If it's not fun, he will say he doesn't like it. Around here lots of babies happen this way. People—meaning men—say this. But the effect falls on you, *meaning women, doesn't it? If the man doesn't wear [a condom] then doesn't the result fall on the woman? But I don't use any of this. Not a pill, not a condom. So tell me, doesn't the effect fall on me? Don't I reap these troubles?"*

Going on, she evokes the physicalities of a kind of mutual consumption that motherhood can constitute "You have babies and your body is destroyed, isn't it? If the babies come fast/early, then the effects fall on your body.... If you don't use anything, if you can't read, can't write, then it is like prostitution, you plow your own furrow. Look, I'm telling the truth, the woman decreases. She eats her own foolishness."

In January the arrests come. According to village talk, her husband and some others robbed a rickshaw-walla down the road and, in the course of the robbery, someone woke the sleeping man, who defended himself with a knife. In the scuffle, he was killed. Pushpadevi's husband and the others escaped into the fields behind Lalpur, "the way all the thieves get away from the police." I miss the next part, being in Lucknow at the time. The Bhabhis tell me that a few weeks later a local man purchased a television and VCR and consummated their use outside a nearby temple. The men went to see, and the police showed up.

The man known as "Jawan" (soldier) is arrested too; his wife is now alone in this village where she has not even affinal kin, having "run" here with her husband after their love marriage in another village. Jawan, too, is not from Lalpur. He is Pasi, and knows some people here; she is a Bakshur, a different Dalit jati, and does her best to pass as Pasi. She is often at Pushpadevi's house.

She seems to hold up, but after the arrests Pushpadevi begins to deteriorate. She visits her husband in prison twice in the next three months. "How long will they be there?" I ask.

"Who knows. These days everything is by money." Later, when I ask about her husband's work and fields, she says, "My husband, he is a thief. He does this work. What can I say?" Jawan's Wife, and the wives of other men, do not admit their husbands' guilt, though they may not directly deny it either. Pushpadevi, perhaps as a measure of her feelings about her husband, is plain-spoken.

In a group of women jokingly comparing breast sizes, Pushpadevi suddenly says, "Look at what pregnancy does to your body, he didi-ji? Look at the marks on my cheeks." She points to the dark blotches which in pregnancy manuals are called "the mask of pregnancy." "And look at my stomach, and my breasts." She holds up her sari anchal. Women snicker, and her sister-in-law covers her mouth, embarrassed but amused. Pushpadevi waves a dismissive hand at them. "Do I lie? They used to be good and now they sag. We nurse and nurse and nurse. One nurses until a new one comes and takes his place. Some old women, they wear a blouse like this and the breasts fall out the bottom. What's the point? It's babies that do it."

One day when I arrive she and her sister-in-law are talking in hushed voices. The children are off somewhere. Pushpadevi looks at me and says nothing. I know she went to see her husband a few days ago. We talk, and Pushpadevi mentions the Mishrein. "She is a good doctor. She knows so much. About needles, about pills, about making babies fall."

I ask who gives abortions around here, and she says there are none she knows of here. Maybe the Chamarins, she is not sure. "You know, my Nani did baby work like the Chamarins do here, but not this work. It's wrong. And this Nani," she says gesturing over to Shalini's grandmother's house, "She doesn't do it either. But the Mishrein, she takes a stick, like this," she holds up a twig from the ground, "and she wraps some cotton around the end. Good clean cotton. New cotton. She puts some kind of medicine on it and then she puts the whole thing up inside." Pushpadevi demonstrates. "She puts it inside the womb. And the baby falls." She looks at her sister-in-law. "She did this work on me."

"A while ago when you told me you had gone to see her?"

"You understand. But something is wrong. The baby fell, but the road isn't clear."

I ask what is wrong. "A lot of pain in my waist. But what can I do, Didi-ji? My husband is gone, I have these kids. I am going back to see her."

The conversation turns again. Later I ask if now might not be a good time to see a doctor at the hospital and perhaps also have the operation she says she wants. "If it is a matter of cost, then I can help," I say.

Pushpadevi says no, it's not the cost. "How can I get an operation with all these kids to take care of?" She says, anyway, when her husband returns he will know and be angry.

"How will he know?" I ask. "I can take you."

"He will know. Leave it."

After the Pasi baby dies I talk to Pushpadevi about the pain of infant death. "I feel sad about him every day," she tells me, talking of her son. "Every day the thought of him comes into my head." "There seems to be a lot of sadness here," I say. I tell her about Death Without Weeping, describe the situation in Brazil, explain the author's argument as best I can. I take pains not to moralize the argument and to explain the depth of poverty and the protections of distance. "Oh ho," Pushpadevi says. "How awful. How sad for those women. It is not like that here. There is no less pain just *because there is more death. Here a mother's love for her baby is very strong. She prays that it will live, and when it does not there is great pain. For a long time."*

"Does your husband ever get angry at you?" she asks when I visit while my husband is here.

"Sometimes."

"Does he hit you?"

"No, never. Does your husband?"

"He hits me a lot. He beat me even more before I had children. He hits me with his hands, with a lathi, with whatever is nearby. He gets angry easily. Does your husband get angry easily?"

"Not easily, but he does get angry sometimes. Does he beat your children?"

"Sometimes, not often. Mostly he beats me. Once he beat me very badly because I asked if I could have an operation."

"Sterilization?"

"Sterilization. I said I wanted to have an operation so I could have no more children. He beat me hard that time. That was when she was born." She points to her third oldest daughter, laughs, then abruptly stops. "And since that time, look how many more. After her I wanted to stop. He wouldn't let me have an operation, and then the man needs it every night. Since her there have been three more.

"But my marriage was a love marriage," she says after a pause, and without hint of the irony too often supplied by Western associations of love with choice. Here, love marriages are often felt to be ill-fated. Mothers worry about the love marriages their daughters might make for the risks they involve, the likelihood of uncertainty and sorrow. As Pushpadevi speaks, several of her children look up from their play, listen haphazardly then go back to their tasks. "We met because my cousin lives in this village. I came to visit her once."

"How old were you?"

"How should I know? I guess I must have been twelve, thirteen, fourteen, fifteen, no, I was fifteen, I was not younger than fifteen. My husband was also very young. He was all smooth—he didn't have a beard or a moustache then. We loved each other. I went home and told my parents I was getting married, and they were very angry. My mother said not to marry that boy, but I did. And look at me now."

A young, unfamiliar, and heavily pregnant woman walks by the house, returning from the fields. She ducks under the veranda roof to speak with Pushpadevi. This is her maike, she tells me; she has returned to have her

*baby. I ask if this is her first. She says no, very softly, and something else I
can not hear, then turns away. As the woman speaks with Jawan's Wife,
Pushpadevi whispers to me, "She has had four babies. But all are finished.
Some right away, some later. This is the fifth time." When she returns to conversation with Pushpadevi, Pushpadevi tells her that there are certain things
she must do to ensure this baby's survival. "Something is grabbing it. Who
knows what, but you must be very careful. Go and get a* taviz *made, wear
it always, carry it near you, with some iron. Or do this. Get a small ball
made of* gobar *[cow dung], and have this man in Bahraich blow some magic
into it. Get one for the baby as well—give it to the baby to wear around its
neck. There is a man in Bahraich who will do this for you."*

"What does he blow into it?" I ask.

*"Who knows? Some kind of spell. There are ghosts that will grab a baby,
you know. Some ghost has grabbed all of that woman's babies."*

"Why do they desire babies? Why do they grab them?"

"They just grab them."

"But what do they want with a baby?"

*"They want its life, its soul. Ghosts have to take birth somehow also,
isn't it?"*

*Simultaneous with this conversation, there is hushed and heated mur-
muring about "the jeep" that has been making noisy rounds through villages.
All morning people have been coming into the Bhabhis'* angan *to say that
a "*pakaran *[seizure, arrest] jeep" from the district revenue office is "coming
to grab/arrest (*pakarna*) people" forcing them to make payments on loans.
I ask Bari Bhabhi if they would take away people's belongings in lieu of
payment. "What belongings?" she scoffs. "They will take the person away.
Who has anything to give?"*

*Dev runs into my room in the morning asking to borrow my motorcycle
for the day. When he returns with it well after nightfall, he recounts that the
pakaran jeep crossed his path and the men threatened to arrest him, but he
pleaded that he had a guest and they let him go.*

*The "jeep" is back in the afternoon and driving by the Pasi neighbor-
hood. Pushpadevi says that most of the men in the neighborhood have run
away to avoid the* tehsil *collection. One guy, someone says, was "grabbed"
because he could not come up with the five thousand rupees ($125.00) that
were demanded. Everyone is shocked at the amount and insists she must
have gotten the number wrong. "No, it was five thousand."*

*Talk comes to a standstill. We all watch as the jeep, with its grabbing
officials, bounces by in a plume of dust. When it turns onto the path into
the fields, women speak in low voices about who owes how much. Pushpadevi nods at me to turn off my tape recorder. There is vulnerability in the
air.*

Chakkar

How do we make sense of the incomprehensible? How is it possible to speak, as Pushpadevi does, of a child's death from a disease for which prevention is both known and withheld? How is it possible to hear the signs of "choice" and "will" speak as the source of suffering—love marriages, operations, pills and needles, or to hear concern about avoided medical techniques silenced because ultimately "they are good"? Law, or the crosscutting signifiers that constitute a multiplicity of law(s), and the structuring of desire within such morally weighted structures, may be part of the tangible ways such illegibility speaks to the shaping of death and suffering.

For Pushpadevi and for many women, both life and pregnancy are a *chakkar*—either a whirlwind or a turn around the park, revolving entrapment or an amazing ride, something by which one is moved or a source of raw effort, like an obsession. Part of the *chakkar* are the dilemmas posed by reproduction, especially in places like Sitapur, where the dialectic and ironic tension between infant loss and overreproduction characterizes having babies (cf. Scheper-Hughes 1987). As well as signaling larger demographic trends, this tension is part of a broader dynamic underlying poverty and rurality—that between abundance and loss, plenty and lack (also noted in Stewart 1996, and Mbembe 2001 in reference to the postcolony). In Sitapur, discourses pull in these two directions until one wonders if it is ever possible to speak of the richness of rural life without also mentioning its losses. Upon my arrival in Lalpur, for the first few weeks of initial encounters, I often got the same introduction to *dehati* life: "You get everything in the country. Wheat, rice, fodder, sugar, vegetables too." Or: "Everything takes birth here." "In *dehat* there is a lot of everything: a lot of vegetables, grains and pulses; a lot of festivals, religious holidays; a lot of gods and goddesses; a lot of children. Every house is full." Often the contrast between this imagined life of abundance and the conditions of lack in which many live were made explicit as a contrast between the abundance of food, religion, and children, and the lack of signs of enfranchisement, of participation in the state and its law, of being part of what modern India has to offer: "We have so much, what we lack is money." "We have all kinds of things: wheat, rice, vegetables, lentils, but what we lack, what you people in cities have, is *suvidha* (amenities, facilities, means)." On several occasions pleasurable debate erupted in these terms: one person tells me about the abundances of rural life and another pipes up that life is not as easy in the country as in cities, and then another mediates: "The things you get in cities you don't get in the country, and the things you get in the country you don't get in the city." Yet something remains: Rakesh, the younger Chamarin's son, once said, with no detectable romanticism, "Unlike in your America, here people live day by day, without anything extra."

My conversations with Pushpadevi seldom strayed far from this divided dynamic of life with abundance but "nothing extra," as she sought me out for advice on contraception as well as to witness her grief and outrage at the lacks in her life. Because our conversations were often truncated or diverted, Pushpadevi's story came to me in bits and pieces over time. It was woven into questions she had about my life, about America, about a range of "others." She asked and re-flected in ways others did not—about sex, bodies, the way sex can ruin a life. Her comments made other women laugh and cover their mouths, to which Pushpadevi often retorted, "What's there to be ashamed about? There's no shame here." She asked me to teach her coarser words for body parts in English, and taught me a range of curses and obscenities. As I describe in Chapter 4, she herself grew wilder and wilder, less and less *sidha* (straight), as events in her life took over. When I left Lalpur I suspected she was pregnant. In our last encounter I gave her money for the sterilization operation she said she wanted, or whatever she deemed necessary.

The mad contrast between excess and lack, between abundance and loss, is, like the contrast between blame and blamelessness, al-ways at stake in talking, even for a moment, about childbearing and the *chakkar* of a life. Within the *chakkar,* desire—and love—have par-ticular straits; Pushpadevi's stories illustrate the Freudian contrast between desire and law, or the way, as Das says, "The lover of the night ... becomes the law giver of the morning" (1989: 323). The straits of law and love may be as specific and located as the notion of *jati* (understood as something like "caste" and also as something like "genus"). Conflicts over "what is at stake" (Kleinman 1999) may in-volve longings lodged on overlapping, overflowing concepts of well-being—narratives of "empowerment," emancipation, life, and health. Yet, at the same time, powerful "others," things and forces—deper-sonalized "ghosts" and "jeeps," or God or "the one above"—exist just beyond what "we" might grasp, yet always in danger of grasping "us."

In such a context, there are (at least) two running sources of sor-row: infant death and exclusion. But "exclusion," in this and other contexts, demands specificity. In Lalpur, caught up in the flows of both casted and caste-neutral utterances characteristic of intervention talk,

I sensed that other forms of social exclusion looked a lot like contemporary forms of "untouchability." In other words, in institutional and quasi-institutional languages grappling with death and "certainty," forms of marginality condensed around moralities and practices—especially ones associated with desire, sexuality, and reproduction—that mapped onto the well-policed boundary between "untouchability" and the rest. This has everything to do with state and state-like forms of power and intervention.

In writings on violence and political unrest, Begonia Aretxaga described the figuring of law in spaces in which the state simultaneously enters and recedes from view (2003). Recognizing the state as an imaginary as well as bearing tangible grips, she described a "political madness" in which one can no longer speak in terms of modernity or development or similar fantasies of places yet to be ordered, but must address histories of disorder as the production of "altered states" (Aretxaga 2000). Such "madness," she said, involves a basic exclusion, the presence of *something* on which the state must constantly feed: "Those who are excluded are included through their exclusion. These exclusions are always present as a potentiality, a sine qua non of the law and the state as embodiments of its form" (2003: 407). With Pushpadevi, we can take this "sine qua non of the law" to the porous boundary of the state, toward power that involves homes and subjects, the interiorizations associated with "privatization." Intervention, then, becomes more than a commentary on becoming ("development," or again, places yet to be ordered). It is a mode of production, a feature of everything it means to be part of the promises and legitimacies of citizenship. Here, the "maddening" quality of transnational power is not a coded way of evoking "the West," but a way to address structures of desire that move across conceptual as well as geopolitical domains.

To return to the quality of abundance, stories told *about* the "Third World" are often coded morality fables about excess and lack. (Or, thinking in terms of Dionysian excess versus Apollonian restraint, they are *always* stories about excess, if lack is excess in another register.) In this element of discourse, apparent in scandal and rumor, mimetic orientalisms are part of the way excess and lack stand for certain ways of being. Nineteenth-century discourses on and fears about hyper-sexuality (Malthusian fears, the sexual savage, etc.) described by Foucault (1978) and related concepts of self and other formed out of colonial encounters, European class dynamics, and bourgeois sensibilities (Stoler 1995, McClintock 1995) are continually reinscribed, multiplied, and involuted in languages of othering in rural India. The already circular *chakkar* of poverty and life may involve scandals reiterating themselves even as they create the realities they often (mis)read.

As have other feminist critics of development, I find the language games of intervention to be critical. This chapter is about that intersection of language and lived experience in which discursive technologies shape conditions of living for those imagined as "targets." Such techniques provide moral frameworks and social visions that offer both conflict and certainty or, in Kriemild Saunders' phrase, "ordeal[s] of the undecidable" (2002: 15).[1] Just as concepts of individuality and self-determination guiding the WID movement have orientalist leanings that render "tradition" the root of female oppression (Apffel-Marglin and Simon, 1994; Morsy 1995), shifts in policy and conflicts between broad and relative values of science and technology create crises of affect. In taking development outside "west and the rest" (or "traditional" or "local" vs. "Enlightenment") dichotomies (Mohanty 1991), we see that development structures are not easily removed from the local socialities against which they are imagined to stand. In the process, it may become clear that the "maddening states" in which citizenship lives in flows of language and affect involve a state experienced as mythical, and a myth of the state that gives "living shape to (and as) coded signs of identity" (Greenhouse1999: 104). Thinking with those coded entities and identities, that is, thinking with caste and its everyday manifestations, or about the distinctions carved at the boundary of untouchability, we receive a mandate to consider the unbearable undecidable part of political subjectivity.

Thus, it may not be enough, in this case, to point to inclusion/ exclusion. We must ask what this dynamic does to people who inhabit that threshold at which inclusion is, by definition, exclusion. In other sites and spaces, it is possible to see the literal quality of exclusion in the exceptions written into the conditions of sovereignty— the cordoning off of the camp (Agamben 2005), institutions established to dump off the unwanted, places to which people are left for no other purpose than to die (Biehl 2005). But there may be something unresolved, shreds of hope, even, in the despairing ways the threshold between exclusion and inclusion is negotiated in noninstitutional spaces (homes, in other words), and the ways it is dealt with in terms of protection. Death may be not only the end product of exclusion, but also the result of efforts toward survival, the result of love.

Dehati birth, or Modernity is a rumor

My time in Lalpur overlaps with a massive effort to immunize children in Uttar Pradesh against polio. Many of my interactions in Lucknow are with folks involved in this effort. My stay also overlaps with rumors of rumors trailing behind (and preceding) the camps and clinics in which the polio drops are given. Manjari comes to see the Bhabhis one afternoon, and they ask how her work is going. She tells them about the polio program, among other things—not something she is directly involved in. "I heard about this problem they're having. People are saying the polio drops are poison, that they'll make the child who gets them infertile. It was an old Muslim couple that started it. But they found them and put them in jail."

Choti Bhabhi agrees, "They really should put them in jail, for saying things like that, no?"

The story is another half-hollow familiarity I will come to know by heart. I hear it in NGO trainings and offices, at dinner parties in Lucknow, in idle conversations with acquaintances. I see it in the newspaper. The logics of difference at work depend on specific anxieties and social preoccupations— Caste? Class? Or Community? According to some, Muslims had started the rumor; according to others, it was people from "Scheduled Castes" (i.e., "untouchables"); and according to others, it was "illiterate peasants" or "rural people" who spread such fear. "It is," one journalist in Lucknow tells me, "just incomprehensible the way some people resist efforts to improve their lives."

Stories about Third World craziness have a global currency: the tale of the rumor finds its way to the front page of the New York Times Sunday edition on 19 January 2003. And such things seem to speak "from" the "local," but have transcultural currency as well—after leaving Lalpur, I become aware of similar accounts from immunization campaigns all over the world. Riding in a taxi to the airport in Boston, a story on NPR talks about Moroccan women saying vaccinations will make their kids infertile. The driver, about whom I only know what I can infer from the name on his card, laughs and shakes his head as he listens. "Those people," he says.

Ideas about modernity emerge in rumors. Tales of medical non-compliance in the developing world are widespread. They are also longstanding. As David Arnold (1993) points out, resistance to bio-medicine in India—by upper castes and classes in particular—was part of the way medicine became a shifting sign of colonial power, on the one hand, and, later, resistance to colonialism, on the other. But the colonial picture is intriguingly different to the contemporary one, even as it offers tantalizing clues to the way power and legitimacy are part of the picture of "noncompliance": upper castes and

classes resisted interventions, especially those associated with vaccinations, on often religious grounds and within a protective ethic,
while lower castes and classes were at once more "available" to colonial forces and also somewhat more receptive (Arnold 1993).

Though contemporary noncompliance tales offer local explanations for failures of intervention, rumors and meta-rumors, the things
people say about the things people say, jar the listener with disrupted
teleologies of progress that are about something other than "culture" or "belief." In a politically loaded circulation of affect, they describe a blurry boundary between observations about the preciously
local ("cultural realities" of caste and religious tension in India) and
the ironically global (what is true about "the poor," "the uneducated,"
and the "traditional" everywhere). They point, if not always directly,
to the affective economies that shape access to health care, exempli-
fying the unstable space between "ignorance" and "fear," and the
way the body's futures are the currencies with which such emotions
are bartered. They provide hints of the way large-scale health campaigns can be repositories for political anxieties (Arnold 1993; Nichter
1990). The continual return to reproduction and fertility as sites of
vulnerability is telling in these rumors. At the hinge point of biopower—the moment at which surveillance of individual bodies segues
into surveillance of populations—fertility makes difference integral to
relationships with institutional authority. This is so in a case in which
difference is already entangled with moral legitimacy, creating convergences of vulnerability and blame. "Rural birth" emerges as a particular kind of entity within this convergence.

The gaps opened up by distrust may speak to a particular kind of
modernity. In rumors about the mistrust and willful negligence of
others, something like modernity emerges in the site of its own disruption, produced alongside caste-like sensibilities and assertions of
blame. However, this disruption is not made in relation to a single
"beyond," a single "modern" other or self. In other words, these are not
Westward-aimed gazes. More importantly, these are not stories with
a particular interest in "modernity" as such. Put baldly, women in Sitapur didn't talk about "modernity," "the modern," or "being modern"
much at all. Other signifiers took the place of longing (and disgust)
modernity might otherwise occupy: references to the urban, mobile,
educated, use of institutions, and bodily practices. Points of contrast
were most salient: rural/urban, educated/uneducated, one who goes
to a doctor/one who does not, one who uses family planning/one who
has many children, *upar log* (upper people)/*niche log* (lower people).
While these categories might fill a similar niche as "modernity," they

empty it of its unitary nature, its cachet as a sign in circulation and its ability to be a *thing* (unlike the fetishized way the "modern" circulates in urban discourses). In a way that speaks to dislocated forms of "medicalization," many urban transplants (nonelites) return to give birth in "the village," settings far away from hospitals, but where they preach hygiene and call upon "doctors" to give injections to stimulate labor.

Amma, now widowed, can sit in the outer veranda without concern about the rules of purdah *that applied to her in her recent married days. She sometimes calls me over to listen to her complaints of her body's aches and pains. "Oh, it is truly* Kali yug,*" she says, bringing the current epoch of chaos and disintegration in which we all exist into her own bodily fibers, "My legs pain so much, and my back hurts as well. Everything disintegrates." Chachi, Naseem's Mother, comes by often to talk with her. She calls the aging, disintegrating Amma "dulhan," bride.*

On one such visit, Chachi asks, "In America are all babies are born by operation?" I am still learning the taxonomy of this vague, generous term— mythical in precisely the way Barthes described, in its ability to accommodate so many signifiers. But here it is fairly clear, for once, that she is referring to caesarians.

"A lot of babies are born this way, but not all, not even the majority. They try for a normal delivery and if it's necessary they do an operation," I say.

"Here," Chachi says, "those with money go to Munniabad to have operations. Hospitals do more operations to get the money."

Amma adds, "If a needle is given during the pains then both the mother and baby lose their strength and of course an operation will have to happen after that."

*Again, the agent is not so clear—*sui, *needle, can refer to so many things. But Amma is more specific here than usual—the injection to give the pains, as opposed to the one that takes it away, the latter being all but unavailable, and also not really desired, by women around here.*

"The hospitals give the sui *and then the woman becomes weak and then they do the operation to get money.... Sometimes the injection is administered when the baby is about to be born and they still give the injection. But I think that if there is time then the injection shouldn't be administered," Chachi says, more to Amma than to me.*

Amma explains, "Here babies are usually born without an injection. They say babies die in the villages, but babies die in hospitals too."

Just as modernity is diffused into its signs, marginality can be diffused into everything it means to be *dehati* (of the countryside). In reference to the urban, *dehati's* marginality is written into a praxis-oriented sense of location. *Dehati* birth means a range of things. First, it involves the choice to give birth in the village, at home. It may mean a return to the village from the city, or a form of embodiment particular to *dehati* women, in which, as Tulsiram put it, "Here women don't need doctors. Birth is just nature doing its work, but if there is money then the family will take the woman to the hospital. Women here have babies easily because they do all the housework, heavy work like grinding grain and work in the fields. So their *sharir* [body or vagina] is loose."

Amma also said, "Here women do so much work so their channels [*nas*—also veins, nerves, openings] stay loose and they have babies easily. When village women are in labor they have fewer problems. You take it easy and the problems are less. They cut the corn, they sweep, they grind with the grinding stone, they cut grass, some go here, some go there, some do this work, some do that."

The embodied convergence of work, morality, location, poverty, and desire for medical intervention means that "operation," "needles," "hospital," and "*angrezi davai*" ("English"—or Western—medicine), while they cannot be lumped together in terms of "medicalization," might converge as points in opposition to the *dehati* female body. Static-seeming notions of "big people," "city folk," and "rich people" filter through this convergence. So do things like "cities" and "hospitals." Medical technologies and objects—needles, pills, and operations—also circulate alongside labor and movement through these ways of putting down stakes. When women say they "gave birth without a single needle," it can be unclear which kind of drugs they are talking about. A more general sense of lacking need for intervention characterizes a context where pain-relieving medication is seldom given during labor to rural women, but labor induction via oxytocin is frequently part of births within and outside of institutions. A drug meant to bring on rather than abate pain, oxytocin/pitocin's figuring in narratives indicates that ideas about needles and "loose" bodies intersect with notions of pain and endurance. As has been oobserved in Tamil Nadu, pain is considered necessary for birth, associated with the force needed to push the baby out, such that use of pain-abating medication is counter-intuitive (Van Hollen 2002). Similarly, in rural Uttar Pradesh, the ability to endure pain and work hard to get the baby out distinguish urban from *dehati* birth and the births of the rich from those of the poor.

Dehati is, itself, a fragmented idea. Like "peasantry" it consists not only of a range of sectors, but includes ideas *about* difference and differentiation, challenging idealizations of "countryfolk" as a unified body (Chatterjee 1994: 167). As Choti Bhabhi told me, in a value-neutral tone, restrictions on eating apply in *dehat* but not cities because, for one thing, "There is a lot of discrimination here." At the same time that "discrimination"—as both perceptive and protective modality—is a defining feature of rural life, it is also, she said, made necessary *by* certain aspects of *dehati* life—the openness of homes, the mobility of people through households. Differences can be subsumed into the broad reach of "them," or "those people." Like other caste-Hindu women, Choti Bhabhi differentiated "us" from "them" on the grounds of reproductive practice, sometimes explicitly referring to "them" as "SCs," "people from lower castes" (*niche jat log*), Muslims (*Musalman log*), and "Pasi-Chamar," and sometimes leaving the category open with a broad reference to *niche log*—lower people. According to common stereotypes, Muslims are notoriously resistant to family planning. This view, as much sentiment as "social fact," is part of NAFPA trainings and is discussed among Mahila Seva Sansthan workers, and easily slips into the folds of derogatory speech. Like other bland, repeated stereotypes, such statements incorporate ways of morally loading difference into a single matrix that converges on reproductive practice.

Death is written into these discourses as well, into population as much as into the flow of a single life.

Manjari and I visit a nearby ANM. I ask if I can spend a day with her, or interview her for my research, and she looks a bit annoyed and says, well, no, not really. We can talk, but I can't mention her name or her town or bring my tape recorder. I have to come on a day when she won't be busy. "The government won't like me talking to you," she says, nervously eyeing the tape recorder in my pocket (which is normally turned off anyway).

We drink tea, and Manjari and the ANM talk about the difficulty of family planning work. Manjari mentions that in America the government doesn't have family planning programs because "everyone takes on responsibility themselves." The ANM says, "Here [family planning] is bad because there are so many Muslims, and Muslims don't do anything to stop the children from coming. On top of that they lie about how many children they have. One came in recently, and when I asked how many children she had she said three, two boys and one girl, even though it was written in her record that she has seven. Another one I knew had two said she only had one. I said, 'What, did one of them die?'"

She laughs, and Manjari looks uncomfortable. "Oh hey, we shouldn't say these things." She changes the topic to her group of CBDs. Talk comes around to Preeti. "Anyway," the ANM says, "All Pasis are thieves."

One evening Manjari tells the Bhabhis how difficult it is to persuade people to use birth control. "People don't want to have fewer children," she says, "They have the wrong ideas about things." She and the Bhabhis joke, sharing stories that mirror explanations given in trainings. "They think they must have four in case two don't survive," Choti Bhabhi laughs.

"Or that there must be four sons to carry a parent's body to the cremation ground," Bari Bhabhi says.

Bari Bhabhi once told me that the village used to be mainly "upar log" (upper people), "Not all of these people. Now look how many Pasis there are—from here to there." I ask if they moved here from other villages.

"No," she says, "All those people, all those houses, that is all just a few families. Those people won't go for operation. They keep having children on top of children. So from one person you get so many. And if a woman dies, a man will marry again and have more kids."

Choti Bhabhi agrees. "We people believe in only having two children. They have a bunch. They never stop."

One afternoon, when I return from visiting Pushpadevi, Bari Bhabhi asks if "anything happened" in "that place." "Was a baby born?"

I say no, but that two are about to be born, within fifteen days or so, I have been told.

"Are," she says, "What do those people know? They have no idea when a baby will come. We people can say within three or four days, but those people can't even say Chaith, Baisakh [months on the Hindu calendar]."

Consumption

Ideas about knowledge, action, sexuality, accounting and a relationship to death create swaths of modernity and marginality in which "them" and "us" can be alternately vague or specific. Along with these factors of reproductive life are matters of consumption—what one takes into one's home and one's body, what one puts into the bodies of one's children and, by extension, into the corporate body of the family. Put in basic terms, according to many caste-Hindu women, some feed their children properly and others do not. When Dilip (Rohit's younger brother) gets sick, we discuss the look of his diarrhea, what might be given to help him, whether he should be taken to "show the doctor." Bari Bhabhi waves her hand to indicate "over the wall," and said, "Those people give their babies no '*upar-walli ciz*' (upper things)."

I ask what this means. "Like Cerelac [a commercial baby cereal], wheat, semolina, rice, lentils. They just feed their babies milk for a

long, long time, and give no *upar-walli ciz* so their children don't shit
as much, because what kind of shit can there be from just milk? Look
at this one next door, that boy—he is three years old. Only when
the new *bitiya* [daughter] came did he stop drinking his mother's
milk. He has hardly eaten a roti."

Upar-walli chiz has a range of meanings, some precise, some general. The term is most often used as a point of contrast to breast
milk. *Upar-walla* means "something from above" (the term can refer to God, though in these contexts it did not have religious connotations). *Upar-walla dudh*, upper milk, in contrast with breast milk
(*dudh*, or *Ma-ka-dudh*) refers to cow's milk. Sometimes the term is
used interchangeably with *"packet-walla dudh"*—milk that comes in
plastic bags. But *upar-walli chiz*, upper *thing*, refers to solid foods as
well as to things that can be bought or exchanged, to a particular
mode of consumption as well as to things consumed.

"Those people," however, is not a reference to a group, though,
more often than not, it is meant to apply to "untouchables" or Muslims, and replaces the specificity of *jati* terms and the undeniable sting
of words for "untouchable" (a name or the derogatory term *achhut*).
It refers to ways of being that encompass habits and praxes bearing
the stain of caste but extending to class and beyond. The Bhabhis
spoke of a branch of the Srivastav family in the same terms used for
"niche log." They described a convergence of medicine, cleanliness,
industriousness, and morality, on one side, and laziness, dirtiness, and
lack of grooming on the other, drawing on the stuff of untouchability to describe the moral failings of caste-Hindus. Talking one afternoon about Pinki, the Bhabhis' seven-year-old niece, who had been
ill, the Bhabhis said that everyone in her household had a blistery
rash that could be helped by bathing in water with *neem* leaves, Bari
Bhabhi said, "But they won't do anything about it."

I mentioned that that Pinki's sister had told me Pinki was refusing
to take medicine, and that they had called a doctor to give an injection. She had also said they might take Pinki to see the Mishrein.

The Bhabhis laughed. "What medicine? They don't give any medicine. And look at the way they live. Everyone is filthy; they all have
that rash. Do you think there is any medicine in that house? They
won't even go and get the *neem* to soak in."

I asked if the fever might be malaria. Bari Bhabhi said scornfully
"No, it is not. How could she get malaria? It is because they live in
such a dirty way."

Later, Choti Bhabhi compared Pinki's baby sister with Jawan's
Wife's baby to emphasize through irony how dirty Pinki's family

was. "Jawan's Wife's baby always looks very clean. With *kajol* under the eyes and oil on its body. But look at that baby. She is so dirty. They never put oil or anything on her."

To listen for what lies beyond banal stereotyping, we must think at the same time about ethics of protection and those of consumption that orient what contemporary caste and contemporary bourgeois longing are, simultaneously, about. Here, we recall first that caste in Sitapur (and beyond) is not only, or even primarily, a matter of birth, but of consumption. *Jati* boundaries are made by the sharing of food and restrictions on food sharing, as well as through labor and marriage (but not necessarily sex, the other kind of *kam* [work], the other *batchit* [conversation]). In everyday terms, the *jati* of the newborn is ambiguous, as is the nature of its "untouchability" (though unambiguous is the fact that newborns *are* "untouchable"). Its untouchability is different from the sociopolitical untouchability of Dalits, as the newborn is outside *all* social bonds, ties, and flows. Caste-like marginality extends to other modes of consumption; when caste is a product of consumption, there seems to be a slender gap between the idea that caste comes into the body via literal consumption and that it is a part of more metaphoric notions of consumption in the idiom of behavior and commodities. Through such logic, in the process of distinguishing "*upar*" from "*niche*," women's (at times nasty) talk is similar to the kinds of things said in policy documents, trainings, and the stuff of rational authority, in that its moments of unclarity allow *jati* categories to shift into discourses no longer explicitly about caste. These discourses rely on other signifiers: cleanliness and hygiene, use and disuse (and misuse) of certain kinds of foods and goods, use and disuse of institutions.

Bari Bhabhi, with tempered sensitivity, says, "It's true that everything the government did [during the Emergency], all the forcing people to get operation and giving them a battery [radio] in return was wrong, but still people should know that all of this is for their own good, it is not something being forced on them, but something which is good for them." Moral utterances, like those associated with fertility and fertility control programs, link person to population in a logic far less precise than the grid-like quantifications and valuations of "biopower" (Foucault 1978) or "stratified reproduction" (Ginsburg and Rapp 1995: 3), though the result is the same: the lives of some are fostered over the lives of others. At the same time, ethoses of consumption orient moralities familiar to the "dividual" self of a casted universe, in which women cordon off others via restrictions on food transactions to, on the one hand, protect the sanctity of the family and, on the other, establish a zone of the disgusting "other."

This slips easily into the ethoses of consumption associated with locating oneself amid flows of commodities and "choices" in how one lives one's life. In both, care is a morality of consumption praxes as much as consumption praxes establish boundaries between us and them on a range of overlapping grounds. Consumption is another site of slippage between caste and class. Individual failures to "do what is good for them" segue into the questionable morality of the group, establishing broad moral categories that incorporate "untouchables," Muslims, the uneducated (I return to this category below), and the poor into a field of marginal—and visceral—otherness on the basis of a logic of reproduction.

The dirty and the good

Morality is taught to caste-Hindu children in terms of a basic difference between the dirty and the good that maps onto concepts of consumption on the one hand and sexuality and overreproduction on the other. Older children, and some adults, played a game with Rohit that could bring him to tears. Rani, his older cousin, was especially unrelenting. She said, "Rohit is a dirty boy," and Rohit insisted, "Rohit is a good boy." Rani repeated, "Rohit is a dirty boy," and Rohit said, again, that he is a "good boy." The game continued until someone stepped in to say, "Rohit is a good boy," or until Rohit began to cry, at which point Rani held him and said soothingly, "Rohit is a good boy."

Differences between the dirty and the good are made clear for Rohit and for the Dalit children who play in and around the house, as well as in chidings to children not to do something because it is a *gandi bat*—a dirty thing. Amma scolded Rohit with, "Go clean your face! Look how dirty you are. You have become a Pasi boy." When Rohit looked as though he was losing his struggle to contain tears, she said more gently, "We will clean your face and then you will be a good boy."

Untouchability threatens in other ways too. A Pasi woman teased Rohit, "Who's your daddy? Your daddy is a Pasi man, no? Your daddy is a Pasi man!" As she laughed, Rohit looked around in confusion and says "My daddy is good. My daddy is a Srivastav."

"Upper" means "clean" means "good" means "us," and discrimination carries its double meaning in Hindi as well as in English—the perceptive quality of knowing difference, and the moralized quality of preserving difference, but it often entails the ability not only to differentiate by *jati* and kin, specifically, but to recognize the crucial line between "untouchable" and the rest—"us." Choti Bhabhi, speaking with the authority of more education (than any other woman in the village, at least) and familiarity with the city in which her husband and siblings all live, told me, "Here there are different kinds of people. *Upar log*—like us—Srivastavas, Vermas, Yadavs, and others [all caste-Hindus, but not necessarily from the upper echelons]. It's okay to take food they have cooked. Then there are *niche log,* like Muslims and Pasis, and you can't eat food they have cooked." That critical distinction, for her, is also one of hygiene and praxis that segues into the vegetarian/moral valencies of "pollution" and "sin." I shouldn't eat from Chachi's house because, she says, they "live in filth," but they live in filth "because they are Muslim and eat beef."

But this is about more than caste as a universal frame. "The village," she said, to clarify, "Is not like the cities, where you can eat what anyone has cooked because people live in cleanliness. In the village some people are dirty, don't live cleanly, and some people are clean. You can't eat from everyone's house." When she sees the food that *"niche log"* eat she feels like throwing up.

In rural communities it seems to be women's job to police the boundaries of households, kin groups, and caste, while it may be men's place to overlook distinctions and forge bonds between households and *jatis.* When Dev is brought in to slaughter the rooster bought for New Year's dinner, he does so behind the house, then eats the food off to the side of the family's lineup of plates, scooping it off plastic ware given by Choti Bhabhi from a special cupboard. After the meal, as he washes his dishes at the government hand pump in the outer yard, Jawahar comes over, pats him on the back in a warm half-embrace, and offers his hand to shake. I cannot hear what they are saying, but the interaction suggests both apology and gratitude (on the part of Jawahar). Dev tells me that before he married, Jawahar often ate in his house. For Choti Bhabhi, though, the matter arises out of an ethos of protection very much a part of a bourgeois sensibility about the urban and the rural, hygiene and appearances, what it means to protect one's own. At the same time, what it means to "do right," to serve one's purpose may be part of the allocation of labor across the life cycle and its orientation, where more bourgeois and slightly more well-off women are concerned, toward doing your part to continue life into the future—a deeply held ethos of "progress."

Naseem is hanging around the house. It is afternoon and the Bhabhis are joking with him about the way he never does any work. "Look, we can give you some work to do," Bari Bhabhi says, "Though everyone around here is

poor. Or why don't you go to Lucknow with your brother and work there?"
She turns to me and says, "Bhaiya [Jawahar] arranged for him to get a rick-
shaw so he could work in the city, but he just came home."

    Naseem laughs. "My health wasn't good. That's hard work! It was hard
to get customers. I like it better here anyway."

    "You are like an old man," Bari Bhabhi laughs. "Useless."

    "It's good to be an old man."

    Choti Bhabhi says, "I never want to be old. I think that once I pass maybe
forty or so I want to die."

    "Why? I hope I live for a really long time," I say, laughing, but perplexed.
Naseem agrees with me. "Of course!"

    "After that you are useless. You do your work, you have your babies, you
watch them get big, then your work is done. Your use is finished. What's the
point after that? It doesn't feel good to be useless. I think it would be better
to just die."

    To belong is to be useful, that much I have heard before. But so too, it
seems, is utility part of what warrants being alive in this way of reckoning
death and resolving the future.

Rejections

It is not the case that upper-caste women who deride lower-caste and
-class women for not using medicines pride themselves for relying
on medical intervention. Many women, across caste, class, and religious lines, reject biomedicine on a range of grounds—the inherent
strength of the *dehati* female body, a preference for "enduring" illness, and the unsuitability of "hot" medicines. Even as caste-Hindus
argue that certain people do not engage institutions for health care,
nearly all the women with whom I spoke, upper and lower caste,
Hindu and Muslim, expressed some level of reticence about hospitals,
medicines, and operations. Upper-caste women choose home births
too; educated women reject birth control pills. Yet, as caste-Hindu
women see it, their own rejection of such things is different from that
of women in the most despised categories. For caste-Hindus, the morality of suspicion is linked with the strength, virtue, and savvy of
dehati women. But the *immorality* of suspicion conferred on *"niche
log"* is linked with ignorance, laziness, dirtiness, thievery, and other
moral failings. The action is the same, but the former morality evades
the latter immorality.

    That untouchability and morality are coproducts of consumption
means that the symbolics of food sharing are drawn along the same

lines as heavily valued moral domains like "dirtiness" and "laziness."
In that slippage "pollution" is left behind, though the same boundaries are drawn, as these values segue into value-neutral languages
of progress—"hygiene" and its lack, "education" and "ignorance," willful mistrust. Such slippages describe a morality of participation, hing-
ing less on a lack of engagement with health care institutions as on
the right kinds of engagement—and the right kinds of resistance.
Women who prefer not to use Western medicines may still use oxytocin and visits to the doctor as signs of affiliation with institutional
authority and the rational consciousness such affiliation signifies. In
the same spirit, they deride others for the same rejections, reiterating a zone of noncompliance already established by interventionist
logics: the "Muslims" and "illiterate people" and "SCs" who spread
rumors, the way "those people never get a needle," "*niche log* never
take their babies to the doctor" "those people never get an operation."
"Those people" may speak to a different form of difference than that
associated with *jati*, strictly speaking, but the social categories it and
its disparaging qualifiers assert are the same.

While women of all castes and classes have reservations about institutional birth, just as women of any caste, class, or religion might
express desire for health care and family planning, or sneak away
from husbands to get sterilization operations in their *maike* (as did the
sister of Meena, an upper-caste schoolteacher in Lalpur), the paired
statements, "those people never go to hospitals" and "I never use
medicine," are neither contradictory nor hypocritical. They produce
a specific moral domain (one that appears from one angle "naturalized," but, from another involves the way the *social* nature of caste
slips into the social scientific quality of "observed inequalities"). These
moralities, according to those who see caste discrimination as a basic—
and necessary—quality of rural life, give rurality a unique purchase
on modernity. In *dehat*—a realm of differing, the space of "discrimination"—in the state programs from which and though which similar utterances flow, caste can be subsumed into other categories to
reappear as part of discourses on progress.

Ideas about how one does or should go about having babies (or
not) stitch caste, class, and gender into a contemporary vision of "untouchability." Where "untouchability" is at once a specific mode of
jati-based exclusion and submerged into broader means of exclusion, it is likewise diffused into ideas about belonging and deservedness—the stuff of citizenship. Meanings of caste are made legible to
national and global ideas, simultaneously produced and erased as intrinsic to the idea of "progress." As such, untouchability is crafted *in*

relation to institutions (not as radically different, premodern, or anti-institutional) just as it is integral to citizenship in terms of political mobilization and constitutional law. It takes shape in a modernity-like matrix in which moral domains are imputed onto particular female bodies. Perhaps this poses a different mode of disruption of modernity's purchase on the real, or perhaps it demonstrates the capacity for exclusion that intervention, in the name of modernity, comes equipped with. Either way, it occurs less through rupture or flawless logic, less by defying the ordering principles of biopower or by unfolding directly from them, than through the convergence of moral domains that are capable of sustaining one another. Such disruptions can hardly be valorized. They suggest close attention to the way "modernity" can swoop marginality into its claims to the opposite. They are part of the ongoing creation of crisis and loss.

Heat and education

Consumption is not only a matter of what is consumed, but of the relationship between the object and that which consumes it. The concept of "heat" brings together what might seem disparate realms— the symbolics of caste and the choice to consume allopathic medicine—as, through its etiologies, moral domains intersect with bodily ontologies and embodied social categories. They also help us bring into more clarity the fuzzy boundary between class and caste. "Heat" may be part of the "suitability" of drugs and interventions (Nichter 1980, 1990; Van Hollen 1998: 206), but its etiologies and moral weight may not be the same across caste and class lines, just as its ability to map onto biomedicine might offer an embodied mode of postcolonial, transnational critique. "Heat" can have a political dimension, being part of the specificity and contextuality of the Indian body. As Lawrence Cohen notes, heat is likewise socialized in the process of aging and its emergent affects (and insanities): "Heat, particularly in the context of the life cycle, may be read as the externalization of power." The "thermodynamic sociality" (Cohen 1999: 155) of the hot brain in the aging man is part of the way that the aging person and the aging body embody family conflict and structures (and breaches) of care.

Thus, in labor, birth, and aging, as well as in broad etiologies of healing and eating, heat indexes the body in a web of social relations that are infused with power. At the same time, in Sitapur and the context of family care and child rearing, heat is part of a morality of consumption that reflects the status of caregiving, often in reiterated moralized idioms. While it is inappropriate to eat hot things while pregnant (except at the end when hot substances encourage the baby to come out), it is considered good for children to be fed hot foods, and foods appropriate to the time of year and bodily conditions. Thus, children should not eat cold foods (such as oranges, lemons, bananas, or yogurt) during the cold season or when they have a cold, and should not eat hot foods when they have a fever. For Choti Bhabhi, consumption of hot and cold foods was another convergence of caste, class, and morality: "*Niche log* never feed their children warm things. They only eat cold things."

Allopathic medicine, considered hot, falls into the hot-cold etiology of health, consumption, and morality, such that people who "don't feed their children hot things" also fail to give them medicines. But women like Choti Bhabhi also reject medicines on the basis of heat. I once make the mistake of associating the hot/cold distinction in medicines with relative strength and the difference between prescription and "over-the-counter" drugs. When I mentioned to Bari Bhabhi that I can get some cream in Munniabad for Rohit's rash, she said, "*Are,* don't give medicine just like that. Take him to show the doctor. That medicine will be too hot."

I said, "This is a *halka* (light) medicine we use at home on babies' rashes."

Choti Bhabhi said, "No, I don't want any of that *khub garam garam* (very hot) medicine. I will take him to get an injection." I argued that the topical cream was "less hot" than an antibiotic injection, but realized that without the distinction between prescription and over-the-counter medication I could not make the case. Once again, it was difficult to locate "modernity" and its others.

Heat merges with class and caste categories in other ways. In the field with Tulsiram's family at the end of a day of harvesting peanuts, we sat around a fire roasting some of the day's take. Tulsiram's son (about ten years old), was wearing only his underwear (*banian*). I asked him if he wasn't feeling cold, and when he said no, Tulsiram said, "Weak people, small people do not feel the cold. In the middle of winter they can wear only a *banian* and be fine. They have the means. [*Inko suvidha hai.*] *Bare log* [big people] go around in winter with sweaters and hats and gloves and still they shiver from the cold. People like the Lalas [Srivastavs], people who do work with their brains get cold very fast, but people who work in the fields, who are outside all day, who do heavy work, they don't need anything, they stay warm themselves." When I asked what he meant by "weak people," he replied, "Weak people, meaning poor people, they have strength."

Tulsiram, referring to "big," not "upper," equating "weakness" with "poverty" and poverty with "strength," and locating the matter of heat and endurance in terms of work and demands placed on the poor, made consumption and praxis matters of class, not caste. Bari Bhabhi too, made a similar comment: People in rural areas "don't feel so cold in the winter because the heat accumulates in their bodies during the times of year when it is warm.... This is because they are out in the sun all summer and the heat collects in their bodies, so in the winter they don't feel cold. But people like you and the *bhaia log* (her husband and his brothers), Srivastav-type people, people who work inside all day and sit at a desk writing, heat never builds up in their bodies and they get very cold in the winter."

Heat is part of consumption and morality—especially when it comes to whether and how one takes medicines or gives them to one's children. At the same time, the processes by which heat adheres in bodies depend upon the social conditions—and work—of the bodies to which it literally adheres (*lagna*). But it is not only on this basis that Dalit and Muslim women's reference to the heat of birth control pills and medications refer to a political or social location.

One evening, Tulsiram tells the story of his recent trip to Lucknow to a group of men in the outer yard. He had gone by bicycle (a five-hour trip one way) to receive a tankhah *(wage) due to him, and had had to visit a bureaucratic office and find a man named Manish Kumar Srivastav. His story has a lyrical ring, with refrains and repetitions about the small man.*

First I had to find the building. As I do not know the city, it was difficult and took some time. But I asked some rickshaw-wallas and was eventually put on the right road. Once I found the building, I looked up and saw that it was huge, huge. A building of many, many floors. At least ten. I had to find a man called Manish Kumar Srivastav, A cashier of some kind. I had this piece of paper with his name on it in my pocket, but I looked up at that building and thought, How will I find him? I began by asking a guard on the ground floor, "Where can I find Manish Kumar Srivastav?

He said to me, "How do I know where some cashier called Manish Srivastav is? Can't you see how many floors there are in this building? And on every floor there are twenty offices at least."

But I said to the guard, "Brother, please help me. I am a dehati man. I am illiterate. How will I find this man without help?"

The guard said, "In this building there must be many Manish Srivastavs"—and it was true, there must have been fifteen Manish Srivastavs—he said, "How am I supposed to know which one you need to see?"

So I said that I thought that this Manish Srivastav was a cashier.

The guard said, "You don't even have his address! Don't you see what a big building this is?"

I thought to myself that I will have to search the whole building for this cashier, and that will take days. Being illiterate, being a man from the country, I will have to look into every corner to see if I can recognize him for myself. The guard told me, "Go start looking," so I went. I went into an office where there was a woman and I asked her if she knew Manish Srivastav. I thought she would be more helpful because she is a woman.

And she said, "No, I do not know any Manish Srivastav. Don't you have his address?"

I told her, "No, I am a dehati man, I am illiterate, I am a small man. What do I know about big government offices?" She sent me to another office, and I asked someone else, "Do you know where Manish Srivastav's office is?" This time it was a young man, and he said he did not know. I asked him for help, I said, "I am a dehati man, I am illiterate, please help me find him. He is a cashier and I am here to get my tankhah." He sent me to a guard on the next floor. I went to him, but he sent me away. Then, by chance, a woman heard me talking to the guard, and she said, "There is a Manish Srivastav working on the seventh floor. Go see if that is the one. He is a cashier."

I said, "I am a dehati man, I am illiterate, please come show me where he might be." So with her kindness we went to the seventh floor and asked someone there, "Do you know a Manish Srivastav?" He said, "I am Manish Srivastav. What do you want?" But he was the wrong one! I asked him to help and explained that I am looking for this man who is a cashier and will give me my tankhah. And again this man said, "How can I help you without an address?" But I thought, "I am here on the seventh floor, I cannot go back now." So I said, "Please brother, I am poor, I am illiterate, I have come all the way from Sitapur on my bike. Please help me find this man." This man took me to someone else, who took me to the right office, but Manish Srivastav had gone home! The next morning, this morning, I went back and found him. He said he had been waiting for me, but went home when I did not arrive. But then everything was fine and I came back.

According to Susan Wadley, in north India "understanding" is a key element of hierarchy (1994: 4). As a means of gaining understanding, education is part of a shifting set of meanings by which difference is produced. Another imprecise but potentially quantifiable category, it marks persons and orients social relationships. It is tied to reproduction in a range of ways—through population studies linking low fertility to higher levels or education, and as a psychological component in everyday speech, in which more educated women are assumed to have a more responsible, choice-oriented "reproductive strategy." Likewise, among lower-level NGO workers I heard the repeated idea that people in rural communities are, by

definition, uneducated, and thus cannot do the work of development. This, too, refracts through caste. Meena, a local schoolteacher,
said, "It is so sad, there is no one in the village to tutor the children.
Lower-caste people don't make their children study or make them
go to school, and if they want help with their homework the parents can't help them because they are uneducated."[2]

Education is also an after-the-fact explanation. "*Woh anpadh hai*"
(S/he is uneducated) or "*Woh padhe-likhe nahin hai*" (S/he is not educated) are dropped into descriptions of events and persons to qual-
ify behavior. Many assume illiteracy or lack of schooling where it
may not actually be the case. For example, many urbanites assume
that all villagers are "illiterate," "uneducated" or "*jhat*" (ignorant). In
such conversations, "ignorance" slips into "lack of education," becoming both derogatory characterization and social explanation, at times
the *only* explanation for noncompliance. Likewise, in villages, upper-
caste people often assume that low-caste people are "*anpadh*." When
I mentioned once that a Chamar neighbor spoke some English, Bari
Bhabhi said, "No, he is uneducated," though he in fact had a tenth
grade education—more than she. Education is also morality. As Rani
put it, explaining why low-caste people cannot be trusted, "Educated
people are more honest." Indeed, in another turn, education is associated with *less* caste discrimination, even as in Lalpur it was the most
highly educated women who were the most visibly, verbally casteist
(or at least education does not prevent many from making poisonous comments about low castes—often precisely on the grounds of
lack of education).

But education, like other signs of authority, can be space for critiques that hollow out morality and "discrimination." In his reference to the political position of "weak people" and "small people,"
Tulsiram made his lack of education part of political maneuvering.
He had run (and lost) in a recent election for the position of *gram
pradhan,* and was considered a leader in the Pasi community. A highly
respected man whose knowledge about agriculture and local history
was often referred—and deferred—to, Tulsiram frequently acted as
mediator between rural people and institutions. In part this was due
to his experience with hospitals. His son, badly burned as a toddler,
had undergone a series of intensive surgical procedures in Lucknow
hospitals. Tulsiram spent months in hospitals with his son, and described the social and bureaucratic alleys he had had to navigate to
get the surgery at low cost. When people in Lalpur needed to go to
hospitals, Tulsiram often went along to help them interact with doctors and negotiate bureaucracies.

In spite of this experience—or because of it—Tulsiram referred to himself as "a small man." Reflecting something similar to what Cohen describes as an embodied social status in the idiom of "weakness" and its way of linking labor and social standing among Dalits, especially (1999), Tulsiram conflated education with political power and equality in broad statements on agency in which the individual and the group (and the weaknesses of each) were not easy to distinguish. Education, in his speech, tended to reiterate ironies of *jati* in which the changeable and unchangeable of the social shifted around. In a riddle of a political theory, he once said to me, "Upper/high people don't have caste." This statement caused me to question what *upar-log* might mean to him, as the term *upar log* incorporates caste and class. Might careful doublespeak allow inequalities to come to the fore without naming sites or origins? Rhetoric of "smallness" showed a different kind of slippage between value-neutral social categories such as "education" and "literacy" and morally loaded categories of knowledge, participation, consumption, and caste—making the matter about access, perhaps, rather than choice, about the exclusion written into the inclusion. Tulsiram referred to upper-caste people as *upar log* and *upar jat log*—how, then, could upper-caste people be without caste? I began to think that Tulsiram did not perceive himself as an exception—a Dalit who "made it"—but rather that he carefully deployed certain realities to create his own brand of relationship with authority.

But what is the nature of this relationship, especially in relation to the circularity of stereotype and "social fact," and to the histories of labor and oppression Tulsiram knew so well? ("I have only read one book," he told me, "And it was about your Muslim president." "Our what?" I asked. "Your Muslim president. Your Ibrahim." Tulsiram, though he never mentioned it as such, had read writings by or about Ambedkar, who commented on Lincoln.) For some historians, the notion of "community" has been seen as central to peasant consciousness (Guha 1983), located "directly ... at the opposite pole to a bourgeois consciousness" dominated by notions of individual actors operating on the basis of will (Chatterjee 1994: 163). Solidarity formation for peasants, it has been suggested, was "paradigmatically" different from that of the bourgeoisie; where the bourgeoisie form "alliances on the basis of common interests," peasants engaged "bonds of solidarity that [already] tie them together" (163).

But this polarity comes into question in a contemporary world that continues to engage its imaginary; the embodied straights of "access" described by Tulsiram and in which bourgeois leanings reiterate notions of "peasant consciousness" (as lack) yet themselves demonstrate a convergence of "community" orientation (in terms of caste) with bourgeois aspirations and promises of enfranchisement. Though scholarly arguments about community consciousness were made in a different context (in reference to nineteenth-century peasant uprisings), the idea that "peasant consciousness" takes shape *in opposition* to bourgeois rationality and individualism resonates with the enunciations of low-caste *dehati* men and women. But it does so with a tinge of irony. In voices like Tulsiram's, self-defined "small people" situate their subjectivity on the grounds of marginalization, but as *trying to get in.* "Peasant consciousness"—whether *"dehati,"* or "lower," or "small"—has long been hollowed out, its solidity and thickness laced with irony, exaggeration, and instrumentality. Tulsiram's story felt much like a song. Its elements were parodic of rationality's Weberian embodiment in big buildings, upper-caste bureaucrats with the same name, mazes of offices and floors. The notion of "strategic essentialism" taken up by many postcolonial scholars (Spivak 1995) suggests that reifications can be used to critique, in essence, themselves, especially in the "pursuit of" political interest (Gupta 1998: 229). Heard literally, Tulsiram's story reiterates the "community consciousness" of peasant identity as other to bourgeois rationality. But heard with an ear for the silly and the strange, and, indeed, an ear for caste, its points of parody make the nonbourgeois story as much about access and the crafting of the margins. Why, it asks, must some things be *so difficult?*

The logic of needles II

In the shifting vagaries—things pointed to and turned away from— of "big people," "small people," "upper people," "lower people," "we people," and "those people" is a sense of what enfranchisement might mean. Also present is something about the affective nature of what we think of as "access." I use the term affect here rather than emotion, taking up the definition used by philosopher Amelie Rorty (1988), because it points to the threshold at which emotion feeds into attitude, involving as much an orientation to the world as a "feeling." Medical care, and access to it, are central parts of this picture, making Pushpadevi's illegible statements and conflicted desires fundamentally stories about the way the promises and hegemonies of medical care can overlap.

Complexities of medicalization in Sitapur, where medical practices are not bound to the "clinic," reiterate Mark Nichter's argument
that, "Medicalization is not just the prerogative of the medical (psychological and medico-legal) professions and it is engaged for reasons
other than social control. It is embraced by people for a variety of
reasons" (1998: 327). As Gertrude Fraser (1998) has shown in relation to the medicalization of birth in African American communities,
the stuff of biomedical management can signify previously denied
enfranchisement, even where its broad reach closes off some of the
"choice" it claims to offer. But for many, enfranchisement is not a
straightforward deal.

*Tulsiram's Wife brings me to Dev's house next door. His wife is there with
her older sister-in-law and their kids. We sit in the hay under the overhang
and swat away the flies. I am trying to figure out which kids belong to which
mother. I ask Dev's Wife's* devrani *how many children she has.*

"I have three brats."

Dev's Wife teases, "No, she has a dozen. Now go get yourself operated on!"

*She replies, with some seriousness, "Ah no. I'm not going to have an op-
eration. If they aren't happening now will they start coming when I'm old?
… But all the big ladies I've seen, they take pills, or they even drink [to stop
having children]. But we people don't even take a needle.… Women these
days, they are looking for doctors. They want to be taken to the hospital and
have all kinds of needles put into them. We people have never been injected
with a* sujja *[big needle].*

Tulsiram's Wife agrees. "I have never been injected. I never needed daktri.*"*

*Dev's Wife laughs and points to her son. "That one, he was born five days
after the first one, and that time I had to go to the doctor!"*

"Yeah, well I had one after six days!" Dev's Wife's devrani *says.*

*Later, Dev's Wife is more serious. "I have two children, one born here,
one born in the hospital."*

*We talk about operations, about the difference between "raw" ones and
"cooked" ones. The raw ones seem clear enough—episiotomies, a little-ish
cut. The cooked ones I am not so sure about. Caesarian? Sterilization? Women
have already told me in ominous voices about the way one often leads to another. Who knows what doctors can do while we are immobile on the table?*

There is another dichotomy to keep straight—the real and the fake.

Tulsiram's Wife tries to explain. "There are asli *(real) and* nakli *(fake)
doctors. If a doctor is genuine and knows what to do then everything will be
fine, but if the doctor is* nakli *then he messes up the operation and she can't
have a baby again. Some go to the doctors and are fine, some go and the* nas
[veins] get cut.…"

Dev's Wife jokes, "Some people have eight children, some people have seven, someone had nineteen children. The pandit's sas, she had so many, she is like a cow, small and very short."

Her devrani bats my arm, "Hey, in the cities they say one girl and one boy. Here we say one dozen."

"If they have three then they think, oh it is a lot," Dev's Wife says.

"In the villages if we have three, people say 'Oh, we only have three, we should have more,'" says Tulsiram's Wife.

Dev's Wife's devrani turns more serious: "They keep telling us, 'Go get an operation. Go get an operation.' Unless we get seven bigha of land from the government we won't get the operation. You're looking for land and every day a child takes birth here, so you want some bigha of land."

In twisting jokes and statements, women blend causalities, mocking my questions and jokingly embracing the idea that rural women produce children at an alarming rate. They describe fake and real doctors, but leave their role uncertain, and express difference in terms of a shifting identification of class, location, big and small, *dehati* and urban. They make fun of the reproductive ways of upper castes and classes (the Pandit's wife, "big women," the rich and the urban) while mocking their own preferred excesses. They joke about the state, just as they referenced the dangers of operation and eschew *sui-sujja* on a range of grounds. They deal with persistent memories of state coercions—the Emergency, the "time of *nazbandhi*"—and the idea that fertility can be exchanged for property, not by rejecting the structure of the exchange, but by shifting its terms. Though mistrust is prevalent, and based on past state misdeeds in far-flung places, loci of coercion are not named in specific terms. The cajoling of state agents is turned into reflection on the state's role in rural poverty, and blame is shifted.

Interventions try to evade the inevitable aura of coercion with phrases implying agency and choice: "target free," "cafeteria approach," and "participatory development." But notions that the body (male or female) can be property—thus alienated—are not easily shaken. In conjunction with now overwhelmingly women-oriented family planning interventions, the possibility of coercion underscores the vulnerability of the female body, located at the juncture of individual, kin-line, and group. Put together with endless commentary on the way *some people* represent everything that stands in the way of progress, women at the margins of a range of hierarchies navigate enfranchisement, surveillance, and coercion. At the same time, they negotiate the mechanisms of power and visions of the freedom each modality represents.

For them, this fraught and absurd situation, in the context of care at once temporary and evasive, creates an affective tension between longing, fear, and resentment. Desiring adequate health care and the belonging that participation in institutions can signify, marginalized women resent the terms by which enfranchisement is said to take place. These include the requirement that they remain representatives of lack and transgression, those upon whom the moral values of "development" exist to be implemented. Such women desire "participation" and "access" but not the provisos with which they come, the terms of the "contract" groups have been "compelled to establish with forms of domination belonging to the structures of modernity" (Das 1989: 313). They may also evade the terms that those concerned with *questioning* those contracts might like to see. Pushpadevi sought emancipation in terms at once modernist and near mystical. She, like other marginalized women, overturned the requirement that "demand" be part of a relationship with institutions by making not fewer demands, but the wrong kinds. Undermining the idea that choice is part of modern female consciousness, she, and others in her social position, described constraints on choice in the sites most representative of it (hospitals, doctors, medical technologies, love marriages).

Naseem's wife looks to be about sixteen, but it is difficult to tell. Her two-ish son was named by Naseem for a popular film star. One day when I stop by for a visit, her own mother is visiting. Chachi—her mother-in-law—is out. Her mother is appropriately reticent for a maike-walli *visiting her daughter's* sasural. *She comes from Bari Bhabhi's* maike, *and we talk about that village, where I have been for a wedding. I ask Naseem's Wife if she went there, went "home," for her baby's birth. "No," she tells me, "It was here."*

"How was it?" I ask, "Who was with you?"

"I didn't get a needle," she says. "No, for three days I endured. He was born into Naseem's mother's hands.... That's all, babies are born like this, But this was in the house. In the hospital it is like this: if you give the "madams" money then they give you a needle to make the pain increase [oxytocin], and if you don't give money then they give you poison. They put poison in the needle. For the poor people. I don't have money, so they demand a thousand, if I give five hundred then they won't do it properly. They may give me poison and I would die. Two thousand, three thousand, five thousand—they take this much for an operation. So who can go? But, now, if the baby is born [at home] then someone or other will come and you will get relief."

Needles—and the stuff they carry—are integral to the push and pull of medical care. For Dalits and Muslims, the metonymic quality of rejecting needles—whether oxytocin or tetanus toxoid—involves the flipside of the status of needles as an icon of biomedical authority. With needles, and especially oxytocin (and its scandals), difference can be a factor of power by which, across chemicals and moral codes, there remains a logic of suppression through reproductive practice. Stories are at the edge of the fantastic, imagining frontiers of the possible within paradoxes of power. Much of women's talk has the same ring as that of their upper-caste neighbors: needles and hot drugs don't "suit" them, their bodies are loosened and strengthened by labor, their subaltern position gives them a healthy dose of suspicion. But their oxytocin stories are darker, with diacritics that speak of the shadows of institutions rather than the light of rationality. Echoing, in a way, the "downward spiral" of birth interventions described by Western natural childbirth advocates, low-caste and Muslim women's fears take that spiral—in which one intervention leads to another, the raw becomes threateningly cooked—even further down. They express a range of fears: that they will receive a needless "operation" (any operation); that if a caesarian is performed a sterilization might be coerced or IUD inserted (a not unfounded concern, see Van Hollen 2002). They fear risks of "operation" in general—the infections, weakness, and ill health that can result, or that interventions for other health concerns are surreptitious efforts to limit their numbers. "The state wants to get rid of the small people;" "The state wants to reduce our numbers"; "The state wants our children to be unable to have children." As Naseem's Wife described, deregulated oxytocin, needles given by "someone or other" in the village, are perceived as *less risky* than institutional deliveries and institutional needles. Where *kaccha* doctors blur distinctions between real and fake, marginalized women utilize the difference, the way that things on the margins of legitimacy allow them to evade structures they fear without forgoing care. This logic of institutionality complicates the accepted parameters of access; it brings the experience of untouchability, in all its diffuse renderings, into the heart of things.

At the same time, marginalized women long for adequate care, visit hospitals and doctors, speak of doctors as skilled. But not only do they subject themselves to the regular ill treatment all women experience in hospitals (scolding and insults from doctors and nurses, symbolic and real swats—one doctor generously showing me around her hospital ward stops in to see a woman moaning in labor, she tells the woman to be quiet and raises her hand as though to hit her;

it may be a familiar gesture including elements of affection, but the pregnant woman winces; this is a problem with global dimensions, cf. Pires et al. 2002), they also submit their bodies—and those of their children—to the threat of disappearance upon which so much about sovereignty is predicated (Biehl 2005; Mbembe 2001). While marginalized women long for the belonging established by the terms of sovereignty, they are terrorized by the ways it is founded on their births.

Fear is a key index of citizenship, of the relationship between self and state that emerges through the allocation of death (Biehl 2001). It does not stand alone, however, and its presence is as much castigated by the powerful as expressed by the marginalized. It is interwoven with specific narratives of self and other, in which untouchability is part of identities formed in relation to institutions, part of persons' self-reckonings vis-à-vis the state. Because it is so embodied, this is a different ground from more overtly group-oriented bases on which persons relate to the state *as* Dalits or Muslims through "reservations" and caste-based political movements. The gendered and embodied relationship to authority is a behind-the-looking-glass form of citizenship to constitutional modes. In constitutional law, difference and group identity are bases for the idea that equality is a goal rather than a fundamental feature of humanity (Nussbaum 2002).[3] But through logics of intervention, exclusion and further differentiation are results of languages aimed toward equality. Social terms set by the power relations through which allopathic medicine circulates as a sign allow the stuff of institutionality to make further marginalization, but on new terms, part of the "contract" for survival.

Casting desire

Even as caste in contemporary India is largely understood as a premodern social formation resonant in modern political configurations, the overedited "staging" of modernity (Mitchell 2000b: 17), even as a condensed social imaginary that holds only limited prescience here, contains, rather than supersedes, "untouchability." "Untouchability"' is reiterated not in any Lamarckian sense—as a remnant of the system—but as an always-remade part of moral and social mappings on which this "effect we recognize as reality" is produced (Mitchell 2000: 17). In reconciling its necessary presence, it is worth quoting Partha Chatterjee at length: "By explaining the innumerable instances of caste practices as ideological manifestations of a premodern social formation, [the argument that caste is mere "superstructure" in Indian society] seems to condemn virtually the entire corpus of traditional cultural institutions in India, both elite and popular. Such undifferentiated advocacy of the "modern" does not sit too well on claims about the identity of the "national." The case is made worse by a growing evidence that the spread of capitalist economic activities or of modern education does not necessarily bring about an end to caste practices" (1994: 173).

In a critique of Louis Dumont's vision of caste as a bounded religious system of internal consistency, Chatterjee asserts that an "immanent critique of caste" must be based in the fact that ideas about caste exist in variance with its actuality (1994: 177), not "sometimes" or "often," but "necessarily," as caste is contested from within its own structures (178). But where childbearing is part of pictures of national progress and individual morality, unified visions of caste (complete with internal contestations) exist simultaneously with fragmented elements that pop up in less-expected discourses. So, to the contrast between ideal and actual caste, we can add the hollowed-out, circulated, and transformed. Chatterjee's juxtaposition of "the fragment" with "the community" in the production of the nation makes it possible to consider both caste *and* modernity in circulation, allowing for a critique along the lines Chatterjee suggests: one "that is at the same time a critique of bourgeois equality" (181).

Through a sociality particular to childbearing, *dehati* women, upper and lower caste, bourgeois and "peasant," are not just points of arrival for development but integral to its sustainability as a meaningful set of ideas. Their subjectivities bypass debates about tradition and modernity that characterize urban popular discourse about rural hinterlands. But convergence is not always friendly; loathing can be modern and bourgeois too. Much as national politics "effect a displacement of the unifying force of dharma" with that of "nation" (Chatterjee 1994: 198), untouchability is instantiated through displacement of its specificities and practices into other terms and forms, vagaries and evasions that slip into yet other affectively weighted utterances. Ashis Nandy describes the way "postcolonial structures of knowledge" are characterized by "a peculiar imperialism of categories" (2001: 61). He writes, "[A] conceptual domain is hegemonised ... so effectively that the original domain vanishes from awareness. Intellect and intelligence become IQ, oral cultures become the cultures of the nonliterate or the uneducated, the oppressed become the proletariat, social change becomes development" (Nandy 2001: 61). So, too, in Sitapur, the process reverberates back and forth across the hegemonic divide: "Lack of education" or "illiteracy" become "stupidity" in the clinical encounter (Chapter 5), Dalit postpartum practitioners become failed dais and failed entrepreneurs (Chapters 1 and 6), "pollution" becomes "lack of hygiene," lack of access becomes bad decisions, and caste privilege becomes "social capital." It is not through bastardized processes of ideology-making in *dehat* that this happens, but through a complex circulation of meanings *unchanged*, shifted and slipped (*not* translated), through the structure and tone and sound of institutional programs as much as through the worlds of "rural housewives" (pace Chapter 3).

On the political stage, moments of replacement coalesce into "the supremely paradoxical phenomenon of low-caste groups asserting their very backwardness in the caste hierarchy to claim discriminatory privileges from the state, and upper-caste groups proclaiming the sanctity of bourgeois equality and freedom … in order to beat back the threat to their existing privileges" (Chatterjee 1994: 198). At the moment, this global structure of neoconservatism entails Hindu-right groups critiquing the "biological essentialisms" of studies finding caste and "Indianness" in DNA, and Dalit organizations claiming genetic markers as evidence of longstanding subordination and their own claim to Indianness. Likewise, universalizing critiques are not so easily put aside by those who find in them powerful statements on the religious and ideological forms of oppression (M. Nanda 2002). Even in political mobilization the stakes of marginalized groups are seldom straightforward; where women's movements have had to ally themselves with state powers they resist (Rajan 1993: 6), some Dalits were, in the past in the troubling position of arguing a better chance of "freedom" under colonial rule. Something similar might be seen at a local level: Dalit and Muslim women assert their difference to demonstrate the discriminatory practices of the state, while upper-caste women (including development workers) take up discourses of education, equality, and medicine to distinguish themselves from various "others" on grounds at once moral and essential. Some make the paradox less paradoxical by hollowing out statements of *both* authority and resistance, revealing the way the production of marginality is embedded in the stuff of a fragmented "modernity"— one already more political and social than the bland and fetishized "modernity" normally allows. Others defy discourses of "choice" and "rights" altogether by evoking terrors of authority, while others resist the imposition of certain critiques by longing for equal treatment and access to care in terms familiar to the most progress-oriented and modernist of feminist discourse.

Van Hollen describes the way didactic and contradictory medical talk demonstrates that discourses of modernity when put into practice are "fundamentally about reifying social difference" rather than conveying knowledge (Van Hollen 1998: 250). Something similar happens outside of institutions as well, when medical practices are invoked, imagined, and talked about as signs of moral quality. But I think the critique, while powerful and apt, might not, in Sitapur at least, take us far enough. The *kind* and *structure* of the way "local moral worlds" take on the sheen of the universal, the visceral feeling of utterances involves an embodied sense of threat that goes beyond social difference and toward forms of embodiment and worlding. It is the dire results that demand our ultimate attention.

As Gupta has pointed out (1998), seemingly self-denigrating eschewing of "traditional" for the "modern" makes uncomfortable hearing for those aiming to acknowledge the "local." Such discomfort unsettles romantic fantasies that require the other occupy a position of resistance—in recognizable forms—to disparaging talk. At the same time, equality talk effaces inequalities by neutralizing them, making them technological and scientific, matters of rational economics, choice and demand, practice rather than essence (Ferguson 1994). In Sitapur, such effacement appears to invigorate inequalities. Where "modernity" is no "seamless real," where it is less important than the nature of praxis, "untouchability" is made (and made stronger) precisely through its own effacement under/into other regimes of common sense. It is not possible to render Sitapur a scene in which reiterated hierarchy is all about institutions, or in which either entrenched aspects of the local absorb or transform the universal, *or* the obliterating march of modernization alters the indigenous. The remarkable fit between the embodied power-scape of medicine and that of untouchability raises important questions about temporal, spatial, and moral categories of modernity, at the same time showing that it is no longer possible to say that "modernity" comes from anywhere other than the "local," or that care and harm are diametrically opposed. Untouchability provides a critical entry into the way technologies of difference can be, from a range of angles, technologies of care. Remarkably, in Sitapur this happens through the absence of a unified or fetishized idea of "modernity," through shifting ways of forging relationships with authority on the ground of the vulnerability of childbearing. Crosscutting marginalities allow us to imagine something beyond "intervention," invoking Foucault, something like "interventionality," a mode of sensation and practice that produces marginality by being evasive about its explicit existence.

To reiterate the more psychoanalytic elements of this language work, in this repression, once again, a certain set of specificities (about identity, about history, about the hatred of the "*achut*") are sublimated to produce means of intervention in the name of equality. The specific labors of Dalit women, like the specific references to located identity that *jati* names can constitute, like the complex multiplicity of factors that bring about a baby's death, like the unbearable weight of grief for rural women—these are suppressed, effaced, turned away from in order to create moral orders and "targets" of intervention: the "dai" as target of hygiene training, "rural women" in need of an emotional upgrade, and a vague other who, through her dirtiness, ignorance, and willful overreproduction collapses a web of social causes into a moral zone that looks an awful lot like what is already associated with "the untouchable." Yet, with repression comes the capacity of eruption. In ways that rural women grapple with the idioms in which they are rescripted, the shiver of recognition (the witchy dai, the ignorant peasant, the "small man," the noncompliant peasant, even the haphazard infanticide) can be a joke, a source of outrage, or a crisis of identification. It is from this point of convergence that a critique of caste, and its immanence in the very sites claiming access to equality, can be made.

The *chakkar* of postcoloniality

It would seem possible to tell this as yet another story about hierarchies, that Indian-est of attributes, the way, according to Louis Dumont, India expresses its humanity and rank always encompasses other narratives (1970). But, continuing an argument begun in the last chapter, this does not, on second glance, seem to me to be a tale of hierarchy; it is, rather, about sensation, revulsion, and establishing deservedness on moral and affective grounds. This is not a case where hierarchy emerges yet again in spaces where it should not appear, but seems to be about the ways discourses precisely about counteracting hierarchy retain exclusion as a feature of citizenship. Likewise, this is not about "Indianness," hierarchical or otherwise, so much as globalized and globalizing logics as they move through households and between neighbors. Thus, when I presented patches of the argument that intervention reiterates untouchability in a conference in New York, the commentator noted a more universal quality to such disparaging talk: "You hear these things in many parts of the world and at many different times: '*Those* people reproduce like animals'." By talking about development and difference in these terms, she implied, we get ensnared in global and historical tangles, and, as a result, in some of the Gordian knots made by thinking about "modernity," as such.

For Foucault, very broadly speaking, modernity occurs as a point of rupture between modes of power—between direct physical repression and repression through self-regulation, techniques of subject formation, and biopower. Biopower, the technology by which life becomes reducible to "explicit calculations" and "knowledge/power [is made] an agent of transformation of human life," marks the moment at which control over death is replaced by the power to foster or disallow life (Foucault 1978: 143). Where biopower hinges on the crafting of subjects through technologies of self, the matter of difference understood in terms tending toward the absolute (social evolution, languages justifying colonial rule, etc.) remains ambiguous, even where the emergence of biomedicine and public health are part of naturalized visions of the body and self of the other (Arnold 1993; Comaroff and Comaroff 1992). If biopower is the *hasiya* of theory, it is also the historically specific cord to be severed.

Scholars considering non-European modernities have critiqued Foucault for not accounting for imperialism in European modes of power (McClintock 1995; Rofel 1999; Stoler 1995). These accounts suggest that anthropologies with a Foucaultian vision of modernity assume that "processes of modernity elsewhere have been identical to those in the West, rather than viewing those processes as the effects of a complex cultural production forged within tangled relationships of (neo)colonialism and uneven transnationalism" (Rofel 1999: 11–12). Difference looks different from the postcolonial point of view because of troubled and deferred longings that are elemental to modernity in the postcolonial world (xxii), sites themselves, circularly, characterized by "a deferred relationship to modernity" (3). In Sitapur, mechanisms of difference at once play upon the notion of "universal" morality while demoting the universal quality of forms of power that constitute modernity. This is true even as techniques of establishing difference give ideas like biopower invigorated purchase in arguably marginal sites. This might be especially the case for the way difference-from-the-modernish is constituted as part of circulations of not only objects of desire and visions of morality, but also of different forms of power and different modes of modernity. The technologies that continue to make self-regulation *the* modern mode of power, rooting biopower and its sister, governmentality, in late capitalist economies and their global(izing) flows have an established place in non-European settings in which the nature of difference might also (perhaps) subvert them. This is the case with difference *from* the West, as has been argued by Partha Chatterjee, Gyan Prakash, Homi Bhabha, and others. And it may also apply to "internal" differences; those who are, as Gayatri Spivak puts it, subalterns to the subaltern (1988a). Indeed, in rural areas, where the state is part of imaginaries of authority involving difference *within* (selves as much as societies) more than difference *from*, obsessions with "Indian" identity so common to urban settings are of little interest. Orientalism is less a master narrative than another mode of difference in circulation. Global discourses on "population" that cast "India's problems" in terms of rampant reproduction ("those people reproduce like rabbits"), oblivious to historical demographic trends and the long-standing productivities that have made the subcontinent a good place to be and reproduce (Drèze and Sen 2002), converge with nationalist discourses of progress in similar Malthusian terms. If not "Indians," broadly speaking, *someone* must be to blame.

Ann Stoler argues that, "In short-circuiting empire, Foucault's history of European sexuality misses key sites in the production of that discourse, discounts the practices that racialized bodies, and thus elides a field of knowledge that provided the contrasts for what a 'healthy, vigorous, bourgeois body' was all about" (1995: 7). To read Stoler's critique into the circulations of morality in Sitapur, racialized and sexualized fantasies about the other can be glimpsed behind the forms of modern subject making Foucault identified (the same objects of knowledge that made the Victorian era a time of exuberantly produced sexualities) (1995). One of these is the Malthusian couple; another is the sexual savage (Stoler 1995:7). If "these people reproduce like animals" has a universal ring to it, like the universal quality of fertility-based fears of vaccination campaigns, we might ask where Sitapur sits in this genealogy of race, sexuality, and empire, the unfolding of colonial and postcolonial "calm violences" (Bhabha 1995). Visceral forms of difference encoded in "family planning" apparatuses and "rural uplift" shift the idea of the sexual savage onto other others, local others with seemingly recognizable praxes and their own senses of the stakes of difference. Postmodern (or extramodern) untouchability, that is also contemporary interventionality, may be a point of reflection of long-standing forms of racism back into the postcolonial world through genealogies of "progress" in India and their often social evolutionary orientations.

David Arnold notes, in the context of nineteenth-century colonial medicine, that while medicine was often reported as perceived locally as a threat to caste sanctity and thus religious piety, it also bore a "certain compatibility with existing social forms and cultural norms in India" (Arnold 1993: 5). A lot has happened in the meantime to make the "certain" compatibility take on a somewhat different shape, including the ways that colonial (and anthropological) forms of biopower themselves shaped "caste" in terms of iconic labor and English obsessions with hierarchy (Das 1995; Dirks 2001). The contemporary shape of that compatibility is, I argue, somewhat different from the compatibilities Arnold described largely in terms of divisions of labor (associating low castes with work involving dissection and cadavers) and the way "western medicine itself bore the taint, the stigma, of the pariah" (1993: 5). Contemporary national and transnational emphasis on the juncture between the "I" and the "we" that fertility represents, alongside the ever-present residue of the coercions of the postcolonial state and the not-far-distant "times of *nazbandhi*," make intervention's dependence on the viscerality of "untouchability" part of contemporary forms of law and citizenship. In these forms, language and legitimacy shape visions of "access" in a context of millennial neoliberalism, privatization, and the intense individualization of accountability. Yet, something about the structures of institutions—or their imaginaries—remains here in the way the "dai," and her own particular "untouchability" are part of the picture. The emergent forms of "untouchability" associated with reproductive health interventions continue to harmonize with a long history of "comfortable fits."

Amid progress's claims to create shared experience (Rofel 1999: 7), breaches between groups' experiences remain, even as they take on new meaning as they are absorbed into ideals of progress as another deferred modernity. The fact that such ideals not only do not ensure a shared experience, but may ensure the opposite makes the deferral all the more poignant. In Sitapur, biopower confronts more directly repressive and vividly hegemonic forms of power. All rural women are caught at the point of slippage between these two forms of power, a slippage always on the horizon in Foucault's accounts. This is best epitomized in the state's schizoid approach to maternal care: overwhelming efforts toward "family planning" and sterilization, and evasive, temporary and shoddy supply of regular health care, maternal or otherwise. Such women are also caught in crises of contemporary Indian interventionality: neoliberal visions of monadic free agents linked via a market versus distinctly postcolonial Indian visions of (and *into which*) group identities and the idea of an *uneven* starting point are written (cf. Kaviraj 2002; Nussbaum 2000). In the affective tensions these situations produce, it becomes possible for doing something to be doing nothing (and vice versa), for the difficulties of getting decent care, even where it is *somewhat* available, to be more than logistical dilemma: part of moral and affective tensions so fraught as to render care nearly out of reach.

Valorizations of "the local" underlying some critiques of development sit uneasily with key symbolics of oppression. These are the structures that make liberal humanism Dalit women's greatest claim to power. And yet, for many women, liberal languages conveying ideals about life and love are less neutral than they seem. Through circulations of talk, "untouchability," too, can be tacked into the girders of universalizing logic. Rather than representing something indelibly local, it is easily accommodated by the most self-proclaimingly "global." How are marginalized women to relate to humanist ideals (that may be their best hope) when those ideals are used to subordinate them?

The suitability of power

In nearly the same breath that Pushpadevi tells me her son died of tetanus she says that none of her children have had injections, "not a single one." "They just don't suit us," she says. How, to ask it again, does one approach such a comment and its place in the larger sory of a life? In going through my notes long after leaving Lalpur, I found that not only were they full of death stories, but that those stories took many forms. Yet, in my efforts to reread, rehear, and grapple with the movements and lacks thereof they contained, I also found that they seemed to fall loosely into two camps: first, stories such as Bari Bhabhi's, recounting desperate and failed efforts to seek out care, the babies born at the margins of or well inside institutional medicine, and second, shorter, less detailed stories in which "it is hard to say what happened, the baby just died," in which "sometimes it is like this," or stories about inaction. While the first stories seemed to offer the ability to counter stereotypes about the fatalism and inaction of rural women, and to offer something like a quiet and desperate heroism, the second kind of story was more challenging. And so, it is with the apparent crisis of inaction, the sites of withdrawal that are also sites of suffering and constraint, that I have tried to find some glimpse of the political (the active) in the very space of its opposite—inaction. It may be here that childbirth becomes political in Arendt's sense, in speaking to the uncertainties of action in a complex world, to the way inaction and action are two sides of the same coin.

The world of talk in which lives unfold, are narrated, are assigned meaning locates those difficult narratives. In particular, the languages surrounding decisions to withhold care, as well as the very terms used to explain them, may tell us something about that political domain, not just to "explain" actions illegible to certain discourses of knowledge, progress, and power, but to articulate the conditions in which language, life, and law collide. For Pushpadevi, as for many others who spoke in terms of the suitability of certain interventions, so much seems to hinge on the space between "I" and "we" charging rural women's discourse. This movement is made possible as much by the biopolitics of intervention as by the structure of Hindi/Awadhi in which first person plural can mean "I" or "we," especially for women speakers. In language games in which notions of "those people" and "we people" efface the specificities from which they derive their meaning, from which they create myths of progress, let us think about the phrase "it doesn't suit us" with an eye toward the flexibility of the "we," the positioning of the self in a flow of layered vulnerabilities.

Some have suggested that women's ideas about incompatibility with biomedicine may have the effect of not allowing generalizable concerns about medical techniques to be raised (Van Hollen 2002). But for Dalit women in particular, "suiting," while it may disallow some critique, refers to embodied political realities. The discourse of "suitability," for marginalized women who are objects of so many forms of blame, may point precisely to the symbolics of that affective tension, to the individual within a group on a "necrographic map" (Mbembe 2003). Marginalized women describe the inappropriateness of medicines as they voice fears that, through political machinations, social engineering, or poor standards of care, birth can be as much a trajectory to obsolescence as coming into being. This "necropolitics" (2003) references both context and memory, enmeshed in and felt through the body. As a speech act, "suiting" may do several things, referencing, even as it buries, social, historical, and individual realities. In the process, it may re-fuse certain deferrals that have already taken place, in which "those people," "the uneducated," and "the ignorant" emerge by deferring the particular referent, becoming code for "untouchable." Re-fusing referents—"we," "I," "me"—to the very places where specificity is evaded, "suiting" might also *refuse* the sublimation of "untouchable" to "uneducated" or "unhygienic." No matter how it does so, for better or for worse, talk of "suiting" breaks down myths of progress—putting a discourse that sounds like individualism and choice in the interest of noncompliance. Because (not in spite) of its ambiguous individualizing, the open-ended causalities of "suiting" overlap with discourses (about, for example, the "heat" of allopathic medicines) already about power, class, and labor.

Women across castes use "suiting" to describe choices in care. But for some, "suiting," like "the hands of God," undermines the certainties that serve as medicine's packaging, *not* biomedical care itself. Critiquing the othering techniques of globalizing health discourses, even as they render biomedicine and health care something they desperately need, marginalized women's reference to "suiting" is mythical itself. More than that, it speaks to a profound crisis of protection and vulnerability. Such is the ordeal in which devastating loss emerges from an unremediable overlap of threat with the subjunctive quality, not so much of illness or healing (Good 1994), but of care itself. This is part of the way, as Chatterjee, Chattoo, and Das put it, voices on the margins critique state power yet are "essential to the functioning" of biomedicine, are "disempowered" by the very "regime" in which they bear a deep stake (1998: 190). Where death stories distribute causality and culpability, "suiting" and its guise of inaction evoke a beyond space in which even morality cannot be constituted. Such breadth makes infant death untouchable, out of reach to moralizing discourses that constitute rural women as backward fatalists for failing to recognize their own losses.

While there may be debate about the *meaning* of such statements, there can be little doubt, at least in Sitapur, about the visible effects of what brings them into being. In the muddle of action and inaction, the breadth of "suitability" speaks to the terrible result of the "crossed purposes" and "ordeals" of citizenship. Undeniably part of the picture of "withholding" care within the ongoing effort of maternal care, "suiting" may open up meaning even as it closes off life. Thinking about "talk" is no mere exercise in analysis. There are terrible stakes to language and meaning. Pushpadevi tells me she thinks about her son every day, and will mourn his loss forever.

Where scarcity can neither be dissociated from regimes of death and colonial strategies of rule-through-disorder (Mbembe 1992) nor from intimate pleasures of administering therapeutics and being part of authoritative scripts, where boundaries between state and non-state, real and spurious are blurred and cast anew, technologies such as needles, pills, and operations—like anything one puts into or takes out of the body—can be shifting signs in the motion back and forth between healing and harming that characterizes biomedicine as a whole. We can now say with some conviction that the regulation of life so characteristic of biomedical and state interventions (at least as ideals) involves the ability to allow some to die (Biehl 2001; Das 2002); many disappear "in the interaction of modern human institutions" (Biehl 2001: 134). But in Sitapur, as subjects and objects of knowledge, history, and intervention, rural women hardly disappear, even as they sometimes also fail to fully appear on biopower's grids. To argue their disappearance would miss the point that it is in the subtle promises and hopes, the spaces where care is really care, and healing happens, that subjectivities are fraught with the constant possibility of failure. In Sitapur, people are not "left to die;" they remain present to the eyes of institutional authority, though the particular trappings of this visibility, this kind of citizenship, involve terms that make survival tenuous. The *threat* of disappearance, felt so acutely at the point of childbearing, the point between body and the population, remains for many a part of the conditions of progress in which and by way of which hope is also constituted.

Where political subjectivities may bespeak presence amid threat of disappearance, they are also formed through very real losses. The convergence of biopower with failure, of social taxonomies with structural violence and despair, the way that the regulation of life points to the way death cannot (but will anyway) be spoken—these may be part of what makes infant death happen where and how and when it does. If interventionality bears at the same time powers of homogenization and differentiation, by virtue of the moral imaginaries that constitute "*dehat*," "the village," "the target," and "the cause," through this web of exclusion and inclusion, some people, by the nature of their conflicting stakes in institutionality and their place in circulations of talk become repositories of a range of deferrals. The busy mess of progress—in the form of biopower, perhaps, but also disrupted and seamed, crosshatched with memories of other forms and imaginaries of power—leaves plenty of room for death. Whether rejecting or despairing or remoralizing those deferrals, women seem to be grappling with the way death is a factor of a hollowed-out legitimacy.

In *dehat*, experiences of birth and death make citizenship part of survival, "not just an abstract index of 'belonging' to a community or class, but an idiom expressive of highly varied, (even crossed) purposes, needs, absences, and desires" (Greenhouse 1999: 105). "Access to resources," as part of the picture of citizenship, must be considered at levels of subjectivity that take us beyond the idioms of "choice" and "demand"—or "culture"—that pervade intervention talk. At the same time, the simultaneous production of "untouchability" and "progress" is something more than an irony of globalization or the craziness of the local. When medical techniques, ersatz or otherwise, lead as much to death and fear as to life and healing, the nature of law and life has banality and dire consequence. As such, we must take incomprehensible acts and utterances seriously, not as burlesque or paradox or postmodern irony, but as part of conscious and earnest efforts to fill gaps, to remedy abuses, to shake up the parodic aspects of *legitimate* things, and to offer care.

Amid circulations of lack, there remains something to be said about its opposite—abundance, or even excess. For the rural poor, we might think of excess as found in the dying (as scandal would have it). But perhaps it lies in what Michel de Certeau described as "the marvelous and ephemeral excess of surviving" (1984: 198). The incomprehensible things "those people" do: noncompliance, reliance on fake doctors, withholding immunizations, even, perhaps, use of concepts of "suiting"—these have little to do with the absence or presence of "knowledge," or the good or bad of "tradition." And they can, indeed, be dangerous, involving a complex of fear and hatred that hold many at bay. But they do so in a context of protection and care, care offered where it is felt to be denied or dangerous. What then do we make of the real and the fake, the active and the passive, the healing and the harming?

EPILOGUE

A final moment to pause on the urgencies of the body… My ex-periences of being pregnant in Lucknow and in New Jersey were much as women had told me they would be—that is, contra-puntal to the things I saw, experienced, and heard in Sitapur. In Lucknow I went to an obstetrician at a clinic where all appointments were made for the same two-hour slot, and waiting women sat in the doctor's central office together with other patients and their fam-ilies. We all waited together, and conferred with the doctor in front of everyone. Pictures of beautiful babies on the wall gave us some-thing to gaze upon, as we spoke in turn to the doctor. Whether it was an STD, pregnancy, abortion complications, a yeast infection, we heard all about it—and pretended not to hear. Downcast gazes (my own and others) made me think we all felt embarrassed together, for ourselves and for each other, and also relieved if our reason for being there was "innocent"—pregnancy within the bounds of mar-riage, for instance.

In this clinic, serving mostly middle-class Lucknowites, my words, too, became subtle, vague, whispery. I wanted some relief from the nausea, some confirmation that things were okay in spite of all the vomiting, some assurance that those pills wouldn't be "dangerous," but my "symptoms" weren't as interesting to the doctor as the tim-ings and measurements of the pregnancy itself. Visits, even very early on, were dominated by ultrasound and its measuring and graphic capabilities. This, in a context in which daily papers provided news and assessment of the latest scandal—ultrasound being used to get rid of unwanted female fetuses. I was given a sonogram at every visit, and referred to another clinic each time for more comprehen-sive scans on newer, better machines. Visibility was everything for the charts and became all but everything for me as well. I asked once if the fetus was a boy or a girl, and the doctor said, "One can

see but one cannot say," so I tried to come up with various subter-
fuges to get an answer from the many technicians and tried in vain
to interpret the signs in the printout. My husband needed proof of
my pregnancy to give the housing office at our university; I sent
him an ultrasound rather than go through the trouble of getting a
letter from the doctor. What better proof than that? It was hard,
though, to make out just what that blotch of white in a field of black
really was. The frequency of the scans disturbed me, but I got hooked
on those little grainy heartbeats and kicking legs. I emailed a friend
in the United States who was aghast at my failed feminist values:
"Don't you know how dangerous it can be? Don't you think they are
taking something away from you?" I had to write back, no, I really
felt that I was getting something out of the exchange.

During this time I left Lalpur for stretches to do archival research
in government libraries. The *jankari* I got turned out to be not worth
a whole lot in the end, and I came to wish I had stayed put. I missed
Lalpur, but in that mustily cozy office in the deep interiors of the state
parliament building, among the female library workers and shadowy
stacks, I learned about the incompatibility of my pregnant body, self,
and experience to the timings, smells, feel, and social structure of
state bureaucratic sites, while also experiencing some of the more
pleasant socialities brought into being by being pregnant among
chatty, friendly, helpful young women. I missed the festival of Holi
in Lalpur due entirely to my pregnancy. I had braced myself for the
raucousness, having experienced Holi several times in different locations already, but instead of throwing colored powders, singing
songs, and noting interactions between women, men, and children
of different caste communities in Lalpur, instead of making the afternoon rounds for *milan* (to meet with friends) I had long promised,
I spent the day of festivity and social reversals in and out of sleep,
and migraine- and nausea-induced stupor in a darkened bedroom
at a friend's house in Delhi.

When I finally, once and for all, left Lalpur for good, my departure played out very much like a *bidai*, in terms of movements, the
shape of preparations, the presence of so many onlookers, friends,
and the curious, to watch me away. I spent days distributing my
stuff, deciding what the Bhabhis would keep (they had dibs on most
stuff, but respected my need and desire to divide the offerings and
my interest in giving as much as I could to the families who had lost
everything in the fires), what I could give to others, what I would
take with me, what I would leave behind with friends in Lucknow,
what would make it only as far as Delhi, and what would make the

final journey. I had hired a van to take me back to Lucknow, and it waited patiently as the day drew on. I bathed in the *angan* (but behind a curtain), changed into clean clothes, packed everything, let Choti Bhabhi help me with the *sindhur* and bindi so important to my self-presentation as a good wife, and eventually, in a small circle of children and women, moved into the outer yard where, amid tears and embraces I finally forced myself into the van. I tried to touch Bari Bhabhi's feet, but she said, "*Are*, what are you doing?" and pushed away my hands.

Counterpoint continued to sound long after I left "the field." I had long conversations with my midwives about placentas, about what happens when the baby takes its first breath and the blood flow to the umbilical cord is cut off, about whether and why it might be better to cut the cord before the placenta comes out. They suggested my husband cut the cord when my daughter was born. I said I thought this was dumb and involved overly Freudian symbolics. In the course of my own "needle-free" labor, I took little comfort from anything. Yet, repeating over and over in my head "What's there to tell? It's like this: there's a lot of pain" did far more for getting me through it than any breathing exercises I had learned. When my daughter was born, in our home in graduate student housing, I asked the midwives to seal the placenta in a Tupperware container I had bought for that purpose before throwing it in the dumpster. They said it would be a waste of a good container. "We'll just tie it up in a plastic bag."

"But some dog will get it and pull it on the road, and everyone will know it is mine. They've heard all my yelling," were the words that came from my mouth. They laughed and thought I was crazy, but obliged when they saw a raccoon crawling out of the trash when they left at 3:00 A.M.

Five months after that, I got into a conversation with an Indian doctor while waiting for a plane in Heathrow airport. She noticed the way my daughter liked to sleep with a blanket pulled over her face, something I always had to explain to people in the states, but not to her; she knew that babies in Indian villages often sleep fully under blankets. But that got us to talking about Sudden Infant Death Syndrome (SIDS). "There is less SIDS in India," she told me, and listed possible cultural practices that might make this so. Less use of high-tech diapers that hold in the urine and its vapors, perhaps, or more open air. At the time I was deeply caught up in indexing and analyzing my notes, and finding far more "death stories" than I had realized I was hearing in Lalpur, and grappling with how I felt about and thought about stories of babies dying for "no reason at all" or because "sometimes it is like this." Her comment was jarring. "Babies don't die this way in India," she said referring to the unexplainable quality of SIDS. "There is always some reason."

And as I wrote things "up" (or down), I was getting to know my new daughter, and also getting to know myself as a mother. I was not one for "new baby instruction books" and actually enjoyed the onslaught of unsolicited advice, but in the chaos of my days and nights I found, in my writing, comfort in structuralist symmetries—I discovered new "rules" to the "division of labor" hiding in my notes, I took shelter in the binaries and symbolics and liminalities of the placenta and the lotus. But as Eve got bigger and she and I (re)entered the social world, I moved away in my writing from "dais" and sors and into *angan* social life. It was then that I found the first-person singular creeping in to my writing. Someone in a reading group commented that this is okay, "The reader's eye is always drawn to the 'I'," he said. But I also came to think, especially as I rewrote many subsequent versions, that something more than a necessary solipsism of style might be part of the shift in my tone. I had begun rereading my diaries, not just my "notes." Sometimes the anger and frustration and Malinowski-esque melancholy in those morning jottings was almost too much to bear.

In Lalpur I had long been frustrated over the way so much of my time was taken up by being interviewed, by unwanted visits, by my efforts at conversation and even "interview" diverted by questions about lives in other places. I noted these things diligently in my notebooks until it became so repetitive that I abandoned that effort to the emotional waste bin of my diary. Questions lessened over time, of course, but never quite went away. They, too, were written into the discourses of life. Pushpadevi pushed me about the knowledge I might be hiding, the unreachable (yet not outlandish) desires I might be capable of finally, once and for all, fulfilling; Bari Bhabhi and Choti Bhabhi, and other women too, wanted to know about life in intimate detail but more because of what I might reinforce about their own approach to things or "knowledge" I could offer. All of the repeated conversations I had about *me* (not "them") in Sitapur, the things that seemed to take up so much precious time, the way I was "interviewed" much more, if I were to enumerate hours and minutes, than I did the "interviewing" have made it hard to put aside the context in which *jankari* was attained, or bloomed (to engage a more organic, less consumerist metaphor)—what anthropologists call the situatedness of that production of knowledge. Alterity, for better or worse, became central to my account.

But a persistent sense of the inherent foreignness of the "I" (not just the "other," part of what it means for something to "just not suit"), for women as well as for myself, also made it necessary to consider the subtleties of just what "othering" and "selfing" might be about, how it also involves "worlding," how it sits in everyday negotiations of desire and annoyance and aversion and love. There are many different kinds of difference, and it bears noting that, broadly, all those questions about how things were done in "my place," the things that filled my notes and my time were, from women at least, so often about marriage, sexuality, babies, bodies. (These are the things women are always interested in anyway, right? the grouchy old man in me kept saying.) It was only very recently, in yet another revision of old-feeling words, and another spin through those awful diaries, that I began to think that in the focus and force of all those questions lay a deep concern about the things people do to bodies in homes and institutions. The ways husbands and wives relate to one another, parents relate to children and children to parents, how doctors relate to patients and about the things that are done to us in the name of healing, how we touch and probe and pierce and feed one another. So much of this I found myself, in more academic languages, charting in and through—often boringly stereotyping—idioms of difference and efforts to hold things (people, groups, institutions, powers) at arm's length. But at the same time, in the concerns about and amusement at what might happen somewhere else, I felt something else that has been more difficult to pin down or write down; that is, what I notice now, at the "end" of it all, is that so many questions were about how people "treat" each other, how we get care, how we give it. To reiterate what one woman said, "A home without children just doesn't feel good; a house should be full." In writing about the ways childbearing can tell us something about the dire conditions and straits of contemporary life in a given context, this persistent sense of abundance and care, of deep and expansive love, has, ironically, been the hardest to capture.

NOTES

Notes on Chapter 1

1. Though I italicize most Hindi and Awadhi words here, I do not do so with the term "dai." This is for two reasons. First, the term has entered into English usage in India, especially in public health circles where its meaning as "traditional midwife" operates largely as a discursive construct. Second, because I frequently have to pluralize the term, as is often done in English, I use the anglicized pluralizations—adding an *s*—that are more pleasant to the ear for non-Hindi speakers.

2. As has been shown elsewhere in India, *jajmani* relationships determine local status according to control over agricultural products, but do not map onto ideological hierarchies of ritual purity for which high-caste Brahman priests represent the pinnacle; Brahman priests receive food goods from lower-caste families according to the *jajmani* system (see Raheja 1988 for the disarticulation of ideological hierarchy from economic status and prestige).

3. According to some, the use of the term to refer to all postpartum workers refers to a time when only those of the *dhanuk jati* performed this labor. In this time of hardship, some said, people from other "untouchable" castes have had to take up the work *mazburi se* (out of necessity). Other informants contradicted this view. (I found no evidence of Muslim women performing such work in the communities where I conducted fieldwork.)

4. One can begin with the contrast made by Louis Dumont between the group-oriented, nonindividuated "homo hierarchicus" of India and the individual, self-oriented egalitarian man of Europe (Dumont 1970). In India, he says, although individual identities may be asserted from time to time, they are always subsumed by larger shared identities, just as politics are always encompassed by religion, and market interactions encompassed by caste. For Dumont the tension between identities is the point of contrast between India and other parts of the world. Sev-

eral schools of thought have been built around critiquing this view, producing, among others, the theories about the "transactional" and fluid nature of the self (Daniel 1984; Inden and Nicholas 1977; Marriott 1968; Marriott and Inden 1977; Raheja 1988). This contrast shows up in other ways for those with a more psychological approach to Indian forms of identity, who suggest that in India identity is largely a relational matter of "synthesizing" one's inner world with broader social groupings (Kakar 1981: 2). This is considered especially the case for Indian women, whose identity is described as "wholly defined by her relationship to others" (Kakar1981: 56). In India, some have suggested, "I-ness" is subordinated to "we-ness" (Roland 1988: 225), and culture based on tensions not between the individual and the group, but between different forms of group identities. In other approaches, the tension between individual and group identities is seen as a cultural narrative underlying symbolic structures and motivating historical processes—"opposite and irreconcilable principles of organization" (Heesterman 1985: 13). Many have challenged these arguments as essentializing and orientalist. Others have noted that notions of abstract individuality may be downplayed, and self-interest and private expressions of individuality coexist alongside group and relational identities as elements of social life not necessarily in tension (Mines 1994).

5. An argument about contrasts in kinds of birth work based on the opposition of distinct ways of being must be followed by certain caveats. Care must be taken to determine which signs index individual and group identities; we must not assume, for example, that demand for higher payment is read in opposition to or as a threat to *jajmani* relationships, or that emotion is a sign of individual rather than group processes (Fruzetti and Ostor 1982; Trawick 1992).

6. This does not make postpartum work unusual in the scope of *jajmani* relationships. As anthropologists have discussed in other *jajmani* exchanges, rather than undermining the fixity of *jajmani* structures, bartering may be a central component of *jajmani* (Parry 1994).

7. While this statement coincides with untouchable men's accounts, past and contemporary, Dumont contradicts himself here. Though he argues that caste is a religious system of rights and obligations based on ideologically valueless notions of pollution and purity, he also rightly argues that work *effects* social identity in such a stigmatizing way—"infamy"—that communities often abandon such work in order to gain legitimacy. Pollution, then, is hardly the valueless stuff of harmonious, nonexploitative hierarchy.

8. These observations are drawn from records held in the archives of the Central Intelligence Department (CID) of Uttar Pradesh, collected by Ramnarayan Singh Rawat and very generously shared with me.

9. Similarly, in Delhi, Vijay Prasad (2000) has documented the way sweepers, organized into urban work forces by the British, also asserted claims

to adequate compensation and working conditions, things which continue to elude them

10. CID, Police Abstract of Intelligence, Uttar Pradesh, 1922.
11. CID, Police Abstract of Intelligence, Uttar Pradesh, 24 March 1922.
12. CID, Police Abstract of Intelligence, Uttar Pradesh, 9 October 1926.
13. CID, Police Abstract of Intelligence, Uttar Pradesh, 20 May 1922.
14. CID, Police Abstract of Intelligence, Uttar Pradesh, 7 August 1926.
15. CID, Police Abstract of Intelligence, Uttar Pradesh, 14 April 1923; 10 June 1933.
16. CID, Police Abstract of Intelligence, Uttar Pradesh, 18 October 1946.
17. CID, Police Abstract of Intelligence, Uttar Pradesh, 10 June 1933.
18. By the 1940s, more disparate political activity coalesced into larger and established movements as debates focused on the end of colonial rule and untouchables' relationships with Congress and the Muslim League (see Rawat 2000). As diverse strains of action came together within coherent ideologies (such as those in support of Ambedkar), the matter of birth work, as far as I can tell, falls out of the record of political mobilization.
19. This is in no small part related to transformations in patterns of land ownership, such that at present some Chamars of Lalpur own land in quantities comparable to that of upper castes once considered "land owning" and many are educated to the same level as upper-caste persons. Where their primary work had been agricultural labor, not hide tanning, before, (though work included hide tanning) it was even more so now, and the social stature of educated and prominent men such as the Schoolteacher—who was a schoolteacher, after all—was felt by many of the community to have raised the political and economic status of the group as a whole. These changes did not, however, appear to have affected the ways women interacted with one another, or patterns of food sharing and marriage taken to be the markers of ideological caste barriers.

Notes on Chapter 2

1. In Buddhist iconography and text the lotus is the manifestation of perfect wisdom, and, rather than representing the abundance and generative energy of the physical realm, symbolizes the apex of spiritual enlightenment (Zimmer 1946: 98).
2. Ferro-Luzzi, noting "unorthodox" uses of the lotus to represent masculinity, also suggests the gender "interchangeability" of the symbol of the lotus in the way it is able to stand for both the *lingam* and the *yoni*, as part of the "paradoxical interchange" of male and female symbols in Indian myth" (1980: 46).
3. I do not wish to suggest that the fetus is unsocial, but rather that for those women I spoke with its sociality is limited to the mother and to

communication with her via personal, hidden, and private means: dreams, sudden and strong desires and aversions. The sociality of the fetus has been explored in other contexts for the ways that it is enhanced and transformed by "new" technologies (Franklin 1997; Rapp 1999; Strathern 1992) such as, in the case of India, ultrasound.

4. There may be other socialities such as those of the spirit or consciousness of the infant before and after it enters into the fetal body (Goslinga-Roy, personal communication).

5. Some women noted that if a house has a concrete foundation the family will dispose of boys' placentas in trash heaps, water sources, or fields, a drawback of the conveniences of concrete and cinder block.

6. There is a legal dimension to this as well. In 2001 the Indian Supreme Court made a ruling stating that married women (even if divorced and living with their parents) cannot, for the purposes of inheritance and land ownership, be considered members of her parents' family. According to news reports, the court stated that the same would not be true of sons as a son's right to his parents' property could be considered "a normal phenomenon with regard to the family in society" (Times of India News Service, 2001).

7. Chawla notes that in certain parts of Rajasthan the dai is referred to as "mother, *vaid* (doctor), and butcher" (2002).

8. The role of Chamars as "midwives" has been considered anomalous in treatises on caste, an exception to rules of pollution-based hierarchy (cf. Dumont 1970: 136). However, if postpartum workers are seen outside of the limiting concept of "midwifery," it is in the specificity of their tasks that they perform work explicitly related to notions of "untouchability."

9. An equally vivid image is conveyed in the oft-repeated statement (also reflected in colonial documents) that "local dais" routinely smear the umbilical stump with cow dung (*gobar*).

Notes on Chapter 3

1. A version of this chapter (Development Without Institutions: Ersatz Medicine and the Politics of Everyday Life) first appeared in *Cultural Anthropology* 19, no. 3 (August 2004).

Notes on Chapter 4

1. A range of studies of visuality in biomedicalized birth include A. Adams 1994; Cartwright 1998; Duden 1993; Georges 1997; Mitchell and Georges 1998; Oakley 1984; Petchesky 1994; Rapp 2000; Rothman 1986; Weir 1998.

2. Woodburne notes that "the name and the shadow are considered parts of the person," and that a way to ward off a woman's malevolent gaze is to repeat her name while tossing pepper into a fire (1981: 58).
3. This is not the case when talking about a new object or a skill. A new motorcycle or television requires that the owner share auspiciousness by displaying the object and distributing sweets, though sharing sweets may involve effort to ward off envy (Foster 1972). Likewise, many birth workers proudly advertise their abilities. This speaks to the difference between acts and things, and the varying degrees of susceptibility of each (especially where caste enters the picture). Birth workers' skills may be valued but not coveted. In the case of the pregnant body—a site of many acts and things—there are graver risks to account for.
4. Again, veiling becomes iconic. Literature on veiling is vast. Some have considered it less a mode of oppression than as encompassing complex and enunciative modes of subjectivity for women. Considering meanings of veiling for "women of cover" (Abu-Lughod 2002), they critique the association of veiling with antimodernism and the assumption that, given the "choice," Muslim women "should" prefer to unveil (Abu-Lughod 1986, 2002; Brenner 1986; El Guindi 1999; Papanek 1982; Zuhur 1992). Like scholars in South Asia, these scholars address the overdetermination of veiling-as-oppression and consider ways veiling can be a point of resistance to Western hegemonic ideologies, a mode of self-protection, and a sign of respectability and elite status.
5. Margaret Sanger's visit to India and conversations with Gandhi on the matter of birth control did involve the question of social evolution (Ahluwalia 2000).

Notes on Chapter 6

1. For the purposes of this section, in order to distinguish primary texts from secondary ones, when using terms or phrases from the four primary texts I use italics. I use quotation marks when quoting secondary sources. Words I mean to emphasize will be underlined. The use of italics to mark primary source material is also used to distinguish language specifically used in those texts from terms whose meanings I aim to problematize by putting them inside quotation marks. Thus, "modern" is a reference to a term whose givenness I am calling into question, whereas *modern* refers to a term used in one of the primary sources.

Notes on Chapter 7

1. This is not to undermine the substandard quality of the rural education system, but to emphasize the moralized quality of such generalizations.

It is not irrelevant that people talk *more often* in these terms than in terms of the faults of the educational system.

2. This can in part be attributed to the fact that untouchability underlies Indian constitutional law, as the Constitution was largely drafted by Dalit activist Ambedkar.

WORKS CITED

Abu-Lughod, Lila. 1986. *Veiled Sentiments: Honor and Poetry in a Bedouin Society.* Berkeley: University of California Press.

———. 2002. "Do Muslim Women Really Need Saving?" *American Anthropologist* 104, no. 3: 783–90.

Adams, Alice. 1994. *Reproducing the Womb: Images of Childbirth in Science, Feminist Theory, and Literature.* Ithaca, NY: Cornell University Press.

Adams, Vincanne. 1998. *Doctors for Democracy: Health Professionals in the Nepal Revolution.* Cambridge: Cambridge University Press.

Agamben, Giorgio. 2005. *States of Exception.* Kevin Attell, trans. Chicago: University of Chicago Press.

Agarwal, Bina. 1988. "Neither Sustenance Nor Sustainability: Agricultural Strategies, Ecological Degradation and Indian Women in Poverty." In *Structures of Patriarchy: the State, the Community and the Household in Modernising Asia,* ed. Bina Agarwal, 83–120. London: Zed Books.

Ahluwalia, Sanjam. 2000. *Controlling Births, Policing Sexualities: A History of Birth Control in Colonial India, 1877–1946.* Ph.D. dissertation. University of Cincinnati.

Anagnost, Ann. 1995. "A Surfeit of Bodies: Population and the Rationality of the State in Post-Mao China." In *Conceiving the New World Order: The Global Politics of Reproduction,* eds. Faye D. Ginsburg and Rayna Rapp, 22–41. Berkeley: University of California Press.

Apffel-Marglin, Frederique. 1996a. "Introduction: Rationality and the World." In *Decolonizing Knowledge: From Development to Dialogue,* eds. Frederique Apffel-Marglin and Stephen Marglin, 1–40. Oxford: Clarendon Press.

———. 1996b. "Rationality, the Body, and the World: From Production to Regeneration." In *Decolonizing Knowledge: From Development to Dialogue,* eds. Frederique Apffel-Marglin and Stephen Marglin, 142–82. Oxford: Clarendon Press.

Apffel-Marglin, Frederique, with Purna Chandra Mishra. 1991. "Death and Regeneration: Brahmin and Non-Brahmin Narratives." In *Devotion Divine: Studies in Honor of Charlotte Vaudeville,* eds. Diana Eck and Francoise Thallison. Paris: Ecole Francaise d'Extreme Orient.

Apffel-Marglin, Frederique, and Suzanne Simon. 1994. "Feminist Orientalism and Development." In *Feminist Perspectives on Sustainable Development,* ed. W. Harcourt, 26–45. London: Zed Books.

Appadurai, Arjun. 1996. *Modernity at Large: Cultural Dimensions of Globalization.* Minneapolis: University of Minnesota Press.

———. 1980. "Response to 'The Female Lingam: Interchangeable Symbols and Paradoxical Associations of Hindu Gods and Goddesses.'" *Current Anthropology* 21, no. 1: 54.

Arendt, Hannah. 1998. *The Human Condition.* Chicago: University of Chicago Press.

Aretxaga, Begoña. 2000. Out of Their Minds? On Political Madness. Paper presented to Harvard University, Department of Social Medicine, Cambridge, MA. December 1.

———. 2003. "The Maddening State." *Annual Review of Anthropology* 32: 393–410.

Arnold, David. 1993. *Colonizing the Body: State Medicine and Epidemic Disease in Nineteenth-Century India.* Berkeley: University of California Press.

Banerjee, Biswajeet. 2001. "Veterinary Injection Supplied for Human Use in PHCs." *Times of India: Lucknow.* April 30.

Barthes, Roland. 1972. *Mythologies.* Annette Lavers, trans. New York: Noonday Press.

———. 1981. *Camera Lucida.* Richard Howard, trans. New York: Farrar, Strauss and Giroux.

Bataille, Georges. 1985. *Visions of Excess: Selected Writings, 1927–1939.* Allan Stoekl, trans., with Carl R. Lovitt and Donald M. Leslie, Jr. Minneapolis: University of Minnesota Press.

———. 1991. *The Accursed Share,* vol. I. Robert Hurley, trans. New York: Zone Books.

Bateson, Gregory. 1958. *Naven.* Stanford: Stanford University Press.

———. 1972. *Steps to an Ecology of Mind.* New York: Ballantine Books.

Berreman, Gerald D. 1991. "The Brahmanical View of Caste." In *Social Stratification,* ed. D. Gupta, 84–92. Delhi: Oxford University Press.

Bhabha, Homi. 1994. *The Location of Culture.* New York: Routledge.

———. 1995. "In a Spirit of Calm Violence." In *After Colonialism: Imperial Histories and Postcolonial Displacements,* ed. G. Prakash, 326–44. Princeton, NJ: Princeton University Press.

Bhagavad Gita. Eliot Deutsch, trans. Lanham, MD: University Press of America, 1968.

Biehl, João. 2001. "Vita: Life in a Zone of Social Abandonment." *Social Text* 68 19, no. 3: 131–49.

———. 2005. *Vita.* Berkeley: University of California Press.

Biehl, João, with Denise Coutinho and Ana Luzia Outeiro. 2001. "Technology and Affect: HIV/AIDS Testing in Brazil." *Culture, Medicine, and Psychiatry* 25: 87–129.

Bierlich, Bernhard. 2000. "Injections and the Fear of Death: An Essay on the Limits of Biomedicine among the Dagomba of Northern Ghana. *Social Science and Medicine* 50, no. 5: 703–13.

Boddy, Janice. 1989. *Wombs and Alien Spirits: Women, Men and the Zar Cult in Northern Sudan.* Madison: University of Wisconsin Press.

Boon, James A. 1999. *Verging on Extra-Vagance: Anthropology, History, Religion, Literature, Arts... Showbiz.* Princeton, NJ: Princeton University Press.

Borst, Charlotte G. 1995. *Catching Babies: The Professionalization of Childbirth, 1870–1920.* Cambridge, MA: Harvard University Press.

Bosniak, Linda. 2000. "Citizenship Denationalized." *Indiana Journal of Global Legal Studies* 7, no. 2: 447–509.

Bourdieu, Pierre. 1977. *Outline of a Theory of Practice.* Richard Nice, trans. Cambridge: Cambridge University Press.

Brenner, Suzanne. 1994. "Reconstructing Self and Society: Javanese Muslim Women and 'the Veil.'" *American Ethnologist* 23, no. 4: 673–97.

Briggs, George W. 1920. *The Chamars.* Delhi: Low Price Publications, 1990.

Caraka-Samhita (text with English translation). 1980. Priyavrat Sharma, trans. Jaikrishnadas Ayurveda Series no. 36. Varanasi: Chaukhambha Orientalia.

Carstairs, G. Morris. 1958. *The Twice-Born.* London.

Cartwright, Elizabeth. 1998. "The Logic of Heartbeats: Electronic Fetal Monitoring and Biomedically Constructed Birth." *Cyborg Babies: From Techno-Sex to Techno-Tots,* ed. Robbie Davis-Floyd and Joseph Dumit. 240–54. New York: Routledge.

Chakrabarty, Dipesh. 1992. "Postcoloniality and the Artifice of History: Who Speaks for 'Indian' Pasts?" *Representations* 37.

Chakravarti, Uma. 1997. "Whatever Happened to the Vedic Dasi? Orientalism, Nationalism, and a Script for the Past." In *Recasting Women: Essays in Indian Colonial History,* eds. Kumkum Sangari and Sudesh Vaid, 27–87. New Brunswick, NJ: Rutgers University Press.

Chatterjee, Partha. 1993. *The Nation and its Fragments: Colonial and Postcolonial Histories.* Princeton, NJ: Princeton University Press.

Chatterjee, Roma, Sangeeta Chattoo, and Veena Das. 1998. "The Death of the Clinic? Normality and Pathology in Recrafting Aging Bodies." In *Vital Signs: Feminist Reconfigurations of the Bio/logical Body,* eds. Margaret Shildrick and Janet Price, 171–96. Edinburgh: Edinburgh University Press.

Chawla, Janet. 1994. *Child-bearing and Culture: Women Centered Revisioning of the Traditional Midwife: The Dai as a Ritual Practitioner.* New Delhi: Indian Social Institute.

———. 2002. "Hawa-Gola and the Mother-in-law's Big Toe: On Understanding Dais' Imagery of the Female Body." In *Daughters of Hariti: Childbirth and Female Healers in South and Southeast Asia,* eds. Geoffrey Samuel and Santi Rozario. New York: Routledge.

Chawla, Janet and Sarah Pinto. 2001. "The Female Body as the Battleground of Meaning." In *Mental Health from a Gender Perspective,* ed. Bhargavi Davar. New Delhi: Sage.

Clifford, James. 1988. *The Predicament of Culture: Twentieth-Century Ethnography, Literature, and Art.* Cambridge, Massachusetts: Harvard University Press.

Cohen, Lawrence. 1998. *No Aging in India: Alzheimer's, the Bad Family, and Other Modern Things.* Berkeley: University of California Press.

———. 1999. "Where It Hurts: Indian Material for an Ethics of Organ Transplantation." *Daedalus* 128, no. 4: 135–65.

———. 2004. "Operability, Availability, and Exception." In *Global Assemblages,* eds. Aihwa Ong and Stephen Collier, 79–90. New York: Blackwell.

Comaroff, Jean. 1985. *Body of Power, Spirit of Resistance: The Cultural and History of a South African People.* Chicago: University of Chicago Press.

Comaroff, John, and Jean Comaroff. 1992. *Ethnography and the Historical Imagination.* Boulder, CO: Westview Press.

Coomeraswamy, Ananda K. 1993. *Yaksas: Essays in the Water Cosmology,* ed. Paul Schroeder. Delhi: Oxford University Press.

Coutin, Susan. 1999. "Citizenship and Clandestinity among Salvadoran Immigrants." *Political and Legal Anthropology Review* 22, no. 2: 53–63.

Csordas, Thomas J. 1994a. "Introduction: The Body as Representation and Being-in-the-World." In *Embodiment and Experience: The Existential Ground of Culture and Self,* ed. Thomas Csordas, 1–26. Cambridge: Cambridge University Press.

———. 1994b. "Words from the Holy People: A Case Study in Cultural Phenomenology." In *Embodiment and Experience: The Existential Ground of Culture and Self,* ed. Thomas Csordas, 269–90. Cambridge: Cambridge University Press.

———. 1997. *The Sacred Self: A Cultural Phenomenology of Charismatic Healing.* Berkeley: University of California Press.

Daniel, E. Valentine. 1984. *Fluid Signs: Being a Person the Tamil Way.* Berkeley: University of California Press.

Das, Veena. 1976. "The Uses of Liminality: Society and Cosmos in Hinduism." *Contributions to Indian Sociology* 10: 2.

———. 1979. "Reflections on the Social Construction of Adulthood." In *Identity and Adulthood,* ed. Sudhir Kakar, 89–104. Delhi: Oxford University Press.

———. 1982. *Structure and Cognition: Aspects of Hindu Caste and Ritual.* Delhi: Oxford University Press.

———. 1983. "Language of Sacrifice." *Man* 18, no. 3: 445–62.

———. 1989. "Discussion: Subaltern as Perspective." In *Subaltern Studies VI: Writings on South Asian History and Society,* ed. Ranajit Guha, 310–24. Delhi: Oxford University Press.

———. 1995. *Critical Events: An Anthropological Perspective on Contemporary India.* Delhi: Oxford University Press.

———. 1997. "Language and Body: Transactions in the Construction of Pain." In *Social Suffering,* eds. Arthur Kleinman, Veena Das, and Margaret Lock, 67–91. Berkeley: University of California Press.

———. 2002. "Pharmaceuticals in the Register of the Local: Urban Poverty and Health in Delhi, India." Paper presented to the Center for Health and Well-Being, Princeton University, Princeton, NJ. November 4.

———. 2003. "Technologies of Self: Poverty and Health in an Urban Setting." *Sarai Reader 2003: Shaping Technologies,* 95–102. Delhi: Sarai.

Davis-Floyd, Robbie. 1987. "Obstetric Training as a Rite of Passage." *Medical Anthropology Quarterly* 1, no. 3: 288–313.

———. 1992. *Birth as an American Rite of Passage*. Berkeley: University of California Press.

Davis-Floyd, Robbie, and Elizabeth Davis. 1996. "Intuition as Authoritative Knowledge in Midwifery and Home Birth." *Medical Anthropology Quarterly* 10, no. 2: 237–69.

de Certeau, Michel. 1984. *The Practice of Everyday Life*. Berkeley: University of California Press.

Delaney, Carol. 1992. *The Seed and the Soil: Gender and Cosmology in a Turkish Village*. Stanford, CA: Stanford University Press.

Desjarlais, Robert. 1992. *Body and Emotion: The Aesthetics of Illness and Healing in the Nepal Himalayas*. Philadelphia: University of Pennsylvania Press.

Devine, John. 1996. *Maximum Security: The Culture of Violence in Inner City Schools*. Chicago: University of Chicago Press.

Dirks, Nicholas B. 1994. "Ritual and Resistance: Subversion as a Social Fact." In *Culture/Power/History: A Reader in Contemporary Social Theory*, eds. Nicholas B. Dirks, Geoff Eley, and Sherry B. Ortner, 483–503. Princeton, NJ: Princeton University Press.

———. 1998. "In Near Ruins: Cultural Theory at the End of the Century." In *In Near Ruins: Cultural Theory at the End of the Century*, ed. Nicholas Dirks, 1–18. Minneapolis: University of Minnesota Press.

———. 2001. *Castes of Mind: Colonialism and the Making of Modern India*. Princeton, NJ: Princeton University Press.

Donnison, Jean. 1988. *Midwives and Medical Men: A History of the Struggle for the Control of Childbirth*. London: Historical Publications.

Douglas, Mary. 1975. *Implicit Meanings: Essays in Anthropology*. New York: Routledge.

Drèze, Jean, and Amartya Sen. 2002. *India: Development and Participation*. Delhi: Oxford University Press.

Duden, Barbara. 1993. *Disembodying Women: Perspectives on Pregnancy and the Unborn*. Cambridge, MA: Harvard University Press.

Dumont, Louis. 1970. *Homo Hierarchicus: The Caste System and Its Implications*. Mark Sainsbury, Louis Dumont, and Basia Gulati, trans. Chicago: University of Chicago Press, 1980.

Eck, Diana L. 1985. *Darsan: Seeing the Divine Image in India*. Chambersburg, PA: Anima Books.

———. 1987. "Rivers." In *The Encyclopedia of Religion*, ed. Mircea Eliade, 425–27. New York: Macmillan and Free Press.

El Guindi, Fadwa. 1999. *Veil: Modesty, Privacy, and Resistance*. Oxford: Berg.

Escobar, Arturo. 1994. *Encountering Development: The Making and Unmaking of the Third World*. Princeton, NJ: Princeton University Press.

Fanon, Frantz. 1967. *Black Skin White Masks*. Trans. Charles Lamm Markman. New York: Grove Press.

Farmer, Paul. 1999. *Infections and Inequalities: The Modern Plagues*. Berkeley: University of California Press.

Feldhaus, Anne. 1993. *Water and Womanhood: Religious Meanings of Rivers in Maharashtra*. New York: Oxford University Press.

Ferguson, James. 1994. *The Anti-Politics Machine: "Development," Depoliticization, and Bureaucratic Power in Lesotho*. Minneapolis: University of Minnesota Press.

Ferro-Luzzi, Gabriella Eichinger. 1980. "The Female Lingam: Interchangeable Symbols and Paradoxical Associations of Hindu Gods and Goddesses." *Current Anthropology* 21, no. 1: 45–68.

Fitzgerald, Rosemary. 1997. "Rescue and Redemption: The Rise of Female Medical Missions in Colonial India During the Late Nineteenth and Early Twentieth Centuries." In *Nursing History and the Politics of Welfare*, eds. Anne Marie Rafferty, Jane Robinson, and Ruth Elkan, 64–79. London: Routledge.

Fitzgerald, Rosemary. 2001. "'Clinical Christianity': The Emergence of Medical Work as a Missionary Strategy in Colonial India, 1800–1814." In *Health, Medicine and Empire: Perspectives on Colonial India*, eds. Biswamoy Pati and Mark Harrison, 88–136. Delhi: Orient Longman.

Forbes, Geraldine. 1994. "Managing Midwifery in India." In *Contesting Colonial Hegemony: State and Society in Africa and India*, eds. Dagmar Engels and Shula Marks, 152–72. London: British Academic Press.

Foster, George M. 1972. "The Anatomy of Envy: A Study in Symbolic Behavior." *Current Anthropology* 13, no. 2: 165–202.

Foucault, Michel. 1975. *The Birth of the Clinic: An Archeology of Medical Perception*. A. M. Sheridan Smith, trans. New York: Vintage.

———. 1977a. *Discipline and Punish*. Alan Sheridan, trans. New York: Vintage Books.

———. 1977b. *Power/Knowledge: Selected Interviews and Other Writings, 1972–1977*. Colin Gordon, Leo Marshall, John Mepham, and Kate Soper, trans. New York: Pantheon Books.

———. 1978. *The History of Sexuality, Volume I: An Introduction*. Robert Hurley, trans. New York: Random House.

———. 1991. "Governmentality." In *The Foucault Effect: Studies in Governmentality*, eds. Graham Burchell, Colin Gordon, and Peter Miller, 87–104. Chicago: University of Chicago Press.

Franklin, Sarah. 1997. "Making Sense of Missed Conceptions: Anthropological Perspectives on Unexplained Infertility." In *Situated Lives: Gender and Culture in Everyday Life*, eds. Louise Lamphere, Helena Ragone, and Patricia Zavella, 99–109. New York: Routledge.

Fraser, Gertrude. 1995. "Modern Bodies, Modern Minds: Midwifery and Reproductive Change in an African American Community." In *Conceiving the New World Order: The Global Politics of Reproduction*, eds. F. D. Ginsburg and R. Rapp, 42–58. Berkeley: University of California Press.

———. 1998. *African American Midwifery in the South: Dialougues of Birth, Race, and Memory*. Cambridge, MA: Harvard University Press.

Freud, Sigmund. 1963. *General Psychological Theory: Papers on Metapsychology*. New York: Simon and Schuster.

————. 2003. *The Uncanny.* David McClintock, trans. New York: Penguin Classics.

Fuller, C. J. 1989. "Misconceiving the Grain Heap: A Critique of the Concept of the Indian Jajmani System. In *Money and the Morality of Exchange,* eds. J. Parry and M. Bloch. Cambridge: Cambridge University Press.

————. 1992. *The Camphor Flame: Popular Hinduism and Society in India.* Princeton, NJ: Princeton University Press.

Fuller, C. J., and Veronique Bénéï, eds. 2001. *The Everyday State and Society in Modern India.* London: Hurst and Company.

Fuss, Diana. 1992. "'Essentially Speaking': Luce Irigaray's Language of Essence." In *Revaluing French Feminism: Critical Essays on Difference, Agency, and Culture,* eds. Nancy Fraser and Sandra Lee Bartky, 94–112. Bloomington: Indiana University Press.

Gailey, Christine. 1987. *Kinship to Kingship: Gender Hierarchy and State Formation in the Tongan Islands.* Austin: University of Texas Press.

Georges, Eugenia. 1998. "Fetal Ultrasound Imaging and the Production of Authoritative Knowledge in Greece." In *Childbirth and Authoritative Knowledge: Cross-Cultural Perspectives,* eds. Robbie Davis-Floyd and Carolyn F. Sargent, 91–112. Berkeley: University of California Press.

Ginsburg, Faye. 1989. *Contested Lives: The Abortion Debate in an American Community.* Berkeley: University of California Press.

Ginsburg, Faye, and Rayna Rapp. 1995. "Introduction: Conceiving the New World Order." In *Conceiving the New World Order,* 1–19. Berkeley: University of California Press.

Good, Byron. 1994. *Medicine, Rationality, and Experience.* Cambridge: Cambridge University Press.

Goslinga-Roy, Gillian. 2002. Paper presented at Annual Conference of the South Asian Studies Association, Madison, WI.

Government of India. 2000. *Women's Health—Towards Empowerment: District Level Training Module.* New Delhi: Ministry of Health and Family Welfare.

————. 2001. *National Family Health Survey.* New Delhi.

Greenhouse, Carol. 1999. "Commentary." *Political and Legal Anthropology Review* 22, no. 2: 104–9.

————. 2001. "Ethnography and the State: Questions and Challenges in the Military Order of November 13, 2001." Paper presented to the Department of Anthropology, Princeton University, Princeton, NJ. April 25.

Greenough, Paul. 1995. "Intimidation, Coercion and Resistance in the Final Stages of the South Asian Smallpox Eradication Campaign, 1973–1975." *Social Science and Medicine* 41, no. 5: 733–645.

Gross, Rita M. 1977. "Menstruation and Childbirth as Ritual and Religious Experience in the Religion of the Australian Aborigines." *Journal of the American Academy of Religion* 45: 4.

Guha, Ranajit. 1983. *Elementary Aspects of Peasant Insurgency in Colonial India.* Delhi: Oxford University Press.

———. 1985. "Chandra's Death." In *Subaltern Studies V: Writings on South Asian History and Society,* ed. Ranajit Guha. Delhi: Oxford University Press.

Gupta, Akhil. 1998. *Postcolonial Developments: Agriculture in the Making of Modern India.* Durham, NC: Duke University Press.

———. 2001. "Governing Population: The Integrated Child Development Services Program in India." *States of Imagination: Ethnographic Explorations of the Postcolonial State,* eds. Thomas Blom Hansen and Finn Stepputat, 65–96. Durham, NC: Duke University Press.

Hansen, Thomas Blom, and Finn Stepputat, eds. 2001. *States of Imagination: Ethnographic Explorations of the Postcolonial State.* Durham, NC: Duke University Press.

Haraway, Donna. 1989. *Primate Visions: Gender, Race, and Nature in the World of Modern Science.* Routledge: New York.

Hardt, Michael and Antonio Negri. 2000. *Empire.* Cambridge, MA: Harvard University Press.

Harrison, Mark. 1994. *Public Health in British India: Anglo-Indian Preventive Medicine, 1859–1914.* Cambridge: Cambridge University Press.

———. 2001. "Medicine and Orientalism: Perspectives on Europe's Encounter with Indian Medical Systems." In *Health, Medicine and Empire: Perspectives on Colonial India,* eds. Biswamoy Pati and Mark Harrison, 37–88. Delhi: Orient Longman.

Heesterman, J. C. 1985. *The Inner Conflict of Tradition: Essays in Indian Ritual, Kinship and Society.* Chicago: University of Chicago Press.

Hertz, Barbara, and Anthony Meacham. 1987. *The Safe Motherhood Initiative: Proposal for Action.* Washington, DC: The World Bank.

Inden, Ronald B. 1990. *Imagining India.* Bloomington: Indiana University Press.

Indo-Asian News Service. 2003. "With Rising Polio Cases, India Dashes Global Hopes." http://in.news.yahoo.com/030208/43/20whw.html. February 8.

Irigaray, Luce. 1985. *Speculum of the Other Woman.* Gillian Gill, trans. Ithaca, NY: Cornell University Press. (Originally published in 1974.)

Jackson, Michael. 1989. *Paths Toward a Clearing: Radical Empiricism and Ethnographic Inquiry.* Bloomington: Indiana University Press.

Jacobson, Doranne. 1977. "The Women of North and Central India: Goddesses and Wives." In *Women in India: Two Perspectives,* eds. Doranne Jacobson and Susan Wadley, 17–112. Delhi: Manohar.

———. 1989. "Golden Handprints and Red-Painted Feet: Hindu Childbirth Rituals in Central India." In *Unspoken Worlds: Women's Religious Lives,* eds. Nancy Auer Falk and Rita M. Gross, 59–71. Belmont, CA: Wadsworth Publishing Company.

Jacobson, Doranne, and Susan Wadley. 1977. *Women in India: Two Perspectives.* Delhi: Manohar.

Jay, Martin. 1993. *Downcast Eyes: The Denigration of Vision in Twentieth-Century French Thought.* Berkeley: University of California Press.

Jayakar, Pupul. 1990. *The Earth Mother: Legends, Goddesses, and Ritual Arts of India.* New York: Harper and Row.

Jeffery, Patricia, and Roger Jeffery. 1996. "Delayed Periods and Falling Babies: The Ethnopsychology and Politics of Pregnancy Loss in Rural North India." In *The Anthropology of Pregnancy Loss: Comparative Studies in Miscarriage, Stillbirth and Neonatal Death,* ed. Rosanne Cecil, 17–28. Oxford: Berg.

Jeffery, Patricia, Roger Jeffery, and Andrew Lyon. 1989. *Labour Pains and Labour Power: Women and Childbearing in India.* London: Zed Books.

Jeffery, Roger, and Patricia M. Jeffery. 1993. "Traditional Birth Attendants in Rural North India: The Social Organization of Childbearing. In *Knowledge, Power and Practice: The Anthropology of Medicine in Everyday Life,* eds. Shirley Lindenbaum and Margaret Lock, 7–31. Berkeley: University of California Press.

Jordan, Brigitte. 1993. *Birth in Four Cultures: A Cross-cultural Investigation of Childbirth in Yucatan, Holland, Sweden and the United States.* Prospect Heights, IL: Waveland Press.

Jordanova, Ludmilla. 1989. *Sexual Visions: Images of Gender in Science and Medicine between the Eighteenth and Twentieth Centuries.* Madison: University of Wisconsin Press.

Juergensmayer, M. 1980. "What if Untouchables Do Not Believe in Untouchability?" *Bulletin of Concerned Asia Scholars* 12, no. 1: 22–28.

Kakar, Sudhir. 1981. *The Inner World: A Psycho-Analytic Study of Childhood and Society in India.* Delhi: Oxford University Press.

Kapferer, Bruce. 1979. "Mind, Self, and Other in Demonic Illness: The Negation and Reconstruction of Self." *American Ethnologist,* Vol. 6, no. 1: 110–133.

Kaviraj, Sudipta. 2000. "Modernity and Politics in India." *Daedulus* 129, no. 1: 137–61.

Ketler, Suzanne. 2000. "Preparing for Motherhood: Authoritative Knowledge and the Undercurrents of Shared Experience in Two Childbirth Education Courses in Cagliari, Italy." *Medical Anthropology Quarterly* 14, no. 2: 138–58.

Khare, R. S. 1984. *The Untouchable as Himself.* Cambridge: Cambridge University Press.

———. 1992. "From Kanya to Mata: Aspects of the Cultural Language of Kinship in Northern India." In *Concepts of Person: Kinship, Caste and Marriage in India,* eds. A. Ostor, L. Fruzzetti, S. Barnett, 143–71. Delhi: Oxford University Press.

———. 1996. "Dava, Daktar, and Dua: Anthroplogy of Practiced Medicine in India." In *Social Science and Medicine* 43, no. 5: 837–48.

———. 1998. *Cultural Diversity and Social Discontent.* New Delhi: Sage.

Kinsley, David R. 1986. *Hindu Goddesses: Visions of the Divine Feminine in the Hindu Tradition.* Berkeley: University of California Press.

Kleinman, Arthur. 1999. "Experience and Its Moral Modes: Culture, Human Conditions, and Disorder. In *The Tanner Lectures on Human Values,* 357–420. Salt Lake City: University of Utah Press.

Kleinman, Arthur, Veena Das, and Margaret Lock. 1997. "Introduction." In *Social Suffering*, eds. Arthur Kleinman, Veena Das, and Margaret Lock, ix–xxvii. Berkeley: University of California Press.

Kligman, Gail. 1995. "Political Demography: The Banning of Abortion in Ceaucescu's Romania." In *Conceiving the New World Order: The Global Politics of Reproduction*, eds. Faye D. Ginsburg and Rayna Rapp, 234–55. Berkeley: University of California Press.

———. 1998. *The Politic of Duplicity: Controlling Reproduction in Ceaucescu's Romania*. Berkeley: University of California Press.

Kolenda, Pauline. 1978. *Caste in Contemporary India: Beyond Organic Solidarity*. Menlo Park, CA: Benjamin/Cummings.

Krieger School of Arts and Sciences. 2002. "Reinventing a Discipline." Johns Hopkins University. http://www.jhu.edu/ksas/website/aboutksas/publications/update/fall00

Kristeva, Julia. 1989. *Black Sun: Depression and Melancholia*. Leon S. Roudiez, trans. New York: Columbia University Press.

Kumar, Kapil. 1984. *Peasants in Revolt*. Delhi: Manohar.

Kuriyama, Shigehisa. 1999. *The Expressiveness of the Body and the Divergence of Greek and Chinese Medicine*. New York: Zone Books.

Lacan, Jacques. 1998. *On Feminine Sexuality the Limits of Love and Knowledge: The Seminar of Jacques Lacan, Book XX Encore 1972–1973*. Bruce Fink and Jacques-Alain Miller, trans. New York: W.W. Norton and Company.

Lal, Maneesha. 1994. "The Politics of Gender and Medicine in Colonial India: The Countess of Dufferin's Fund, 1885–1888." *Bulletin of the History of Medicine* 68, no. 1 (Spring): 29–66.

Langford, Jean M. 1999. "Medical Mimesis: Healing Signs of a Cosmopolitan 'Quack'." *American Ethnologist* 26, no. 1: 24–46.

———. 2002. Fluent Bodies: Ayurvedic Remedies for Postcolonial Imbalance. Durham, NC: Duke University Press.

Leavitt, Judith Walzer. 1986. *Brought to Bed: Child-Bearing in America 1750–1950*. Oxford: Oxford University Press.

Levi-Strauss, Claude. 1963. *Structural Anthropology*. New York: Basic Books.

Lewin, Ellen. 1993. *Lesbian Mothers: Accounts of Gender in American Culture*. Ithaca, NY: Cornell University Press.

Lock, Margaret. 1993. *Encounters with Aging: Mythologies of Menopause in Japan and North America*. Berkeley: University of California Press.

Maglacas, A. Mangay, and John Simons, eds. 1986. *The Potential of the Traditional Birth Attendant*. Geneva: World Health Organization.

Maloney, Clarence. 1976. "Don't Say 'Pretty Baby' Lest You Zap It with Your Eye: The Evil Eye in South Asia." In *The Evil Eye*, ed. C. Maloney, 102–48. New York: Columbia University Press.

Mandelbaum, David G. 1988. *Women's Seclusion and Men's Honor: Sex Roles in North India, Bangladesh and Pakistan*. Tucson: University of Arizona Press.

Mani, Lata. 1985. "Contentious Traditions: The Debate on Sati in Colonial India." *Cultural Critique* 7: 119–56.

Marglin, Stephen. 1990. "Towards a Decolonization of the Mind." In *Dominating Knowledge: Development, Culture, and Resistance,* eds. Frederique Apffel-Marglin and Stephen Marglin. Oxford: Clarendon Press.

Marriott, McKim. 1968. "Caste Ranking and Food Transactions: A Matrix Analysis." In *Structure and Change in Indian Society,* eds. Milton Singer and Bernard S. Cohn, 133–71. Chicago: Aldine Publishing Company.

Marriott, McKim, and Ronald Inden. 1977. "Toward an Ethnosociology of South Asian Caste Systems." In *The New Wind: Changing Identities in South Asia,* ed. K. David, 227–38. The Hague: Mouton Publishers.

Martin, Emily. 1987. *The Woman in the Body: A Cultural Analysis of Reproduction.* Boston: Beacon Press.

———. 1991. "The Drama of the Egg and the Sperm: How Science Has Constructed a Romance Based on Stereotypical Male-Female Roles." *Signs* 16, no. 3: 485–501.

———. 1994. *Flexible Bodies: Tracking Immunity in American Culture-From the Days of Polio to the Age of AIDS.* Boston: Beacon Press.

Mayer, Peter. 1993. "Inventing Tradition: The Late 19th Century Origins of the North Indian 'Jajmani' System." *Modern Asian Studies* 27, no. 2: 357–95.

Mayo, Katherine. 1927. *Mother India.* Delhi: Low Price Publications.

Mbembe, Achlle. 2001. *On the Postcolony.* Berkeley: University of California Press.

———. 2003. "Necropolitics," Libby Meintjes, trans. *Public Culture* 15, no. 1: 11–40.

McCartney, Eugene S. 1981. "Praise and Dispraise in Folklore." In *The Evil Eye: A Casebook,* ed. A. Dundes, 9–38. Madison: University of Wisconsin Press.

McClintock, Anne. 1995. *Imperial Leather: Race, Gender and Sexuality in the Colonial Conquest.* New York: Routledge.

McGregor, R. S. 1997. *The Oxford Hindi-English Dictionary.* Delhi: Oxford University Press.

Mehta, Deepak. 2000. "Circumcision, Body, Masculinity: The Ritual Wound and Collective Violence." In *Violence and Subjectivity,* eds. Veena Das, Arthur Kleinman, Mamphela Ramphele, and Pam Reynolds, 79-101. Berkeley: University of California Press.

Mendelsohn, Oliver, and Marika Vicziany. 2000. *The Untouchables: Subordination, Poverty and the State in Modern India.* Cambridge: Cambridge University Press.

Millen, Joyce V., Allen Irwin, and Jim Yong Kim. 2000. "Introduction: What is Growing, Who is Dying?" In *Dying for Growth: Global Inequality and the Health of the Poor,* ed. Jim Yong Kim. Monroe, ME: Common Courage Press.

Mines, Mattison. 1994. *Public Faces, Private Voices: Community and Individuality in South India.* Berkeley: University of California Press.

Minh-Ha, Trinh, T. 1989. *Woman, Native, Other: Writing Postcoloniality and Feminism.* Bloomington: Indiana University Press.

Mishra, Manjari. 2001. "Daais-in-Hurry Inject Death to Rural Women." *Times of India: Lucknow.* March 5.

Mitchell, Lisa, and Eugenia Georges. 1998. "Baby's First Picture: The Cyborg Fetus of Ultrasound Imaging." In *Cyborg Babies: From Techno-Sex to Techno-Tots,* eds. Robbie Davis-Floyd and Joseph Dumit, 105–24. New York: Routledge.

Mitchell, Timothy. 2000a. "Introduction." *Questions of Modernity,* ed. Timothy Mitchell, xi–xxvii. Minneapolis: University of Minnesota Press.

———. 2000b. "The Stage of Modernity." *Questions of Modernity,* ed. Timothy Mitchell, 1–34. Minneapolis: University of Minnesota Press.

Moffatt, Michael. 1979. *An Untouchable Community in South India: Structure and Consensus.* Princeton: Princeton University Press.

Mohanty, Chandra Talpade. 1991. "Under Western Eyes: Feminist Scholarship and Colonial Discourses." In *Third World Women and the Politics of Feminism,* eds. C. T. Mohanty, A. Russo, and L. Torres, 51–80. Bloomington: University of Indiana Press.

———. 2003. "'Under Western Eyes' Revisited: Feminist Solidarity through Anticapitalist Struggles." *Signs* 28, no. 2: 499–535.

Morsy, Soheir. 1995. "Deadly Reproduction among Egyptian Women: Maternal Mortality and the Medicalization of Population Control." In *Conceiving the New World Order: The Global Politics of Reproduction,* eds. F. D. Ginsburg and R. Rapp, 162–76. Berkeley: University of California Press.

Moscucci, Ornella. 1990. *The Science of Woman: Gynecology and Gender in England, 1800–1929.* Cambridge: Cambridge University Press.

Nabokov, Isabelle. 2000. *Religion Against the Self: An Ethnography of Tamil Rituals.* Oxford: Oxford University Press.

Nanda, B. R., ed. 1976. *Indian Women: From Purdah to Modernity.* Delhi: Vikas Publishing House.

Nanda, Meera. 2002. "Do the Marginalized Valorize the Margins? Exploring Dangers of Difference." In *Feminist Post-development Thought,* ed. Kriemild Saunders, 212–24 London: Zed Books.

Nandy, Ashis. 2001a. *An Ambiguous Journey to the City: The Village and Other Odd Ruins of the Self in the Indian Imagination.* Oxford: Oxford University Press.

———. 2001b. *Time Warps: The Insistent Politics of Silent and Evasive Pats.* Delhi: Permanent Black. Narayan, R. K. 1976. *The Painter of Signs.* London: Penguin.

Narayan, Uma. 1997. *Dislocating Cultures: Identities, Traditions, and Third World Feminism.* New York: Routledge.

Newman, Karen. 1996. *Fetal Positions: Individualism, Science, Visuality.* Stanford, CA: Stanford University Press.

Nichter, Mark. 1980. "The Layperson's Perception of Medicine as Perspective into the Utilization of Multiple Therapy Systems in the Indian Context." In *Social Science & Medicine* 14, no. B: 225–33.

———. 1990. "Vaccinations in South Asia: False Expectations and Commanding Metaphors." In *Anthropology and Primary Health Care,* eds. J. Coreil and D. Muil. CT: Westwood Press.

————. 1995. "Vaccinations in the Third World: A Consideration of Community Demand." *Social Science and Medicine* 41, no. 5: 617–32.

————. 1998. "The Mission within the Madness: Self-initiated Medicalization as Expression of Agency." In *Pragmatic Women and Body Politics*, eds. Margaret Lock and Patricia A. Kaufert, 327–53. Cambridge: Cambridge University Press.

Nussbaum, Martha. 2002. "Sex, Laws and Inequality: What India Can Teach the United States." *Daedalus* (Winter): 95–106.

Oakley, Ann. 1984. *The Captured Womb: A History of the Medical Care of Pregnant Women*. London: Blackwell.

Obeyesekere, Gananath. 1981. *Medusa's Hair*. Chicago: The University of Chicago Press.

————. 1988. *The Work of Culture*. Chicago: University of Chicago Press.

O'Flaherty, Wendy Doniger. 1980. *Women, Androgynes, and Other Mythical Beasts*. Chicago: University of Chicago Press.

Orenstein, Henry. 1968. Toward a Grammar of Defilement in Hindu Sacred Law. In *Structure and Change in Indian Society*, eds. Milton Singer and Bernard S. Cohn, 115–31. Chicago: Aldine.

Pandey, Gyanendra. 1997. "In Defense of the Fragment: Writing about Hindu-Muslim Riots in India Today." In *A Subaltern Studies Reader 1986–1995*, ed. Ranajit Guha, 1–33. Minneapolis: University of Minnesota Press.

Pandey, Sandeep. 2006. *Report: Public Hearing on Right to Food in Sitapur*. National Alliance of People's Movements, People's Union for Human Rights, Asha Parivar, Sangatin. Lucknow.

Pandolfo, Stefania. 1997. *Impasse of the Angels: Scenes from a Moroccan Space of Memory*. Chicago: University of Chicago Press.

Papanek, Hanna. 1982. "Purdah in Pakistan: Seclusion and Modern Occupations for Women." In *Separate Worlds*, eds. H. Papanek and G. Minault, ??–??. Columbus, MO: South Asia Books.

Parry, Jonathan. 1994. *Death in Banaras*. Cambridge: Cambridge University Press.

Patel, Vibhuti. 1989. "Sex Determination and Sex Pre-selection Tests in India: Recent Techniques in Femicide." *Journal of Reproductive and Genetic Engineering* 2, no. 2: 139–52.

Pati, Biswamoy, and Mark Harrison. 2001. "Introduction." In *Health, Medicine and Empire: Perspectives on Colonial India*, eds. Biswamoy Pati and Mark Harrison, 1–36. Delhi: Orient Longman Limited.

Petchesky, Rosalind Pollack. 1994. "Fetal Images: The Power of Visual Culture in the Politics of Reproduction." In *The Gender Sexuality Reader*, eds. R. N. Lancaster and M. di Leonardo, 134–52. New York: Routledge.

Pigg, Stacey. 1992. *Inventing Social Categories through Place: Social Representations and Development in Nepal*. Society for the Comparative Study of Society and History.

————. 1996. "The Credible and the Credulous: The Question of 'Villagers' Beliefs' in Nepal." *Cultural Anthropology* 11, no. 2: 160–201.

———. 1997. "Authority in Translation: Finding, Knowing, Naming, and Training 'Traditional Birth Attendants' in Nepal." In *Childbirth and Authoritative Knowledge,* eds. Robbie Davis-Floyd and Carolyn Sargent, 233–62. Berkeley: University of California Press.

Pinto, Sarah. 2006. "Globalizing Untouchability: Grief and the Politics of Depressing Speech." In *Social Text* (April).

Pires, Ana Flavia, Lucas d'Oliveira, Simone Grilo Diniz, and Lilia Blima Schraiber. 2002. "Violence against Women in Health-care Institutions: An Emerging Problem." *Lancet* 359: 1681–85.

Pocock, D. F. 1981. "The Evil Eye: Envy and Greed among the Patidar of Central Gujarat." In *The Evil Eye: A Casebook,* ed. Alan Dundes, 201–10. Madison: University of Wisconsin Press.

Prakash, Gyan. 1999. *Another Reason: Science and the Imagination of Modern India.* Princeton, NJ: Princeton University Press.

Prashad, Vijay. 2000. *Untouchable Freedom: A Social History of a Dalit Community.* New Delhi: Oxford University Press.

Qadeer, Imrana. 1998a. "Reproductive Health: A Public Health Perspective." *Economic and Political Weekly.* October 10.

———. 1998b. "Our Legacy in MCH Programmes." In *Gender Population and Government,* eds. Maitreyi Krishnaraj, Radha M. Sridarshan, and Abusaleh Sharif, 267–89. Delhi: Oxford University Press.

———. 2001. "Impact of Structural Adjustment Programs in Concepts of Public Health." In *Public Health and the Poverty of Reforms: The South Asian Predicament,* eds. Imrana Qadeer, Kasturi Sen, and K. R. Nayar, 117–36. New Delhi: Sage.

Ragone, Helena. 1997. "Chasing the Blood Tie: Surrogate Mothers, Adoptive Mothers, and Fathers." In *Situated Lives: Gender and Culture in Everyday Life,* eds. Louise Lamphere, Helena Ragone, and Patricia Zavella, 110–27. New York: Routledge.

Raheja, Gloria Goodwin. 1988. *The Poison in the Gift.* Chicago: University of Chicago Press.

Raheja, Gloria Goodwin, and Ann Grodzins Gold. 1994. *Listen to the Heron's Words: Reimagining Gender and Kinship in North India.* Berkeley: University of California Press.

Rajan, Rajeswari Sunder. 1993. *Real and Imagined Women: Gender, Culture and Postcolonialism.* London: Routledge.

———. 1999. "The Story of Draupadi's Disrobing: Meanings for Our Times." In *Signposts: Gender Issues in Post-Independence India,* 332–59. Delhi: Kali for Women.

———. 2003. *The Scandal of the State: Women, Law, and Citizenship in Postcolonial India.* Delhi: Permanent Black.

Ram, Kalpana. 1998a. "Epilogue: Maternal Experiences and Feminist Body Politics: Asian and Pacific Experiences." In *Maternities and Modernities: Colonial and Postcolonial Experiences in Asia and the Pacific,* eds. Kalpana Ram and Margaret Jolly, 275–98. Cambridge: Cambridge University Press.

———. 1998b. "Maternity and the Story of Enlightenment in the Colonies: Tamil Coastal Women, South India. In *Maternities and Modernities: Colonial and Postcolonial Experiences in Asia and the Pacific,* eds. Kalpana Ram and Margaret Jolly, 114–43. Cambridge: Cambridge University Press.

———. 1998c. "Uneven Modernities and Ambivalent Sexualities: Women's Constructions of Puberty in Coastal Kanyakumari, Tamilnadu." In *A Question of Silence? The Sexual Economies of Modern India,* eds. Mary E. John and Janaki Nair. Delhi: Kali for Women.

———. 2001. "Rationalizing Fecund Bodies: Family Planning Policy and the Modern Indian Nation-State. In *Borders of Being: Citizenship, Fertility, and Sexuality in Asia and the Pacific,* eds. Margaret Jolly and Kalpana Ram, 82–117. Ann Arbor: University of Michigan Press.

Rao, Mohan. 1999. *Disinvesting in Health.* Delhi: Sage.

Rapp, Rayna. 1988. "Chromosomes and Communication: The Discourse of Genetic Counseling." *Medical Anthropology Quarterly* 2, no. 2: 143–57.

———. 1998. "Real-Time Fetus: The Role of the Sonogram in the Age of Monitored Reproduction." In *Cyborgs and Citadels: Anthropological Interventions in Emerging Sciences and Technologies,* eds. G. L. Downey and J. Dumit, 31–48. Santa Fe, NM: School of American Research Press.

———. 2000. *Testing Women, Testing the Fetus: The Social Impact of Amniocentesis in America.* New York: Routledge.

Rawat, Ramnarayan S. 2002. "Partition Politics and Achhut Identity: A Study of Scheduled Castes Federation and Dalit Politics in U.P. 1946–1948." In *The Partitions of Memory,* ed. Suvir Kaul. Delhi: Permanent Black.

———. 2003. "Making Claims for Power: A New Agenda in Dalit Politics of Uttar Pradesh, 1946–48." In *Modern Asian Studies.* Cambridge: Cambridge University Press.

Robinson, Kathryn. 2001. "Government Agency, Women's Agency: Feminisms, Fertility, and Population Control." In *Borders of Being: Citizenship, Fertility, and Sexuality in Asia and the Pacific,* eds. Margaret Jolly and Kalpana Ram, 36–57. Ann Arbor: University of Michigan Press.

Rofel, Lisa. 1999. *Other Modernities: Gendered Yearnings in China after Socialism.* Berkeley: University of California Press.

Roland, Alan. 1988. *In Search of Self in India and Japan.* Princeton, NJ: Princeton University Press.

Rorty, Amelie. 1988. *Mind in Action: Essays in the Philosophy of Mind.* Boston: Beacon Press.

Rothman, Barbara Katz. 1986. *The Tentative Pregnancy, Prenatal Diagnosis and the Future of Motherhood.* New York: W.W. Norton.

———. 1989. *Recreating Motherhood: Ideology and Technology in Patriarchal Society.* New York: W.W. Norton.

Rozario, Santi. 1998. "The Dai and the Doctor: Discourses on Women's Reproductive Health in Rural Bangladesh." In *Maternities and Modernities: Colonial and Postcolonial Experiences in Asia and the Pacific,* eds. Kalpana Ram and Margaret Jolly, 144–76. Cambridge: Cambridge University Press.

———. 2002. "The Healer on the Margins: The Dai in Rural Bangladesh." In *Daughters of Hariti: Childbirth and Female Healers in South and Southeast Asia*, eds. Santi Rozario and Geoffrey Samuel. New York: Routledge.

Rubin, Gayle. 1975. "The Traffic in Women: Notes on the 'Political Economy' of Sex." In *Toward an Anthropology of Women*, ed. Rayna Reiter, 157–210. New York: Monthly Review Press.

Ruhl, Leslie. 2002. "Dilemmas of the Will: Uncertainty, Reproduction, and the Rhetoric of Control." *Signs* 27, no. 3: 641–63.

Sahlins, Marshall. 1985. *Islands of History.* Chicago: University of Chicago Press.

Samuel, Geoffrey. 2002. "The Daughters of Hariti Today." In *Daughters of Hariti: Childbirth and Female Healers in South and Southeast Asia*, eds. Santi Rozario and Geoffrey Samuel. New York: Routledge.

Sangari, Kumkum, and Sudesh Vaid. 1997. "Recasting Women: An Introduction." In *Recasting Women: Essays in Indian Colonial History*, eds. Kumkum Sangari and Sudesh Vaid, 1–26. New Brunswick, NJ: Rutgers University Press.

Sassen, Saskia. 1998. *Globalization and its Discontents.* New York: New Press.

Saunders, Kriemild. 2002. "Introduction: Towards a Deconstructive Post-development Criticism." In *Feminist Post-development Thought*, ed. Kriemild Saunders, 15. New York: Zed Books.

Scheper-Hughes, Nancy. 1987. "Introduction: The Cultural Politics of Child Survival." In *Child Survival: Anthropological Perspectives on the Treatment and Maltreatment of Children*, ed. Nancy Scheper-Hughes, 1–32.

———. 1992. *Death Without Weeping: The Violence of Everyday Life in Brazil.* Berkeley: University of California Press.

Shulman, David. 1980. *Tamil Temple Myths: Sacrifice and Divine Marriage in the South Indian Saiva Tradition.* Princeton, NJ: Princeton University Press.

Sen, Kasturi. 2001. "Health Reforms and Developing Countries—A Critique." In *Public Health and the Poverty of Reforms: The South Asian Predicament*, eds. Imrana Qadeer, Kasturi Sen, and K. R. Nayar, 137–53. New Delhi: Sage.

Sharma, Harivansh Ray. 1999. *Rajpal Muhavra Kosh.* Delhi: Rajpal.

Sharpe, Jenny, and Gayatri Chakravorty Spivak. 2002. "A Conversation with Gayatri Chakravorty Spivak: Politics and the Imagination." *Signs: Journal of Women in Culture and Society* 28, no. 2: 609–24.

Sontag, Susan. 1976. *On Photography.* New York: Farrar, Straus, and Giroux.

Spivak, Gayatrai Chakravorty. 1988a. "Can the Subaltern Speak?" In *Marxism and the Interpretation of Culture*, eds. C. Nelson and L Grossberg. Urbana: University of Illinois Press.

———. 1988b. *In Other Worlds: Essays in Cultural Politics.* New York: Routledge.

———. 1995. *The Spivak Reader*, eds. Donna Landry and Gerald Maclean. New York: Routledge.

Stewart, Kathleen. 1996. *A Space on the Side of the Road.* Princeton, NJ: Princeton University Press.

Stoler, Ann Laura. 1995. *Race and the Education of Desire: Foucault's History of Sexuality and the Colonial Order of Things.* Durham, NC: Duke University Press.

Strathern, Marilyn. 1992. *Reproducing the Future: Anthropology, Kinship, and the New Reproductive Technologies.* New York: Routledge.

Swantz, Marja-Liisa. 1994. "Woman/Body/Knowledge: From Production to Regeneration." In *Feminist Perspectives on Sustainable Development,* ed. Wendy Harcourt. London: Zed Books.

Taussig, Michael. 1992a. *Mimesis and Alterity.* New York: Routledge.

———. 1992b. *The Nervous System.* New York: Routledge.

———. 1997. *The Magic of the State.* New York: Routledge.

———. 1998. "Viscerality, Faith, and Skepticism: Another Theory of Magic." In *In Near Ruins: Cultural Theory at the End of the Century,* Nicholas Dirks, ed. 221–57. Minneapolis: University of Minnesota Press.

Tharu, Susie. 1998. "Citizenship and its Discontents." In *A Question of Silence? The Sexual Economies of Modern India,* eds. Mary E. John and Janaki Nair, 216–42. Delhi: Kali for Women.

———. 1989. "Response to Julie Stephens." In *Subaltern Studies VI: Writings on South Asian History and Society,* ed. Ranajit Guha, 126–31. Delhi: Oxford University Press.

Times of India News Service. 2001. "SC Says Married Woman Not Part of Her Parents' Family." *Times of India: Lucknow.* April 21.

Trawick, Margaret. 1992. *Notes on Love in a Tamil Family.* Berkeley: University of California Press.

Tsing, Anna Lowenhaupt. 2004. *Friction: An Ethnography of Global Connection.* Princeton, NJ: Princeton University Press.

Turner, Victor. 1974. *Dramas, Fields, and Metaphors.* Ithaca, NY: Cornell University Press.

Unnithan-Kumar, Maya. 2001. "Emotion, Agency and Access to Healthcare: Women's Experiences of Reproduction in Jaipur." In *Managing Reproductive Life: Cross-Cultural Themes in Fertility and Sexuality,* ed. Soraya Tremayne. London: Berghahn.

———. 2002. "Midwives among Others: Knowledges of Healing and the Politics of Emotions in Rajasthan, Northwest India." In *Daughters of Hariti: Childbirth and Female Healers in South and Southeast Asia,* eds. Santi Rozario and Geoffrey Samuel. New York: Routledge.

———. 2005. *Reproductive Agency, Medicine, and the State: Cultural Transformations in Childbearing.* London: Berghahn.

Van der Veer, Peter. 1988. *Gods on Earth: The Management of Religious Experience and Identity in a North Indian Pilgrimage Center.* London: Athlone Press.

Van Hollen, Cecilia Coale. 1998. *Birthing on the Threshold: Childbirth and Modernity Among Lower Class Women in Tamil Nadu, South India.* Ph.D. dissertation, Department of Anthropology, University of California, Berkeley.

———. 2002. *Birth at the Threshold: Childbirth and Modernity in South India.* Berkeley: University of California Press.

Verderese, Maria de Lourdes, and Lily M. Turnbull. 1975. *The Traditional Birth Attendant in Maternal and Child Health and Family Planning.* Geneva: World Health Organization.

Visveswaran, Kamla. 1994. *Fictions of Feminist Ethnography.* Minneapolis: University of Minnesota Press.

Wadley, Susan. 1975. *Shakti: Power in the Conceptual Structure of Karimpur Religion.* Chicago: University of Chicago Press.

———. 1977. "Women and the Hindu Tradition." In *Women in India: Two Perspectives,* eds. Doranne Jacobson and Susan Wadley, 113–40. Delhi: Manohar.

———. 1994. *Struggling with Destiny in Karimpur, 1925–1984.* Berkeley: University of California Press.

Waldman, Amy. 2003. "Distrust Reopens the Door for Polio in India." *New York Times.* January 13, A1.

Weir, Lorna. 1998. "Pregnancy Ultrasound in Maternal Discourse." In *Vital Signs: Feminist Reconfigurations of the Bio/logical Body,* eds. Margaret Shildrick and Janet Price, 78–101. Edinburgh: Edinburgh University Press.

Weismantel, Mary. 2001. *Cholas and Pishtacos: Stories of Race and Sex in the Andes.* Chicago: University of Chicago Press.

Williams, Raymond. 1977. *Marxism and Literature.* Oxford: Oxford University Press.

Wilson, Adrian. 1995. *The Making of Man-Midwifery: Childbirth in England 1660–1770.* London: University College London Press.

Whyte, Susan Reynolds, and J. Van der Geest. 1994. "Injections: Issues and Methods for Anthropological Research." In *Medicines, Meanings and Contexts,* eds. Nina Etkin and Michael Tan, 137–61. Quezon City: Health Action Information Network.

Woodburne, A. Stewart. 1981. "The Evil Eye in South Indian Folklore. In *The Evil Eye: A Casebook,* ed. A. Dundes, 55–64. Madison: University of Wisconsin Press.

World Health Organization. 1992. *Traditional Birth Attendants: A Joint WHO/UNFPA/UNICEF Statement.* Geneva: World Health Organization.

Zimmer, Heinrich. 1946. *Myths and Symbols in Indian Art and Civilization.* New York: Harper and Row Publishers.

Žižek, Slavoj. 1997. *The Plague of Fantasies.* New York: Verso.

Zuhur, Sherifa. 1992. *Revealing Reveiling: Islamist Gender Ideology in Contemporary Egypt.* Albany, NY: SUNY Press.

INDEX

D

dai, x, 5, 29–36, 58, 71, 98, 114,
118, 127, 129, 206, 211–223,
233–43, 280, 282, 285, 294,
299n7, 299n9
as category, ix, 27, 59, 70,
235–37, 242
blame of, 128–29, 218,
payment of, 48, 238
stigmatization of, 44, 61, 191,
216–223
training of, 3, 4, 5, 13, 45, 47,
48, 52, 74, 78, 97, 98, 100,
101, 115, 191, 214–223,
232–37, 243
use of term, viii, 235–37, 241,
296n1
darsan (sight), 27, 143–46, 158,
160–61, 163, 172–74, 176
Das, Veena, 3, 16–17, 35, 62,
86–87, 95, 109, 162, 164,
187, 197–98, 207, 209, 252,
276, 285, 288–89
death, 3, 5, 11, 19, 24, 25, 26, 27,
28, 36, 44, 94–96, 102–103,
104, 105, 129, 146, 154–155,
178–210, 212, 248, 253, 254,
259, 260, 265, 278, 283,
288–90, 293
"bad death," 93
infant death, xi, 1, 2, 3, 19, 20,
22, 27, 154–55, 161, 172,
178–210, 232, 248, 251–252,
282, 288–90
idioms for, 181
narratives of, 27, 32, 178–210,
286, 288, 293
photography of, 154–55
pollution of, 62
statistics of, 181, 192
symbols of, 77, 81, 94
work associated with, 47,
56–57, 59–60, 89, 91
demand, 11, 12, 15, 21, 24, 46,
48, 51, 60, 63, 64, 68, 121,
142, 152, 172, 173, 175, 183,
190–91, 197, 204, 217,

226–28, 233, 234, 240–41,
250, 252, 269, 276, 290
de Certeau, Michel, xi, 3, 25, 26,
124, 182, 188, 207, 209, 290
development, 2, 5, 8, 15–18, 22,
25, 27, 33–34, 35, 36, 49, 66,
106–140, 190–92, 207, 212,
219, 220–21, 234–37, 241–43,
253–54, 275–76, 279, 281,
283, 286
agricultural development, 8
child development, 86
discourses of, 61–62, 67,
190–92, 223–232, 241–243
rural development, 8
Dhanuk (*dhanuk*), 47, 57, 114,
296n3
disbelief, 39, 40, 204
doctors, 3, 8, 11, 12, 13, 16, 17,
18, 25, 26, 28, 32, 49, 52, 53,
76, 101, 109, 110, 11, 112,
113–19, 122, 123, 125, 127–
30, 137, 158, 166, 169, 171,
172, 173, 176, 179, 186–87,
191, 194, 195–96, 199, 200,
204, 205–206, 215, 219, 222,
225, 227, 232, 245, 248,
256–58, 260, 261, 266, 268,
271, 274, 275, 276, 277, 290,
291, 292, 293, 295, 299n7
Dom, 42, 47
Douglas, Mary, 81, 88, 91, 97
Dumont, Louis, 61, 67, 208, 279,
282, 296n4, 297n7, 299n8

E

Eck, Diana, 145–46, 159, 176
education, 7, 8, 11, 13, 18, 26, 65,
67, 98, 114, 118, 119, 120,
121, 123, 124, 125, 138, 139,
212, 214, 215, 227, 229, 233,
234, 237, 241, 246, 264, 266,
267, 270–72, 279–80,
300c7n1, 301n1
Emergency, the, 191, 220, 262, 275
episiotomy, 274
ethnography, 34, 164, 165–66

sterilization, 116, 134, 167–68,
244, 246, 248–49, 252, 260,
262, 275, 277
"suitability" of, 244, 246, 248
outsiders, 9, 68, 116, 117, 125,
153
oxytocin, 108, 127, 128, 129, 130,
258, 266, 276, 277

P
pain, 32, 37, 54–55, 128, 129,
131, 135, 168, 197–98, 209,
248, 257
labor, 31, 37, 42, 49–50, 53,
54–55, 99, 108, 115, 127–29,
170, 186, 211, 233, 244, 246,
257–58, 276–77, 293
of grief, 185–86, 195, 249
postpartum, 40
panchayat, 119, 211
Parry, Jonathan, 59, 62, 63,
92–93, 95, 297n6
Pasi, 6, 47, 63, 73, 89, 181, 195,
247, 248, 250, 260, 271
stereotypes of, 45, 134, 153,
259, 263–64
stigma associated with, 11, 42,
49, 132, 133, 178, 180, 259,
263
pharmaceuticals, 25, 128, 305
photography, 143, 147, 151, 154,
203, 317
pills, *See* goli
placenta, xi, 27, 31, 37–39, 41, 53,
56, 57, 59, 72–105, 113, 115,
143, 179, 191, 233, 293
disposal of, 40, 41, 56, 72–75,
78, 80, 82–88, 93, 95, 100,
104–105, 293, 299n5
malevolent use of, 78, 83, 93
oxytocin (relation to), 128
use in resuscitation, 78
polio, 178, 255, 309, 312, 319
possession (spirit), 73, 83, 94
postpartum
care (*See* postpartum work)
fluids, 79

hemhorrage, 128
massage (*See* massage)
ritual (*See* Chatti puja)
work, 16, 27, 32, 36–49, 52, 53,
56–71, 72, 74, 80, 83, 88–90,
92, 97, 101–103, 114, 222,
296n3
workers 12, 32, 36–49, 52, 53,
56–71, 74, 83, 96–97,
101–103, 114, 115, 185, 280,
296n3, 299n8
pradhan, 118–19, 120, 123, 124,
126, 127, 130, 136, 140, 271
pregnancy, 14, 27, 45, 53, 60, 77,
111, 141–77, 190, 193, 211,
221, 244, 247, 251, 291
privatization, 3, 109, 191, 206,
240–41, 285
protection, 90, 134, 150, 152, 161,
172, 204, 248, 254, 262, 264,
290, 300
puja, 43, 80, 83, 85, 141, 194, 203
purdah, See veiling

Q
quacks, 109, 111, 112, 117, 118,
125, 126, 130, 136–37, 138,
140, 154, 169, 194, 199, 204,
206, 236, 277, 290, 299c3n1

R
rebirth, 77, 95
rejection of biomedicine, 116, 131,
172, 241, 255–256, 265–66,
271, 282, 288, 290
repression, 104, 105, 205, 282,
283, 285
resentment, 69, 276

S
sacred, 58, 80, 81, 92, 94, 96, 97,
102, 131, 217
Safe Motherhood Initiative,
190–91, 224, 227, 228, 229
sarkar (government), 106, 109,
110
scandal, 130, 217, 253, 290

www.ingramcontent.com/pod-product-compliance
Lightning Source LLC
Chambersburg PA
CBHW060025030426
42334CB00019B/2182